Lecture Notes on Mathematical Modelling in the Life Sciences

The rapid pace and development of new methods and techniques in mathematics and in biology and medicine creates a natural demand for up-to-date, readable, possibly short lecture notes covering the breadth and depth of mathematical modelling, mathematical analysis and numerical computations in the life sciences, at a high scientific level.

The volumes in this series are written in a style accessible to graduate students. Besides monographs, we envision the series to also provide an outlet for material less formally presented and more anticipatory of future needs due to novel and exciting biomedical applications and mathematical methodologies.

The topics in LMML range from the molecular level through the organismal to the population level, e.g. gene sequencing, protein dynamics, cell biology, developmental biology, genetic and neural networks, organogenesis, tissue mechanics, bioengineering and hemodynamics, infectious diseases, mathematical epidemiology and population dynamics.

Mathematical methods include dynamical systems, partial differential equations, optimal control, statistical mechanics and stochastics, numerical analysis, scientific computing and machine learning, combinatorics, algebra, topology and geometry, etc., which are indispensable for a deeper understanding of biological and medical problems.

Wherever feasible, numerical codes must be made accessible.

Founding Editors:

Michael C. Mackey, McGill University, Montreal, QC, Canada

Angela Stevens, University of Münster, Münster, Germany

More information about this series at https://link.springer.com/bookseries/10049

Arnaud Ducrot • Quentin Griette • Zhihua Liu •
Pierre Magal

Differential Equations and Population Dynamics I

Introductory Approaches

Foreword by Jacques Demongeot and Glenn Webb

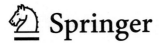 Springer

Arnaud Ducrot
Laboratoire de Mathématiques Appliquées
du Havre
Université Le Havre Normandie
Le Havre, France

Quentin Griette
Institut de Mathématiques
de Bordeaux
University of Bordeaux
Bordeaux, France

Zhihua Liu
School of Mathematical Sciences
Beijing Normal University
Beijing, China

Pierre Magal
Institut de Mathématiques
de Bordeaux
University of Bordeaux
Bordeaux, France

ISSN 2193-4789   ISSN 2193-4797   (electronic)
Lecture Notes on Mathematical Modelling in the Life Sciences
ISBN 978-3-030-98135-8   ISBN 978-3-030-98136-5   (eBook)
https://doi.org/10.1007/978-3-030-98136-5

This Springer imprint is published by the registered company Springer Nature Switzerland AG
The registered company address is: Gewerbestrasse 11, 6330 Cham, Switzerland

Foreword

This book provides an excellent introduction to the mathematical analysis and simulation techniques of ordinary differential equations (ODEs). Moreover, it opens up exciting perspectives on the applications of this widely used theoretical tool, particularly in biomedicine. We will comment below on the genesis of these important applications, namely population dynamics applied to the modeling of epidemic diseases and to morphogenesis.

1. Genesis of population dynamics applied to the modeling of epidemic diseases
  1.1. Introduction of numbers in medicine: the Greeks
  The first numerical table intended for use in medicine appears in a letter from Aristotle to his student Alexander the Great. This letter (undoubtedly apocryphal), called the *Secretum secretorum* (the Secret of Secrets),[1] treats a wide range of topics, including astrology and medicine. Transmitted (in fact probably written) by Rhazes (865–935), a Persian polymath and physician, it describes how to predict whether someone's hour of death has come. The table is a double chart of numbers between 1 and 30, the left column showing death numbers and the right column survival numbers. The founder of algebra, al-Khwârizmî (c. AD 84), and his numerous disciples, including Guillaume d'Auberive (1120–1180) and his Cistercian colleagues Odon de Morimond and Thibaut de Langres, and Shaiykh Bahā'ī (1546–1622), knew the science of numbers and were familiar with the charts of the *Secretum secretorum*, which includes an amazing mix of rules, some simple, such as arithmetic sequences, and some sophisticated, such as those which describe Tutte's equilateral triangle dissection. The medical table was used for centuries by the Greeks and Arabs to calculate a score (based on the numerical value of the letters of an individual's name and their pulse value) which was compared (modulo 30) with the double series of death and survival numbers, especially during epidemics. Before the Christian era, at least forty epidemics followed one another, all of them echoed by the Bible, Thucydides, the Iliad and the Aeneid. Most of these accounts combine various "plagues" under the same term (*pestis*, "scourge"); thus, the "plague of Athens" of 430 BC was probably an epidemic of typhus. The Justinian plague (2nd century AD), dominated by

[1] Bacon, R. *Secretum secretorum cum Glossis et Notulis* (1280). In: Steele, R. (ed) *Opera hactenus inedita Rogeri Baconsi.* Clarendon Press, Oxford, pp. 287—313 (1920).

the bubonic form, struck the entire Mediterranean basin and is therefore considered
the first "real" plague pandemic.

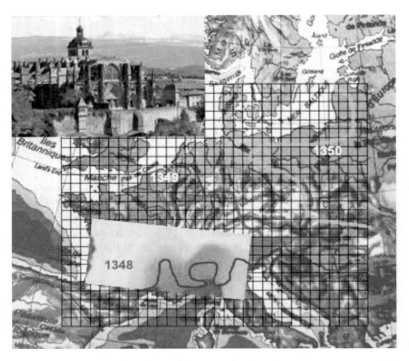

Fig. 0.1: *Representation of the "Black Death" epidemy front waves in central Europe
from the St. Anthony's Abbey records between 1349 (in blue) and 1350 (in green).
Top thumbnail: St. Anthony's Abbey (near Grenoble, France). Bottom thumbnail:
year 1348 front wave in France (in red from the St. Anthony's Abbey records, in blue
from a PDE equation simulation).*

1.2. The beginning of population dynamics: The Middle Ages

The great plague of the Middle Ages, the black plague, was the second. Coming
from India, it reached the Mediterranean and, from there, all of Europe was soon
talking about the pulmonary form. It took more than 25 million victims (between
a quarter and a half of the population) between 1346 and 1353. Another example
concerns social and infectious contagious diseases: St. Anthony's Monastery near
Grenoble was in charge of watching and curing infectious spreads like the Black
Death of 1348 and social epidemics like St. Anthony's fire disease (now called
ergotism, or ergot poisoning). The Antonin congregation was founded in 1095 by
Gaston de Valloire, a nobleman of the Dauphiné, and confirmed by Pope Urban II
in the same year, in gratitude for his son's miraculous cure from St. Anthony's fire
thanks to the relics of Saint Anthony the Great. During the XIVth and XVth centuries,
St Anthony's monastic Order had 640 hospitals and 10,000 brothers in Europe

along the roads to Santiago de Compostela and Jerusalem, watching plague, leprosy, and ergotism. This monastery is also known for having sheltered two illustrious mathematicians, Jean Borrel (1492—1564), also called Johannes Buteo, an algebraist who refuted the circle quadrature theory, and Jean Duchon, inventor of the thin-plate splines theory. The "Black Death" (or plague) watching by St. Anthony's Order had the character of a pandemic study, with dramatic economic and demographic consequences. At least 75 million people died from the disease during the spread of the Black Death. Born in the Caspian area, the wave went through the Mediterranean routes, reaching Marseilles in France and Genoa in Italy at the end of 1347, and spread for five years in Europe before coming back to the Caspian reservoir. Using the St. Anthony's Monastery data, numerous PDE models have been proposed to retro-predict the front waves observed at that time (Figure 0.1), the best being those using viscosities proportional to the altitude.[2]

1.3. Modeling of population dynamics: the Age of Enlightenment

The plague endemic which had started in the Middle Ages continued for three centuries before disappearing after sporadic episodes in Constantinople (1839) and Egypt (1844). At the same time, smallpox killed about 400,000 Europeans each year, including 80% of infected children. This health disaster led to the birth of the epidemiological approach to contagious diseases, making use of real data, which developed during the second half of the XVIIIth century. The seminal article was written by D. Bernoulli in 1760[3] followed by improvements due to R. Ross,[4] A.G. McKendrick[5] and eventually by many others, such as P. Magal and colleagues in the present book. These articles discuss and solve one of the central problems of epidemic modeling, the estimation of parameters in the logistic growth equation governing the observed infectious cases, namely the transmission rate and the initial number of susceptible individuals.

1.4. Pandemics in the XXth century

The third pandemic began with the awakening of the old hearth of Yunnan in South China, from where it reached Hong Kong in 1894. It was there that A. Yersin discovered the germ responsible for the plague, in both rats and humans. Four years later in Calcutta, P.L. Simond demonstrated the transmission of the plague by ship. The passage of infected rats and fleas by steam navigation provided an exceptional means of propagation. The plague reached Suez in 1897; Madagascar and India (where it caused more than 12 million deaths) in 1898; Alexandria, Japan, East Africa, Portugal and then Brazil in 1899; Manila, Sydney, Glasgow and San Francisco in 1900; Honolulu in 1908; Java in 1911; Ceylon in 1914; and Marseilles in 1920. Along with this invasion by sea, other old centers reawakened, such as

---

[2] Gaudart, J., Ghassani, M., Mintsa, J., Rachdi, M., Waku, J. and Demongeot, J. Demography and Diffusion in epidemics: Malaria and Black Death spread. *Acta Biotheoretica* **58**, 277–305 (2010).

[3] Bernoulli, D. Essai d'une nouvelle analyse de la mortalité causée par la petite vérole, et des avantages de l'inoculation pour la prévenir. *Histoire et Mémoires de l'Académie Royale des Sciences de Paris*, 1–45 (1760, 1766) .

[4] Ross, R. An application of the theory of probabilities to the study of a priori pathometry. *Proc. R. Soc. Series A* **92**, 204–230 (1916).

[5] McKendrick, A.G. Applications of mathematics to medical problems. *Proc. Edinburgh Math. Soc.* **44**, 1–34 (1925).

Manchuria which saw in 1910 more than 50,000 deaths from pulmonary plague, in three months of epidemic.

In Book II of his opus "Men Like Gods" (1923), H.G. Wells, inspired by the Spanish flu pandemic, describes a quarantine on the planet Utopia, showing the complexity of a collective response to a viral attack. Patient zero of the Spanish flu was observed in March 1918 in Kansas (USA), and further cases were recorded in France, Germany and the United Kingdom in April. Two years later, a third of the world's population (about 500 million people) had been infected during four successive waves, with deaths estimated to be in the range 17–50 million, that is, a maximum size ten times greater than the present Covid-19 epidemic.

1.5. Population dynamics in the time of Covid-19

In the spirit of Bernoulli, Pierre Magal and his colleagues have developed a coherent approach to epidemic modeling, as described in the present book. Their main contributions concern the estimation of the transmission rate, the evaluation of the number of unreported cases and the initial susceptible population size, as well as the use of the logistic equation to build a robust phenomenological model of the pandemic.

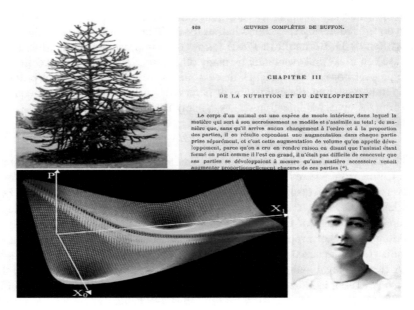

Fig. 0.2: *Top left: growth of the Chilean tree Araucaria. Top right: Buffon's interior mold theory, the first analogy of the present notion of attractor. Bottom left: surface representative of the potential P with its two minima. Bottom right: Maud Menten, co-creator of Michælis–Menten kinetics.*

2. Cell dynamics applied to morphogenesis

In morphogenesis modeling, the notion of attractor (initiated by Buffon) is fundamental. René Thom called the growth of trees a "wave towards the light", maximizing the capture of solar energy through photosynthesis. A very simple model, valid for the growth of the Chilean tree Araucaria (Figure 0.2), can account for the main stages observed in a tree's morphogenesis. At the end of a tree's branches, the local apices promote the synthesis of a plant hormone, auxin, in its meristems, which stimulates local growth and promotes the synthesis of an inhibitor which diffuses, prohibiting the growth of secondary axillary buds. An apex in operation therefore inhibits the other buds of its branch. Modeling this growth uses a gradient ODE defined by a potential P relating the variables X_0 (cell mass of apex) and X_1 (mass of primary axillary buds which succeed it on the branch) with a kinetic term called Michælis–Menten[6] competitive inhibition, expressed by the auxin. Figure 0.2 (bottom left) shows the potential P and its two minima, which correspond to the two stationary states of the ODE, as well as their basin of attraction.

The biological interpretation of these results is as follows: when the apical cells X_0 develop, the auxin they secrete inhibits the axillary buds. The development of the trunk carrying the apex makes the diffusion of auxin more difficult, over an increasing length, which frees the growth of the nearest axillary buds, which have arrived, thanks to the growth of the branch, in contact with the border of the phototropic zone. In turn, these primary axillary buds inhibit the secondary axillary buds that follow them, which will themselves be activated only when the critical distance of diffusion of auxin from the first axillary buds is reached again. An example of the shape that an adult tree will assume through this process is provided by Figure 0.2 (top left).

3. Conclusion

The present book is a beautiful illustration of what can be modeled and simulated using differential equations. Applications in biology (such as morphogenesis) and medicine (such as epidemic diseases) open up a huge field, which is well covered at the end of the book. The numerous mathematical results presented throughout the book, some of which are very original or intelligently revisited, provide the reader and future modeler with all the tools necessary to carry out his own research and add his contribution to the rich and exciting world of dynamical systems and their applications.

Grenoble, France, November 15, 2021 *Jacques Demongeot (UGA, IUF)*

---

[6] Michælis L. and Menten, M.L. Die Kinetik der Invertinwirkung. *Biochem. Z.* **49**, 333–369 (1913).

Foreword

"In my opinion, everything happens in nature in a mathematical way."

René Descartes, 1640

"If you assume continuity, you can open the well-stocked mathematical toolkit of continuous functions and differential equations, the saws and hammers of engineering and physics for the past two centuries (and the foreseeable future)."

Benoit Mandelbrot, 2004

Populations are ubiquitous in nature. All natural beings and natural phenomena can be viewed as populations. A central feature of all populations is their dynamic capacity – their ability to change. The understanding of population dynamics requires mathematical description, mathematical formulation, and mathematical analysis. These mathematical requirements have been central in the history of science.

In "Differential Equations and Population Dynamics I: Introductory Approaches", the authors unite the past and present developments of mathematical population theory and establish a foundation for its future development. Their treatment is designed for new and advanced students and new and advanced researchers in the subjects of this theory. Their emphasis is upon recent and current developments, which are undergoing major advances.

Throughout the book importance is placed on the presentation of meaningful applications to mathematical biology. Many of these applications are of major current interest to scientific researchers. The treatment of population processes in this book is applicable to all population levels – micro-populations in laboratory experiments, in-host population levels in individuals, and general population levels in compartmentalized species. The integration of classical and current research results provides researchers in both theoretical and applied specialties with a valuable resource. Current research in mathematical population dynamics is intimately connected to computer simulations of models and their applications. Numerous illustrative examples are provided, with MATLAB computer codes for their numerical simulations. The assembly of these computer codes is of great value to the scientific research community. The book includes a wealth of well-constructed figures, which illuminate the concepts presented. Each section provides a useful history of works in the topics presented and has instructive exercises for students.

In Part I, Linear Differential and Difference Equations, the general theory of linear differential equations, discrete time equations, and partial differential equations of population processes is developed. The exposition includes the treatment of continuous and discrete age-structured population models, delay equations and continuous time renewal equations, which are very useful in many biological processes. Part I contains a high-level operator-theoretic approach to linear models in the mathematical setting of Banach spaces. The results provide existence, uniqueness, positivity, and stability of solutions in this general context.

In Part II, Nonlinear Differential Equations, the theory of nonlinear differential equations and nonlinear discrete equations is developed. The principle of linearized stability is presented and illustrated with population examples. A treatment of positive and invariant subregions is provided for n-dimensional and infinite-dimensional cases. This section includes a detailed exposition on monotone semi-flows in general settings, with applications to diffusion processes in biological population theory. Examples of the general theory of nonlinear equations are given for diffusive logistic equations, for Bernoulli–Verhulst equations, and for competitive and co-operative Lotka–Volterra equations with multiple species. This material is very applicable to many current mathematical biological studies.

In Part III, Applications to Epidemic Models, recent publications of the authors concerning the COVID-19 pandemic are presented. The connection of models to data is emphasized, which is of major importance for validating projections of the models to future progression of the pandemic. The presentation of numerical simulations is of particular importance for researchers in epidemiology and public health. Because of the complexity and irregularity of typical COVID-19 daily reported cases, finding methods to fit data to models is an extreme challenge for the COVID-19 pandemic. In this section this data fitting problem is analyzed for cumulative reported cases in specific locations. Age-structured models for the COVID-19 epidemic are presented, which is very important for understanding the character of COVID-19 transmission related to age. Valuable numerical simulations for COVID-19 transmission in specific locations are provided, with careful attention to reported data. This section investigates the basic reproduction rate R_0 for COVID-19 epidemics. The basic reproduction rate R_0, which is the number of new infections generated by each current infection, is standard in epidemiology and is very important in assessing the severity of an epidemic disease. The analysis of R_0 for the COVID-19 epidemic in specific locations is carefully connected to reported COVID-19 data in these locations. The results of this section are applicable to all locations and time frames for the COVID-19 pandemic.

This book offers a valuable comprehensive treatment of the current subjects of mathematical population theory. It unites these subjects from the past to the present, and for the future.

Nashville, Tennessee, USA, October 15, 2021   *Glenn Webb*

Preface

This book is divided into three parts. The first part is devoted to linear ordinary differential equations. The second part focuses on nonlinear ordinary differential equations. In the third part, we present some examples of applications to epidemic models. Throughout the book, the concepts are illustrated with examples coming from population dynamics.

The first part contains four chapters. In Chapter 1, we present some examples of linear population dynamics models. These models can take into account age as well as spatial structure (i.e. the population is subdivided according to the age of the individuals or their spatial location). Chapter 2 focuses on the existence and uniqueness of solutions for linear ordinary differential equations. To consider less classical examples of linear systems, we extend Chapter 2 with some examples of differential equations with delay as well as the Volterra integral equation. In Chapter 3, we explore the notion of stability and instability for linear ordinary differential equations. Chapter 4 focuses on the notion of positivity of solutions. We also consider the Perron–Frobenius theorem and we derive several consequences.

In the second part, we start with Chapter 5, which extends the results of Chapter 2 to ordinary nonlinear differential equations. The novelty, compared with Chapter 2, will be the possibility for solutions to blow up after a finite period of time. The problem is illustrated with the one-dimensional logistic equation as well as the Bernoulli–Verhulst model. We also provide some explicit formulas for n-dimensional logistic equations and n-dimensional Bernoulli–Verhulst equations. Chapter 6 is devoted to the notion of linearized equations. Some stability and instability theorems are presented. The problem is again illustrated with the logistic equation. In Chapter 6, we also prove the Hartman–Grobman theorem for a hyperbolic equilibrium. Chapter 7 is focused on the notion of positivity of solutions as well as the invariance of subdomains. In Chapter 8, we consider monotone systems. We start this chapter by considering several types of differential inequalities. This provides a gentle introduction to monotone systems. We illustrate the use of monotone systems theory by considering logistic equations with diffusion.

In the third part, we discuss some recent developments in the application of ordinary differential equation models to real-world epidemiological problems. In Chapter 9, we present a method to compare epidemic models to the number of reported cases of the COVID-19 outbreak in Wuhan, China. Chapter 9 is a first attempt to understand how to identify the parameters of an epidemic model. The unknown parameters include some components of the initial distribution of the model. We also introduce the notion of a phenomenological model to represent the data (here an exponential function). In Chapter 10 we adapt the method to reported cases data decomposed into several age classes. We apply the method to COVID-19 data from Japan. In Chapter 11, we introduce a model which takes into account the data for the daily number of tests and the number of reported cases. In Chapter 12, we return to the single group problem and discuss the use of a phenomenological model to reconstruct data. We match phenomenological models to reported case data to uncover robust trends in the variations of the data and leave out random fluctuations. Then we analyze the phenomenological model to reconstruct the sociological behavior of individuals and to understand how the contacts between individuals change in time. Chapter 13 extends this idea and we show that phenomenological models can be applied to the cumulative reported cases data for France. In Chapter 14, the method is also extended to investigate the predictability of the outbreak in several countries, including China, South Korea, Italy, France, Germany, and the United Kingdom.

PM gave many winter and summer lectures to graduate students, Master's students, and Ph.D. students in Bordeaux and China (Shanghai Jiao Tong University, Beijing Normal University, Lanzhou University). The goal of these lectures was to introduce some aspects of population dynamics and ordinary differential equations and to focus on finite-dimensional results which admit an infinite-dimensional version.

Throughout this book, the last section of each chapter is devoted to additional remarks and notes, in which we will quote some related books where the reader can find more results. We include some of the MATLAB codes used to draw some figures of the book at the end of several chapters.

Le Havre,   *Arnaud Ducrot*
Bordeaux,   *Quentin Griette*
Beijing,   *Zhihua Liu*
Bordeaux, November 2021,   *Pierre Magal*

Contents

Part II Nonlinear Differential Equations

Part III Applications to Epidemic Models

Part I
Linear Differential and Difference Equations

Chapter 1
Introduction to Linear Population Dynamics

1.1 The Malthusian Model

Let $N(t)$ be the number of individuals in a population. Probably the first model to describe the growth of a population is the model of Malthus [246] (1798), which reads as follows

$$\frac{dN(t)}{dt} = \underbrace{b\,N(t)}_{\text{Flux of newborn}} - \underbrace{m\,N(t),}_{\text{Flux of exiting or death}} \tag{1.1}$$

where $b \geq 0$ is the *birth rate* and $m \geq 0$ is the *mortality rate*.

Equation (1.1) must be supplemented by initial data

$$N(t_0) = N_0 \geq 0, \tag{1.2}$$

where $N_0 \geq 0$ is the number of individuals at time t_0.

If we integrate equation (1.1) over the interval $[t, t + \Delta t]$, we obtain

$$N(t + \Delta t) = N(t) + \int_t^{t+\Delta t} b\,N(\sigma)d\sigma - \int_t^{t+\Delta t} m\,N(\sigma)d\sigma. \tag{1.3}$$

When we talk about the *flux* of newborn (respectively the flux of exiting or death), we mean that by integrating in time over the interval $[t, t + \Delta t]$ we obtain

$$\int_t^{t+\Delta t} b\,N(\sigma)d\sigma, \quad \left(\text{respectively } \int_t^{t+\Delta t} m\,N(\sigma)d\sigma \right),$$

the number of newborn individuals (respectively the number of exiting or dead individuals) during the time interval $[t, t + \Delta t]$.

The *growth rate of the population* is defined as $r = b - m$ and we can rewrite the equation as

$$\frac{dN(t)}{dt} = r\,N(t). \tag{1.4}$$

If we assume that $N(t) > 0$ for all $t \geq t_0$, then

© The Author(s), under exclusive license to Springer Nature Switzerland AG 2022
A. Ducrot et al., *Differential Equations and Population Dynamics I*, Lecture Notes on
Mathematical Modelling in the Life Sciences, https://doi.org/10.1007/978-3-030-98136-5_1

$$\frac{N'(t)}{N(t)} = r, \quad \forall t \geq t_0,$$

$$\Leftrightarrow \int_{t_0}^{t} \frac{N'(\sigma)}{N(\sigma)} d\sigma = \int_{t_0}^{t} r \, d\sigma, \quad \forall t \geq t_0,$$

$$\Leftrightarrow \ln(N(t)) - \ln(N(t_0)) = r \, (t - t_0), \quad \forall t \geq t_0,$$

therefore we obtain

$$N(t) = N_0 \exp\left(r \, (t - t_0)\right), \quad \forall t \geq t_0. \tag{1.5}$$

Remark 1.1 By computing the derivative of the formula obtained in (1.5) we deduce that this formula remains a solution whenever $N_0 \leq 0$.

In practice we fix a time step Δt (equal to one year, one month, one day etc . . .) and by using (1.4) we obtain the formula

$$N(t + \Delta t) = N(t) \exp\left(r \, \Delta t\right), \quad \forall t \geq t_0 \quad \Leftrightarrow \quad \ln\left(\frac{N(t + \Delta t)}{N(t)}\right) = r \, \Delta t, \quad \forall t \geq t_0. \tag{1.6}$$

This means that the function $t \to \ln\left(\frac{N(t + \Delta t)}{N(t)}\right)$ is constant in time, and

$$r \, \Delta t = \ln\left(\frac{N(t + \Delta t)}{N(t)}\right) = \ln\left(N(t + \Delta t)\right) - \ln\left(N(t)\right), \quad \forall t \geq t_0. \tag{1.7}$$

Hence r is the log variation of $N(t)$ per unit of time Δt.

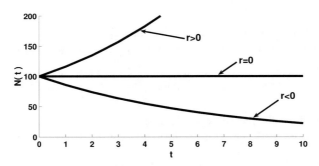

Fig. 1.1: *In this figure we plot $t \to 100 \exp(rt)$ over the time interval $[0, 10]$ and choose $r = 0.15$, $r = 0$ and $r = -0.15$ from the top to the bottom. The MATLAB code used for this figure is presented in Section 1.12.*

This model predicts that

- If $r = 0$ the population size is stationary or constant (in time).
- If $r > 0$ the population size grows exponentially and never stops growing.
- If $r < 0$ the population size approaches 0 as the time goes to infinity. In other words, the population becomes extinct after an infinite time.

1.2 The Time Periodic Population Dynamics Model

The continuous model assumes that the flux of newborns and the flux of death are constant in time. In most wild populations reproduction takes place seasonally, and mortality is also influenced by the seasons (temperature, food availability, etc...). The same is true for humans, who are more susceptible to viruses in winter (for example), so the seasons also matter for human populations. The cells in our body do not have the same activity during the day as they do at night. This is the so-called circadian rhythm.

Therefore it makes sense to consider the following extended version of the Malthusian model

$$\frac{dN(t)}{dt} = r(t)\,N(t), \quad \forall t \geq t_0 \text{ and } N(t_0) = N_0 \geq 0. \tag{1.8}$$

The time-dependent growth rate $r(t)$ can be defined by

$$r(t) = b(t) - m(t), \quad \forall t \geq t_0,$$

where $b(t)$ and $m(t)$ are respectively the time-dependent birth rate and mortality rate.

In Figure 1.2, if the time $t_0 = 0$ corresponds to January 1, the mortality of the animals will reach a maximum and therefore it makes sense to consider a mortality rate having the following form

$$m(t) = \cos(2\pi t) + 1.$$

The births will take place mostly around June, so it makes sense to consider a birth rate having the following form

$$b(t) = 2\,(\cos(2\pi(t + 0.6)) + 1).$$

The birth rate $b(t)$, the death rate or mortality rate $m(t)$ and the growth rate $r(t) = b(t) - m(t)$ are represented in Figure 1.2 (a), (b) and (c) respectively. The solutions of the periodic Malthusian model are represented in Figure 1.3 and in Figure 1.4 with a log scale.

In Figures 1.3 and 1.4 we are using the following formula for the solution

$$N(t) = N_0 e^{\int_{t_0}^{t} r(\sigma)d\sigma}, \quad \forall t \geq t_0.$$

By comparing Figure 1.3 and Figure 1.4 we can see that making some nonlinear transformation on the number of individuals may completely change our understanding of the solution. Indeed it is difficult to say anything about Figure 1.3, which looks complex already, while we can see that Figure 1.4 involves some periodic growth. The same thing could happen for data involving the seasonal growth of populations.

(a)

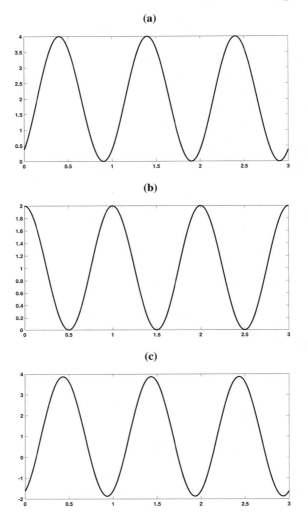

(b)

(c)

Fig. 1.2: *In this figure we plot the birth rate $t \rightarrow b(t) = 2\,(\cos(2\pi(t + 0.6)) + 1)$ in figure (a), the death rate $t \rightarrow m(t) = \cos(2\pi t) + 1$ in figure (b) and we plot the growth rate $t \rightarrow b(t) - m(t)$ in figure (c). The MATLAB code used for this figure is presented in Section 1.12.*

1.3 The Discrete-Time Population Dynamics Model

For the time-periodic population dynamics model, the period Δt could be one day (if we are talking about a cell growing in a dish); one year (if we are considering populations subject to seasonal changes), etc...

In periodic Malthusian models, we can take advantage of the periodicity to summarize the growth by using a single parameter over the whole period of time Δt.

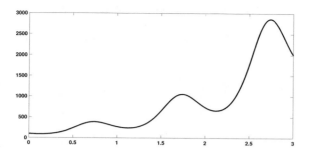

Fig. 1.3: *In this figure we plot*

$$t \to N(t) = 100 \times \exp\left(\int_0^t 2\left(\cos(2\pi(\sigma + 0.6)) + 1\right)\right) - \left(\cos(2\pi\sigma) + 1\right) d\sigma\right).$$

The MATLAB code used for this figure is presented in Section 1.12.

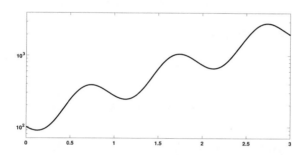

Fig. 1.4: *In this figure we plot*

$$t \to N(t) = 100 \times \exp\left(\int_0^t 2\left(\cos(2\pi(\sigma + 0.6)) + 1\right)\right) - \left(\cos(2\pi\sigma) + 1\right) d\sigma\right)$$

with a log scale for the vertical axis. The MATLAB code used for this figure is presented in Section 1.12.

Remember that

$$N(t) = e^{\int_{t_0}^t r(\sigma)d\sigma}, \quad \forall t \geq t_0 \text{ and } N(t_0) = N_0 \geq 0. \tag{1.9}$$

Assume that $t \to r(t)$ is Δt-periodic, that is,

$$r(t + \Delta t) = r(t), \quad \forall t \in \mathbb{R}.$$

Then

$$\frac{d}{dt} \int_t^{t+\Delta t} r(\sigma)d\sigma = r(t + \Delta t) - r(t) = 0,$$

and the map $t \to \int_t^{t+\Delta t} r(\sigma)\mathrm{d}\sigma$ is constant. We deduce that

$$N(t + \Delta t) = R\, N(t), \quad \forall t \geq t_0,$$

where

$$R = \exp\left(\int_{t_0}^{t_0+\Delta t} r(\sigma)\mathrm{d}\sigma\right).$$

Moreover, by defining

$$t_n = n \times \Delta t + t_0, \quad \forall n \in \mathbb{N},$$

and

$$U_n := N(t_n), \quad \forall n \in \mathbb{N},$$

we have

$$t_{n+1} = t_n + \Delta t \text{ and } U_{n+1} := N(t_n + \Delta t), \quad \forall n \in \mathbb{N}.$$

So we obtain the difference equation

$$U_n = R\, U_{n-1}, \quad \forall n \in \mathbb{N} \text{ with } U_0 = N_0. \tag{1.10}$$

The above equation can be rewritten equivalently as follows

$$U_n = R^n\, U_0, \quad \forall n \in \mathbb{N}, \tag{1.11}$$

where

$$R^n = \underbrace{R \times R \times \ldots \times R}_{n \text{ times}}.$$

The qualitative behavior of the solution is completely determined by comparing R to 1:

- If $R = 1$ the population size is stationary or constant (in time).
- If $R > 1$ the population size grows exponentially and never stops growing.
- If $R < 1$ the population size approaches 0 as the time goes to infinity. In other words, the population becomes extinct in infinite time.

In vitro experiments allow the computation of r and R. For example, the above formula is used to compute the so-called growth rate in cell cultures (in a Petri dish). In vivo, exponentially growing populations can also be observed by looking at an invading population. Otherwise, after the population has become well established, some limitations (for food, space, etc...) will limit the exponential growth and another behavior (with a saturation) will occur.

A natural question to address is the following:

Does a population (without limitation) always grow exponentially?

We can also ask the following question:

Is there a unique growth rate for the population that does not depend on how much time has elapsed since the population was established?

To investigate this question, in the next section we consider a discrete-time age-structured model and we will see what can be kept from the Malthusian models.

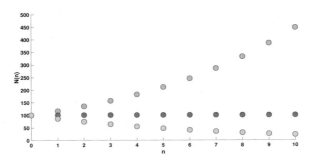

Fig. 1.5: *In this figure we plot $n \to 100 \times R^n$ over the time interval $[0, 10]$ and choose $R = \exp(0.15)$ (green), $R = 1$ (orange) and $R = \exp(-0.15)$ (blue) from the top to the bottom. The MATLAB code used for this figure is presented in Section 1.12.*

1.4 The Discrete-Time Leslie Model With Two Age Classes

In this section, we consider the so-called Leslie model (1945) [199, 200]. The Leslie model is a discrete-time age-structured population dynamics model. When we consider only two age classes, this model reads as follows

$$\begin{cases} N_1(t+1) = \beta_1 N_1(t) + \beta_2 N_2(t), \\ N_2(t+1) = \pi_1 N_1(t), \end{cases} \tag{1.12}$$

for each $t \in \mathbb{N}$ (time in year) with the initial distribution

$$\begin{pmatrix} N_1(0) \\ N_2(0) \end{pmatrix} = \begin{pmatrix} N_1^0 \\ N_2^0 \end{pmatrix}. \tag{1.13}$$

The parameters of the system as well as the state variables are defined below.

- β_1 is the average number of offspring produced per individuals in the first age class (i.e. with age $a \in [0, 1)$);
- β_2 is the average number of offspring produced per individuals in the second age class (i.e. with age $a \in [1, 2)$);
- $\pi_1 \in [0, 1]$ is the probability to survive from the first age class to the second age class;
- $N_1(t)$ is the number of individuals in the first age class at time t. That is, the number of individuals with age $a \in [0, 1)$ at time t;
- $N_2(t)$ is the number of individuals in the second age class at time t. That is, the number of individuals with age $a \in [1, 2)$ at time t.

The total number of individuals in the population at time t is given by

$$N(t) := N_1(t) + N_2(t).$$

The diagram of flux is presented in Figure 1.6. The loop for the first age class corresponds to the individuals that reproduce immediately after their birth. This is possible if we consider some insects like mosquitoes, for example. This model is

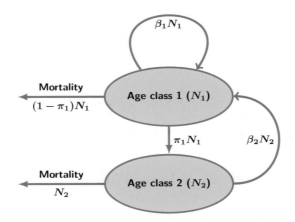

Fig. 1.6: *Diagram of flux for the two age classes model* (1.12).

obtained by using the following description

$$N_1(t+1) = \text{number of offspring produced by the first age during the}$$
$$\qquad\qquad\quad \text{period } [t, t+1]$$
$$\qquad\quad + \text{ number of offspring produced by the second age during the}$$
$$\qquad\qquad\quad \text{period } [t, t+1]$$

and

$$N_2(t+1) = \text{number of individuals in the first age class who survived the period}$$
$$\qquad\qquad\quad \text{of time } [t, t+1].$$

The system (1.12) can be rewritten in matrix form as

$$\begin{pmatrix} N_1(t+1) \\ N_2(t+1) \end{pmatrix} = \begin{pmatrix} \beta_1 & \beta_2 \\ \pi_1 & 0 \end{pmatrix} \begin{pmatrix} N_1(t) \\ N_1(t) \end{pmatrix}, \tag{1.14}$$

where the matrix

$$L = \begin{pmatrix} \beta_1 & \beta_2 \\ \pi_1 & 0 \end{pmatrix} \tag{1.15}$$

is called a *Leslie matrix*.

We observe that

$$\begin{pmatrix} N_1(2) \\ N_2(2) \end{pmatrix} = L \times \begin{pmatrix} N_1(1) \\ N_2(1) \end{pmatrix} = L \times L \begin{pmatrix} N_1(0) \\ N_2(0) \end{pmatrix}$$

therefore by using an induction argument we obtain

$$\begin{pmatrix} N_1(n) \\ N_2(n) \end{pmatrix} = L^n \begin{pmatrix} N_1(0) \\ N_2(0) \end{pmatrix}, \quad \forall n \geq 0,$$

where

$$L^n = \underbrace{L \times L \times \ldots \times L}_{n \text{ times}}.$$

1.4.1 The special case $\beta_1 = 0$

In the special case $\beta_1 = 0$ the Leslie matrix L has the following form

$$L = \begin{pmatrix} 0 & \beta_2 \\ \pi_1 & 0 \end{pmatrix},$$

and it follows that

$$L^2 = L \times L = \begin{pmatrix} \beta_2\pi_1 & 0 \\ 0 & \beta_2\pi_1 \end{pmatrix} = \beta_2\pi_1 \begin{pmatrix} 1 & 0 \\ 0 & 1 \end{pmatrix}.$$

Therefore

$$L^2 = \gamma^2 I,$$

where

$$I = \begin{pmatrix} 1 & 0 \\ 0 & 1 \end{pmatrix} \text{ and } \gamma = \sqrt{\beta_2\pi_1}.$$

By using this observation we deduce that

$$\begin{aligned} L^2 &= \gamma^2 I, \\ L^3 &= L \times L \times L = \gamma^2 L, \\ L^4 &= L \times L \times L \times L = L^2 \times L^2 = \gamma^4 I, \end{aligned}$$

and by induction, we deduce that for each integer $n \geq 0$

$$L^{2n} = \underbrace{L^2 \times L^2 \times \ldots \times L^2}_{n \text{ times}} = \gamma^{2n} I$$

and

$$L^{2n+1} = L^{2n} \times L = \gamma^{2n} L.$$

In this special case the population grows but the direction of the distribution $(N_1(n), N_2(n))$ may change a lot.

By using Figures 1.7 and 1.8 we obtain undamped oscillations for the direction of the population distribution. The population grows like an exponential, but with a large oscillation.

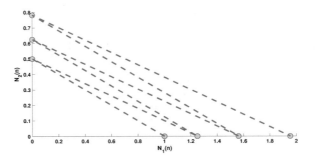

Fig. 1.7: *In this figure we plot* $(N_1(n), N_2(n))$ *where* n *varies from* 0 *to* 6. *The MATLAB code used for this figure is presented in Section 1.12.*

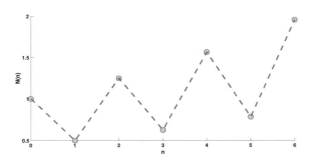

Fig. 1.8: *In this figure we plot* $n \rightarrow N(n) = N_1(n) + N_2(n)$ *over the time interval* $[0, 6]$. *The MATLAB code used for this figure is presented in Section 1.12.*

In this special case, we may try to find some initial distribution that gives a constant direction (i.e. we can look for some non-negative eigenvector). In other words, we look for a non-negative vector $(N_1^\star, N_2^\star)$ such that

$$L \begin{pmatrix} N_1^\star \\ N_2^\star \end{pmatrix} = \gamma \begin{pmatrix} N_1^\star \\ N_2^\star \end{pmatrix},$$

where $\gamma = \sqrt{\beta_2 \pi_1}$. We have

$$L \begin{pmatrix} N_1^\star \\ N_2^\star \end{pmatrix} = \gamma \begin{pmatrix} N_1^\star \\ N_2^\star \end{pmatrix} \Leftrightarrow \begin{cases} \beta_2 N_2^\star = \gamma N_1^\star \\ \pi_1 N_1^\star = \gamma N_2^\star \end{cases} \Leftrightarrow N_1^\star = \sqrt{\frac{\beta_2}{\pi_1}} N_2^\star.$$

Therefore starting from

$$N_1^\star = \sqrt{\frac{\beta_2}{\pi_1}} \text{ and } N_2^\star = 1,$$

the direction of the population distribution does not change over time. In Figure 1.9 we observe that this direction is preserved.

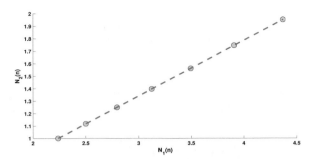

Fig. 1.9: *In this figure we plot $(N_1(n), N_2(n))$ where n varies from 0 to 6. The MATLAB code used for this figure is presented in Section 1.12, in which we use the initial distribution $N_1(0) = \sqrt{\dfrac{\beta_2}{\pi_1}}$ and $N_2(0) = 1$.*

In Figure 1.10 we observe a Malthusian growth with no oscillations around the exponential.

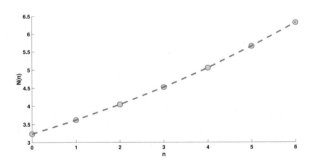

Fig. 1.10: *In this figure we plot $n \rightarrow N(n) = N_1(n) + N_2(n)$ over the time interval $[0, 6]$. The MATLAB code used for this figure is presented in Section 1.12, in which we use the initial distribution $N_1(0) = \sqrt{\dfrac{\beta_2}{\pi_1}}$ and $N_2(0) = 1$.*

1.4.2 The special case $\beta_2 = 0$

In the special case $\beta_2 = 0$ the Leslie matrix L has the following form

$$L = \begin{pmatrix} \beta_1 & 0 \\ \pi_1 & 0 \end{pmatrix}$$

and it follows that

$$L^2 = \begin{pmatrix} \beta_1^2 & 0 \\ \pi_1\beta_1 & 0 \end{pmatrix}$$

and by induction

$$L^n = \begin{pmatrix} \beta_1^n & 0 \\ \pi_1\beta_1^{n-1} & 0 \end{pmatrix} = \beta_1^{n-1}L, \quad \forall n = 1, 2, 3, \ldots.$$

We deduce that

$$L^n \begin{pmatrix} 1 \\ 0 \end{pmatrix} = \beta_1^{n-1} \begin{pmatrix} \beta_1 \\ \pi_1 \end{pmatrix}$$

and

$$L^n \begin{pmatrix} 0 \\ 1 \end{pmatrix} = \begin{pmatrix} 0 \\ 0 \end{pmatrix}.$$

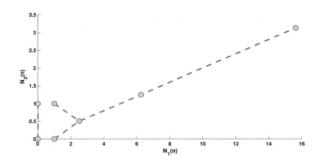

Fig. 1.11: *In this figure we plot* $(N_1(n), N_2(n))$ *where* n *varies from* 0 *to* 6. *The MATLAB code used for this figure is presented in Section 1.12, in which the initial distribution* $(N_1(0), N_2(0))$ *is either* $(1, 0)$, $(0, 1)$ *or* $(1, 1)$. *We use* $\pi_1 = 0.5$ *and* $\beta_1 = 2.5$.

1.4.3 The special case $\beta_1 > 0$ and $\beta_2 > 0$

The case $\beta_1 > 0$ and $\beta_2 > 0$ is considered in Chapter 4, devoted to the so-called Perron–Frobenius theorem (see [275] and [111, 112]). Actually from this theorem, we obtain an asynchronous exponential growth result.

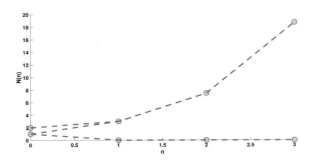

Fig. 1.12: *In this figure we plot* $n \to N(n) = N_1(n) + N_2(n)$ *over the time interval* $[0, 6]$. *The MATLAB code used for this figure is presented in Section 1.12, in which the initial distribution* $(N_1(0), N_2(0))$ *is either* $(1, 0)$, $(0, 1)$ *or* $(1, 1)$. *We use* $\pi_1 = 0.5$ *and* $\beta_1 = 2.5$.

In Chapter 4, we will see that there exists a constant $\lambda > 0$ and two strictly positive vectors $V_r \in (0, +\infty)^2$, a right eigenvector of L (i.e. $LV_r = \lambda V_r$), and $V_l \in (0, +\infty)^2$, a left eigenvector of L (i.e. $V_l^T L = \lambda V_r^T$), with $\langle V_l, V_r \rangle = 1$ such that

$$\lim_{n \to +\infty} \frac{1}{\lambda^n} L^n U(0) = \langle V_l, U_0 \rangle V_r,$$

where $\langle \cdot, \cdot \rangle$ is the Euclidean scalar product.

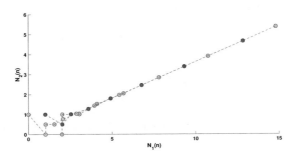

Fig. 1.13: *In this figure we plot* $(N_1(n), N_2(n))$ *where n varies from 0 to 6. The MATLAB code used for this figure is presented in Section 1.12, in which the initial distribution* $(N_1(0), N_2(0))$ *is either* $(1, 0)$, $(0, 1)$ *or* $(1, 1)$. *We use* $\pi_1 = 0.5$ *and* $\beta_1 = \beta_2 = 1.01$.

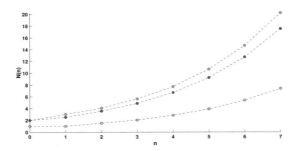

Fig. 1.14: *In this figure we plot* $n \to N(n) = N_1(n) + N_2(n)$ *over the time interval* $[0, 6]$. *The MATLAB code used for this figure is presented in Section 1.12, in which the initial distribution* $(N_1(0), N_2(0))$ *is either* $(1, 0)$, $(0, 1)$ *or* $(1, 1)$. *We use* $\pi_1 = 0.5$ *and* $\beta_1 = \beta_2 = 1.01$.

1.5 The Discrete-Time Leslie Models With an Arbitrary Number of Age Classes

Before describing the general Leslie model, let us consider the Leslie model with three age classes. By using the same notation and the same idea as the model with two age classes we can write the following model

$$\begin{cases} N_1(t+1) = \beta_1 N_1(t) + \beta_2 N_2(t) + \beta_3 N_3(t), \\ N_2(t+1) = \pi_1 N_1(t), \\ N_3(t+1) = \pi_2 N_2(t), \end{cases} \tag{1.16}$$

for each $t \in \mathbb{N}$ (time in year) with the initial distribution

$$\begin{pmatrix} N_1(0) \\ N_2(0) \\ N_3(0) \end{pmatrix} = \begin{pmatrix} N_1^0 \\ N_2^0 \\ N_3^0 \end{pmatrix}.$$

The Leslie system (1.16) can be rewritten in the following matrix form

$$\begin{pmatrix} N_1(t+1) \\ N_2(t+1) \\ N_3(t+1) \end{pmatrix} = \begin{pmatrix} \beta_1 & \beta_2 & \beta_3 \\ \pi_1 & 0 & 0 \\ 0 & \pi_2 & 0 \end{pmatrix} \begin{pmatrix} N_1(t) \\ N_2(t) \\ N_3(t) \end{pmatrix}.$$

Therefore the Leslie matrix corresponding to three age groups takes the following form

$$L = \begin{pmatrix} \beta_1 & \beta_2 & \beta_3 \\ \pi_1 & 0 & 0 \\ 0 & \pi_2 & 0 \end{pmatrix}.$$

The diagram of flux is presented in Figure 1.15. The loop for the first age class corresponds to the individuals that reproduce immediately after their birth (as in some insects, like mosquitoes). The Leslie model can be extended to an arbitrary

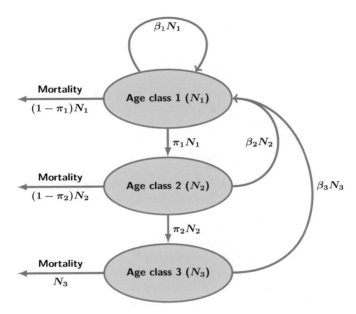

Fig. 1.15: *Diagram of flux for the three age classes model* (1.16).

number of age classes $n \geq 2$

$$\begin{cases} N_1(t+1) = \beta_1 N_1(t) + \beta_2 N_2(t) + \cdots + \beta_n N_n(t), \\ N_2(t+1) = \pi_1 N_1(t), \\ \vdots \\ N_n(t+1) = \pi_{n-1} N_{n-1}(t), \end{cases} \tag{1.17}$$

for each $t \in \mathbb{N}$ (time in years) with the initial distribution

$$\begin{pmatrix} N_1(0) \\ N_2(0) \\ \vdots \\ N_n(0) \end{pmatrix} = \begin{pmatrix} N_1^0 \\ N_2^0 \\ \vdots \\ N_n^0 \end{pmatrix}.$$

The diagram of flux is presented in Figure 1.16. The loop for the first age class corresponds to individuals that reproduce immediately after their birth. The system (1.17) can be rewritten in matrix form as the following vector-valued difference equations

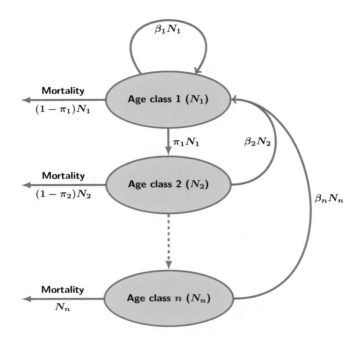

Fig. 1.16: *Diagram of flux for the n age classes model* (1.17).

$$
\begin{pmatrix} N_1(t+1) \\ N_2(t+1) \\ \vdots \\ N_n(t+1) \end{pmatrix} = \begin{pmatrix} \beta_1 & \beta_2 & \beta_3 & \cdots & \beta_n \\ \pi_1 & 0 & 0 & \cdots & 0 \\ 0 & \pi_2 & 0 & \cdots & 0 \\ \vdots & \ddots & \ddots & \ddots & \vdots \\ 0 & \cdots & 0 & \pi_{n-1} & 0 \end{pmatrix} \begin{pmatrix} N_1(t) \\ N_2(t) \\ \vdots \\ N_n(t) \end{pmatrix}, \quad \forall t = 0, 1, \dots . \qquad (1.18)
$$

The corresponding Leslie matrix is the following

$$
L = \begin{pmatrix} \beta_1 & \beta_2 & \beta_3 & \cdots & \beta_n \\ \pi_1 & 0 & 0 & \cdots & 0 \\ 0 & \pi_2 & 0 & \cdots & 0 \\ \vdots & \ddots & \ddots & \ddots & \vdots \\ 0 & \cdots & 0 & \pi_{n-1} & 0 \end{pmatrix} .
$$

Remark 1.2 The above convergence result of the normalized distribution is a consequence of the Perron–Frobenius theorem. This example will be reconsidered in Chapter 4.

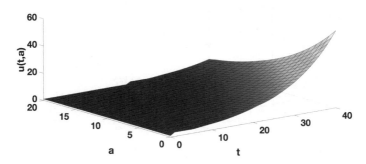

Fig. 1.17: *In this figure we plot a solution* $t \to u(t, a)$ *of the Leslie model with* $a \in [0, 20]$. *The reproduction function is defined by* $\beta(a) = 0.8 * \Delta a$ *if* $a > 5$ *and* $\beta(a) = 0$ *otherwise. The survival rate is* $\pi(a) = \exp(-0.1 * \Delta a)$. *The initial distribution is constant, equal to 1. We observe that it takes 40 years for the distribution of population to grow exponentially.*

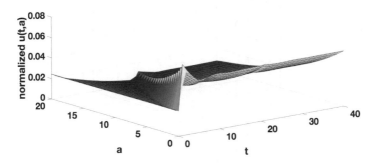

Fig. 1.18: *In this figure we plot a normalized solution* $t \to u(t, a)/\Sigma_{i=0,\dots,20} u(t, i)$ *of the Leslie model* $a \in [0, 20]$. *The reproduction function is defined by* $\beta(a) = 0.8 * \Delta a$ *if* $a > 5$ *and* $\beta(a) = 0$ *otherwise. The survival rate is* $\pi(a) = \exp(-0.1 * \Delta a)$. *The initial distribution is constant, equal to 1. We observe the convergence of the normalized distribution when the time becomes large enough.*

1.6 The Continuous-Time Leslie Models With an Arbitrary Number of Age Classes

Instead of considering a discrete-time age-structured model we can also look at a continuous-time model with a discrete number of age classes as before. By using the same notations and the same model idea as the model with two age classes we can write the following model

$$\begin{cases} N_1(t)' = \underbrace{\beta_1 N_1(t) + \cdots + \beta_n N_n(t)}_{\text{Flux of newborn}} - \underbrace{\mu_1 N_1(t)}_{\text{Exit or death}} - \underbrace{\eta_1 N_1(t)}_{\text{Flux going to class 2}}, \\ N_2(t)' = \eta_1 N_1(t) - \underbrace{\mu_2 N_2(t)}_{\text{Exit or death}} - \underbrace{\eta_2 N_2(t)}_{\text{Flux going to class 3}}, \\ \vdots \\ N_n(t)' = \eta_{n-1} N_{n-1}(t) - \underbrace{\mu_n N_n(t)}_{\text{Exit or death}} - \underbrace{\eta_n N_n(t)}_{\substack{\text{Flux of individuals} \\ \text{getting older}}}, \end{cases} \tag{1.19}$$

for each $t \in \mathbb{N}$ (time in years) with the initial distribution

$$\begin{pmatrix} N_1(0) \\ N_2(0) \\ \vdots \\ N_n(0) \end{pmatrix} = \begin{pmatrix} N_1^0 \\ N_2^0 \\ \vdots \\ N_n^0 \end{pmatrix}.$$

The system (1.19) can be rewritten in matrix form as

$$N(t)' = M\,N(t),$$

where the matrix of the system is the difference of two matrices

$$M = L - D,$$

where L is again a Leslie matrix defined by

$$L = \begin{pmatrix} \beta_1 & \beta_2 & \beta_3 & \cdots & \beta_n \\ \eta_1 & 0 & 0 & \cdots & 0 \\ 0 & \eta_2 & 0 & \cdots & 0 \\ \vdots & \ddots & \ddots & \ddots & \vdots \\ 0 & \cdots & 0 & \eta_{n-1} & 0 \end{pmatrix}$$

and D is the diagonal matrix

$$D = \begin{pmatrix} \mu_1 + \eta_1 & 0 & \cdots & 0 \\ 0 & \mu_2 + \eta_2 & \ddots & \vdots \\ \vdots & \ddots & \ddots & 0 \\ 0 & \cdots & 0 & \mu_n + \eta_n \end{pmatrix}.$$

1.7 A Patch Model With Two Cities

In this section, we follow an idea of Sattenspiel and Dietz [305]. We present a patch model adapted to intercity movement. Our goal is to explain how to derive the parameters of the model in practice.

Our goal is to propose a short-term patch model to describe the movement of individuals during a few months (1–6 months). Therefore we can neglect the vital birth and death dynamic. In the case of an epidemic, we assume that the number of deaths does not significantly change the number of individuals in a given city.

To build our patch model, we make the following assumptions.

Assumption 1.3 We assume that the time spent in city 2 by visitors from city 1 follows an exponential law, and the average length of stay is $1/\rho_{21}$.

Let us start with two cities. Let $U_{i1}(t)$ be the number of individuals from city 1 and either: 1) staying in city 1 if $i = 1$; or 2) traveling in city 2 if $i = 2$. The total number of individuals originating from city 1 is

$$U_1 = U_{11}(t) + U_{21}(t), \tag{1.20}$$

which is assumed to be constant for simplicity. The model is given by

$$
\begin{aligned}
U'_{11}(t) &= -\Gamma_{12}(t) && +\rho_{21}U_{21} \\
U'_{21}(t) &= + \underbrace{\Gamma_{12}(t)}_{\substack{\text{Flux of individuals} \\ \text{traveling to city 2} \\ \text{from city 1}}} && - \underbrace{\rho_{21}U_{21}}_{\substack{\text{Flux of individuals} \\ \text{returning back home}}}
\end{aligned}
\tag{1.21}
$$

In our model $\rho_{21}U_{21}$ is the flux of individuals returning back home to city 1 after a trip in city 2. In order to apply our model we need to determine $1/\rho_{21}$, the average length of stay in city 2 for individuals originating from city 1. Moreover, Γ_{12} is the flux of individuals living in city 1 who are traveling in city 2.

Assumption 1.4 We assume that the number of individuals originating from city 1 who are traveling in city 2 is

$$U_{21} = f_{21} U_{11}, \tag{1.22}$$

where $f_{21} \geq 0$.

Remark 1.5 From (1.20) and (1.22) we have

$$U_1 = (1 + f_{21})U_{11} \Leftrightarrow U_{11} = \frac{1}{1 + f_{21}}U_1,$$

therefore (1.22) is equivalent to

$$U_{21} = \frac{f_{21}}{1 + f_{21}} U_1 = p_{21} U_1.$$

We observe that

$$p_{21} = \frac{f_{21}}{1 + f_{21}} \Leftrightarrow f_{21} = \frac{p_{21}}{1 - p_{21}}.$$

Therefore the parameter f_{21} in (1.22) can be computed by using $p_{21} \in (0, 1)$, which is the fraction of individuals living in city 1 and traveling in city 2.

By substituting $U_{21} = p_{21} U_1$ (on the left-hand side) and $U_{21} = f_{21} U_{11}$ (on the right-hand side) of the U_2-equation into the second equation of (1.21) we get

$$0 = +\Gamma_{12}(t) - p_{21} f_{21} U_{11}(t). \tag{1.23}$$

Therefore we obtain

$$\Gamma_{12}(t) = p_{21} f_{21} U_{11}(t).$$

Hence the patch model describing the movement of individuals living in city 1 must be

$$\begin{cases} U'_{11} = -p_{21} f_{21} U_{11} + p_{21} U_{21} \\ U'_{21} = +p_{21} f_{21} U_{11} - p_{21} U_{21}. \end{cases} \tag{1.24}$$

Remark 1.6 Conversely by summing the two equations of (1.24), we obtain $U_1(t)' = 0$. Moreover, by replacing U_{11} by $U_1 - U_{21}$ in the second equation of (1.24), we obtain

$$U'_{21} = +p_{21} f_{21} (U_1 - U_{21}) - p_{21} U_{21} \tag{1.25}$$

which is equivalent to

$$U'_{21} = +p_{21} f_{21} U_1 - p_{21} (1 + f_{21}) U_{21}. \tag{1.26}$$

Therefore

$$\lim_{t \to \infty} U_{21}(t) = \frac{f_{21}}{1 + f_{21}} U_1 = p_{21} U_1.$$

Similarly,

$$\lim_{t \to \infty} U_{11}(t) = (1 - p_{21}) U_1.$$

The model with two cities

The movement of individuals living in city 1 with 2 cities is described by

$$\textbf{(Individuals from city 1)} \begin{cases} U'_{11} = -p_{21} f_{21} U_{11} + p_{21} U_{21} \\ U'_{21} = +p_{21} f_{21} U_{11} - p_{21} U_{21}. \end{cases} \tag{1.27}$$

The movement of individuals living in city 2 with 2 cities is described by

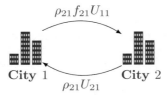

Fig. 1.19: *Movement of individuals originating from city 1 with 2 cities.*

(Individuals from city 2) $\begin{cases} U'_{22} = -\rho_{12}f_{12}\,U_{22} \ +\rho_{12}\,U_{12} \\ U'_{12} = +\rho_{12}f_{12}\,U_{22} \ -\rho_{12}\,U_{12}, \end{cases}$ $\hspace{2cm}$ (1.28)

where U_{12} is the number of individuals originating from city 2 who are traveling in city 1 and U_{22} is the number of individuals originating from city 2 staying in city 2. The total number of individuals in city 2 is

$$U_2 = U_{12} + U_{22}.$$

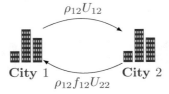

Fig. 1.20: *Movement of individuals originating only from city 2 with 2 cities.*

The model with two cities and without origin distinction

The previous models (1.27) and (1.28) allow more freedom in the movement of individuals. Indeed, such models allow different behaviors for the people who originate from each city. However, to simplify the model, we may wish to reduce the number of parameters. The following reduction procedure can be helpful.

To simplify the previous models (1.27) and (1.28), we write a model without distinguishing the origin of individuals. Indeed, the total number of individuals staying in city 1 at time t is given by

$$U_{1.} = U_{11} + U_{12}$$

and the total number of individuals staying in city 2 at time t is given by

$$U_{2.} = U_{21} + U_{22}.$$

By summing the first equation of (1.27) and the second equation of (1.28) we obtain

$$U'_{1.} = -\rho_{21}f_{21}\,U_{11} + \rho_{21}\,U_{21} + \rho_{12}f_{12}\,U_{22} - \rho_{12}\,U_{12},$$

and by summing the second equation of (1.27) and the first equation of (1.28) we obtain

$$U'_{2.} = +\rho_{21}f_{21}\,U_{11} - \rho_{21}\,U_{21} - \rho_{12}f_{12}\,U_{22} + \rho_{12}\,U_{12}.$$

Assumption 1.7 Assume that $\rho_{21}f_{21} = \rho_{12}$ and $\rho_{21} = \rho_{12}f_{12}$.

Under the above assumption, we obtain a model with two cities without origin distinction

$$\begin{cases} U'_{1.} = -\rho_{12}U_{1.} + \rho_{12}U_{2.}, \\ U'_{2.} = \rho_{12}U_{1.} - \rho_{12}U_{2.}. \end{cases} \tag{1.29}$$

1.8 The model with N cities

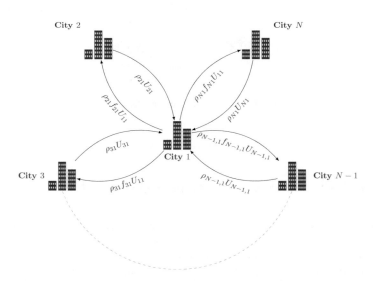

Fig. 1.21: *Movement of individuals originating from city 1.*

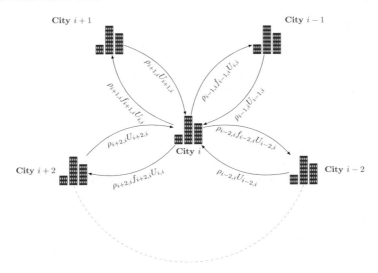

Fig. 1.22: *Movement of individuals originating from city i.*

The model describing the movement of individuals originating from city 1 is

(Individuals from city 1)

$$
\begin{cases}
U_{11}' = -\left(\sum_{i=2}^{N} \rho_{i1} f_{i1}\right) U_{11} + \sum_{i=2}^{N} \rho_{i1} U_{i1} \\
U_{21}' = \quad +\rho_{21} f_{21} U_{11} \qquad -\rho_{21} U_{21} \\
\quad\vdots \qquad\qquad \vdots \qquad\qquad \vdots \\
U_{N1}' = \quad +\rho_{N1} f_{N1} U_{11} \qquad -\rho_{N1} U_{N1}.
\end{cases}
\tag{1.30}
$$

The model describing the movement of individuals originating from city i is

(Individuals from city i)

$$
\begin{cases}
U_{1,i}' = \qquad +\rho_{1,i} f_{1,i} U_{i,i} \qquad\qquad -\rho_{1,i} U_{1,i} \\
\quad\vdots \qquad\qquad \vdots \qquad\qquad\qquad \vdots \\
U_{i-1,i}' = \qquad +\rho_{i-1,i} f_{i-1,i} U_{i,i} \qquad\qquad -\rho_{i-1,i} U_{i-1,i} \\
U_{i,i}' = -\left(\sum_{j=2,\dots,i-1,i+1,\dots,N} \rho_{j,i} f_{j,i}\right) U_{i,i} + \left(\sum_{j=2,\dots,i-1,i+1,\dots,N} \rho_{j,i} U_{j,i}\right) \\
U_{i+1,i}' = \qquad +\rho_{i+1,i} f_{i+1,i} U_{i,i} \qquad\qquad -\rho_{i+1,i} U_{i+1,i} \\
\quad\vdots \qquad\qquad \vdots \qquad\qquad\qquad \vdots \\
U_{N,i}' = \qquad +\rho_{N,i} f_{N,i} U_{i,i} \qquad\qquad -\rho_{N,i} U_{N,i}.
\end{cases}
\tag{1.31}
$$

Assumption 1.8 We assume that each city $i = 1, \ldots, N$ satisfies

$$\rho_{j,i} f_{j,i} > 0, \quad \forall j = 1, \ldots, i-1, i+1, \ldots, N.$$

Due to Assumption 1.8, by using the Perron–Frobenius theorem there exists a unique distribution $p_{1,i} > 0, \ldots, p_{N,i} > 0$ such that

$$p_{1,i} + \cdots + p_{N,i} = 1$$

and satisfying

$$\begin{cases} 0 = & +\rho_{1,i} f_{1,i} \, p_{i,i} & -\rho_{1,i} \, p_{1,i} \\ \vdots & \vdots & \vdots \\ 0 = & +\rho_{i-1,i} f_{i-1,i} \, p_{i,i} & -\rho_{i-1,i} \, p_{i-1,i} \\ 0 = -\left(\displaystyle\sum_{j=2,\ldots,i-1,i+1,\ldots,N} \rho_{j,i} f_{j,i} \right) p_{i,i} & + \left(\displaystyle\sum_{j=2,\ldots,i-1,i+1,\ldots,N} \rho_{j,i} \, p_{j,i} \right) \\ 0 = & +\rho_{i+1,i} f_{i+1,i} \, p_{i,i} & -\rho_{i+1,i} \, p_{i+1,i} \\ \vdots & \vdots & \vdots \\ 0 = & +\rho_{N,i} f_{N,i} \, p_{i,i} & -\rho_{N,i} \, p_{N,i}. \end{cases} \quad (1.32)$$

Definition 1.9 The quantity $p_{j,i}$ is the proportion of individuals moving from city i to city j.

As before we express the parameters $f_{j,i}$ as a function of $p_{j,i}$

$$\begin{cases} f_{1,i} = \dfrac{p_{1,i}}{p_{i,i}} \\ \vdots \\ f_{i-1,i} = \dfrac{p_{i-1,i}}{p_{i,i}} \\ f_{i+1,i} = \dfrac{p_{i+1,i}}{p_{i,i}} \\ \vdots \\ f_{N,i} = \dfrac{p_{N,i}}{p_{i,i}}. \end{cases} \quad (1.33)$$

Remark 1.10 Due to seasonal variation between business trips and personal trips the parameters of the model should vary in time. For example, the proportion $p_{j,i}$ of individuals traveling from city i to city j and the length of stay $1/\rho_{j,i}$ in city j should both vary in time.

1.9 A Diffusion Process Between N Aligned Cities

In this section we consider the heat equation. This equation is commonly used in population dynamics to describe the movement of individuals. It reads as follows

$$\begin{cases} \partial_t u(t,x) = \varepsilon \partial_x^2 u(t,x), \text{ for } x \in (0,1)\,, \\ \partial_x u(t,0) = \partial_x u(t,1) = 0, \\ u(0,\cdot) = \varphi \in L^2\,(0,1)\,. \end{cases}$$

The boundary conditions mean that there is no flux at the boundary.

To write the numerical scheme for this equation (i.e. a discrete version of it) we set

$$u_i^n = u(n\Delta t, i\Delta x).$$

Then the main part of the equation may be written for $i = 2, ..., N-1$ as

$$\frac{u_i^{n+1} - u_i^n}{\Delta t} = \varepsilon \frac{1}{\Delta x^2} \left(u_{i+1}^n - 2u_i^n + u_{i-1}^n \right).$$

For $i = 1$ we obtain

$$\frac{u_1^{n+1} - u_1^n}{\Delta t} = \varepsilon \frac{1}{\Delta x^2} \left[\left(u_2^n - u_1^n \right) - \left(u_1^n - u_0^n \right) \right]$$

and the boundary condition $\left(u_1^n - u_0^n \right)/\Delta x = 0$ gives

$$\frac{u_1^{n+1} - u_1^n}{\Delta t} = \varepsilon \frac{1}{\Delta x^2} \left(u_2^n - u_1^n \right).$$

Similarly for $i = N$ we should have

$$\frac{u_N^{n+1} - u_N^n}{\Delta t} = \varepsilon \frac{1}{\Delta x^2} \left(u_N^n - u_{N-1}^n \right).$$

So we obtain the following explicit numerical scheme for the heat equation for $n \geq 0$

$$u^{n+1} = u^n + \frac{\varepsilon \Delta t}{\Delta x^2} D u^n,$$

with the initial distribution

$$u^0 = u_0 \geq 0,$$

where

$$D = \begin{pmatrix} -1 & 1 & 0 & \cdots\cdots\cdots & 0 \\ 1 & -2 & 1 & & \vdots \\ 0 & 1 & -2 & 1 & \ddots & \vdots \\ \vdots & & \ddots & \ddots & \ddots & 0 \\ \vdots & & & \ddots & -2 & 1 \\ 0 & \cdots\cdots & 0 & 1 & -1 \end{pmatrix}.$$

The numerical scheme may be rewritten as

$$u_i^{n+1} = u_i^n + \varepsilon \frac{\Delta t}{\Delta x^2} \left(u_{i+1}^n - 2u_i^n + u_{i-1}^n \right).$$

So we obtain for $i = 2, \ldots, N - 1$,

$$u_i^{n+1} = \frac{p}{2} u_{i+1}^n + (1 - p) u_i^n + \frac{p}{2} u_{i-1}^n$$

and for $i = 1$

$$u_1^{n+1} = \frac{p}{2} u_2^n + \left(1 - \frac{p}{2} \right) u_1^n$$

and for $i = N$

$$u_N^{n+1} = \left(1 - \frac{p}{2} \right) u_N^n + \frac{p}{2} u_{N-1}^n,$$

where

$$p := 2\varepsilon \frac{\Delta t}{\Delta x^2}.$$

Therefore we can interpret the discrete model as follows. An individual in city i, with $2 \le i \le N - 1$, will move to city $i - 1$ or to city $i + 1$, each with probability $p/2$, or stay in city i with probability $1 - p$. An individual in city 1 or N will move to city 2 or $N - 1$, respectively, with probability $p/2$, or stay with probability $1 - p/2$.

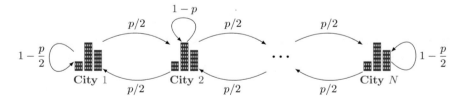

Fig. 1.23: *Diagram of flux for a diffusion process between N aligned cities.*

Definition 1.11 The condition $p = 2\frac{\varepsilon\Delta t}{\Delta x^2} < 1$ is called the *Courant–Friedrichs–Lax condition* (*CFL condition* for short).

Let $\mathbb{1} := (1, \ldots, 1)^T$. Then we obtain

$$D\mathbb{1} = 0 \text{ and } \mathbb{1}^T D = 0^T$$

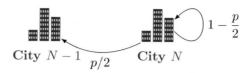

Fig. 1.24: *Diagram of flux of individuals leaving city N.*

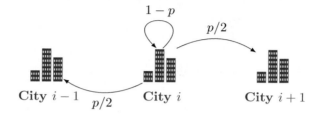

Fig. 1.25: *Diagram of flux of individuals leaving city i.*

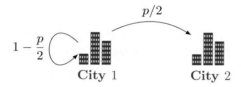

Fig. 1.26: *Diagram of flux of individuals leaving city 1.*

thus

$$\left(I + \frac{\varepsilon \Delta t}{\Delta x^2} D\right) \mathbb{1} = \mathbb{1} \quad \text{and} \quad \mathbb{1}^T \left(I + \frac{\varepsilon \Delta t}{\Delta x^2} D\right) = \mathbb{1}^T.$$

Therefore for each $u_0 \geq 0$,

$$\left\langle \mathbb{1}, u^{n+1} \right\rangle = \left\langle \mathbb{1}, u^n + \frac{\varepsilon \Delta t}{\Delta x^2} D u^n \right\rangle = \left\langle \mathbb{1}, u^n \right\rangle$$

and it follows that

$$\sum_{i=0}^{N} u_i^n = \sum_{i=0}^{N} u_{0i}, \quad \forall n \geq 0.$$

Moreover, as a consequence of the Perron–Frobenius theorem in Chapter 4 we have

$$\lim_{n \to +\infty} u^n = \left(\sum_{i=0}^{N} u_{0i}\right) \begin{pmatrix} 1/N \\ 1/N \\ \vdots \\ 1/N \end{pmatrix}.$$

Figure 1.27 illustrates this convergence result.

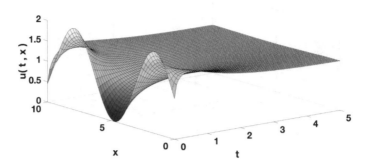

Fig. 1.27: *In this figure we plot a solution of the heat equation with $x \in [0, 10]$. The diffusion coefficient is equal to $\varepsilon = 2$. The initial distribution is equal to $u_0(x) = 1 + \sin(x)$. We observe the quite rapid convergence to the constant distribution.*

Remark 1.12 The above convergence result of the distribution is a consequence of the Perron–Frobenius theorem. This example will be reconsidered in Chapter 4.

1.10 A Discrete Diffusion Process on a Ring of Cities

In this section we again consider the heat equation

$$
\begin{cases}
\partial_t u(t, x) = \varepsilon \partial_x^2 u(t, x), \text{ for } x \in (0, 1), \\
u(t, 0) = u(t, 1), \\
u(0, \cdot) = \varphi \in L^2(0, 1).
\end{cases}
$$

The boundary conditions mean that there is no flux at the boundary.

To write the numerical scheme for this equation (i.e. a discrete version of it) we set

$$
u_i^n = u(n\Delta t, i\Delta x).
$$

Then the main part of the equation may be written for $i = 2, ..., N - 1$ as

$$
\frac{u_i^{n+1} - u_i^n}{\Delta t} = \varepsilon \frac{1}{\Delta x^2} \left(u_{i+1}^n - 2u_i^n + u_{i-1}^n \right).
$$

For $i = 1$ we obtain

$$
\frac{u_1^{n+1} - u_1^n}{\Delta t} = \varepsilon \frac{1}{\Delta x^2} \left[\left(u_2^n - u_1^n \right) - \left(u_1^n - u_0^n \right) \right]
$$

and the boundary condition $u_0^n = u_N^n$ gives

$$\frac{u_1^{n+1} - u_1^n}{\Delta t} = \varepsilon \frac{1}{\Delta x^2} \left(u_2^n + u_N^n - 2u_1^n \right).$$

Similarly for $i = N$ we should have

$$\frac{u_N^{n+1} - u_N^n}{\Delta t} = \varepsilon \frac{1}{\Delta x^2} \left(u_{N-1}^n + u_1^n - 2u_N^n \right).$$

So we obtain the following explicit numerical scheme for the heat equation for $n \geq 0$

$$u^{n+1} = u^n + \frac{\varepsilon \Delta t}{\Delta x^2} D u^n,$$

with the initial distribution

$$u^0 = u_0 \geq 0,$$

where

$$D = \begin{pmatrix} -2 & 1 & 0 & \cdots & 0 & 1 \\ 1 & -2 & 1 & & & 0 \\ 0 & & & & & \\ \vdots & & & & & 0 \\ 0 & & & & & 1 \\ 1 & 0 & \cdots & 0 & 1 & -2 \end{pmatrix}.$$

The numerical scheme may be rewritten as

$$u_i^{n+1} = u_i^n + \varepsilon \frac{\Delta t}{\Delta x^2} \left(u_{i+1}^n - 2u_i^n + u_{i-1}^n \right).$$

So we obtain for $i = 2, \ldots, N - 1$,

$$u_i^{n+1} = \frac{p}{2} u_{i+1}^n + (1 - p) u_i^n + \frac{p}{2} u_{i-1}^n$$

and for $i = 1$

$$u_1^{n+1} = \frac{p}{2} u_2^n + (1 - p) u_1^n + \frac{p}{2} u_N^n$$

and for $i = N$

$$u_N^{n+1} = \frac{p}{2} u_1^n + (1 - p) u_N^n + \frac{p}{2} u_{N-1}^n,$$

where

$$p := 2\varepsilon \frac{\Delta t}{\Delta x^2}.$$

Therefore we can interpret the discrete model as follows. An individual in city i, with $2 \leq i \leq N - 1$, will move to city $i - 1$ or to city $i + 1$, each with probability $p/2$, or stay in city i with probability $1 - p$. An individual in city 1 will move to city 2 or city N, each with probability $p/2$, or stay in city 1 with probability $1 - p$, and an individual in city N will move to city 1 or city $N - 1$, each with probability $p/2$, or stay in city N with probability $1 - p$.

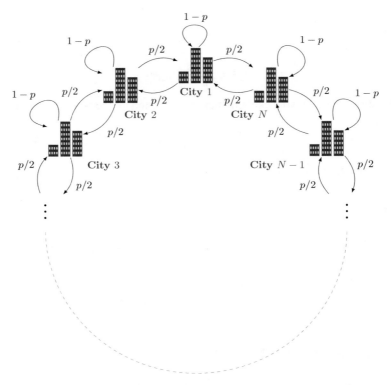

Fig. 1.28: *Diagram of flux for a diffusion process between a ring of N cities.*

Let $\mathbb{1} := (1, \ldots, 1)^T$. Then we obtain

$$D\mathbb{1} = 0 \text{ and } \mathbb{1}^T D = 0^T,$$

thus

$$\left(I + \frac{\varepsilon \Delta t}{\Delta x^2} D\right) \mathbb{1} = \mathbb{1} \text{ and } \mathbb{1}^T \left(I + \frac{\varepsilon \Delta t}{\Delta x^2} D\right) = \mathbb{1}^T.$$

Therefore for each $u_0 \geq 0$,

$$\left\langle \mathbb{1}, u^{n+1} \right\rangle = \left\langle \mathbb{1}, u^n + \frac{\varepsilon \Delta t}{\Delta x^2} D u^n \right\rangle = \langle \mathbb{1}, u^n \rangle$$

and it follows that the total number of individuals is constant

$$\sum_{i=0}^{N} u_i^n = \sum_{i=0}^{N} u_{0i}, \quad \forall n \geq 0.$$

Moreover, as a consequence of the Perron–Frobenius theorem in Chapter 4 we have

$$\lim_{n \to +\infty} u^n = \left(\sum_{i=0}^{N} u_{0i} \right) \begin{pmatrix} 1/N \\ 1/N \\ \vdots \\ 1/N \end{pmatrix}.$$

Figure 1.29 illustrates this convergence result.

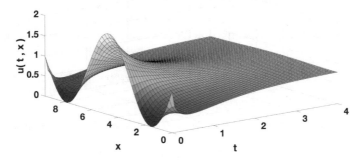

Fig. 1.29: *In this figure we plot a solution to the heat equation with $x \in [0, 3\pi]$. The diffusion coefficient is equal to $\varepsilon = 2$. The initial distribution is equal to $u_0(x) = 1 + \sin(x + \pi)$. We observe the quite rapid convergence to the constant distribution.*

Remark 1.13 The above convergence result of the distribution is a consequence of the Perron–Frobenius theorem. This example will be reconsidered in Chapter 4.

1.11 Remarks and Notes

In this section, we provide some references. The topics mentioned below are so rich, active, and extensive that it would be impractical to provide an exhaustive list. Instead, we have chosen an illustrative selection.

Population dynamics has a long history which starts with Fibonacci in 1202 who, in his book entitled *Liber Abaci* (Book of Calculation) [73], introduced his famous sequence

$$P_1 = 1, \quad P_2 = 2, \quad P_{n+1} = P_n + P_{n-1}, \quad \forall n \geq 0.$$

This turned out to be a special case of the Leslie model with two age classes, introduced in 1945.

As we will see several times in this book, in 1760 Daniel Bernoulli [28] proposed a mechanistic model and a phenomenological model to describe the epidemic of smallpox. We already mentioned the work of Malthus [246] in this chapter. In 1838 Verhulst rediscovered Bernoulli's generalized logistic equation [347].

The so-called Bernoulli–Verhulst equation is a scalar ordinary differential equation that takes the following form

$$N'(t) = \lambda N(t) \left(1 - (N(t)/\kappa)^{\alpha}\right), \quad \forall t \geq 0, \text{ and } N(0) = N_0 \geq 0,$$

where $\lambda > 0$, $\alpha > 0$, and $\kappa > 0$. The Bernoulli–Verhulst equation is studied in Chapter 5, as well as some n dimensional extensions of it.

Ronald Ross was awarded a Nobel prize for his famous work on malaria in 1911 [297, 298, 299, 300]. His work is partly based on the following system of two differential equations. The first equation for $H(t)$, the number of infected humans, is the following

$$H'(t) = \alpha \underbrace{(N_H - H(t))}_{\text{number of non-infected humans}} M(t) - \beta H(t),$$

which is coupled with an equation for $M(t)$, the number of infected mosquitoes,

$$M'(t) = \gamma \underbrace{(N_M - M(t))}_{\text{number of non-infected mosquitoes}} H(t) - \eta M(t).$$

Ross's model was later extended by Macdonald [223, 224, 225] in the 1950s. Therefore, nowadays this model is commonly called the Ross–Macdonald model.

The Lotka–Volterra predator-prey model is a celebrated example of a system of differential equations representing a biological system. It was first developed by Alfred Lotka in 1920 in the context of a plant-herbivorous interaction [215], although a similar system of equations had already been employed by the same author in the context of autocatalytic chemical reactions [214]. Vito Volterra developed a similar model in 1926 independently from Lotka, in the context of a predator-prey model for different species of fishes [185, 350]. The model reads as follows:

$$\begin{cases} \frac{d}{dt}u(t) = u(t)\left(r - \beta v(t)\right), \\ \frac{d}{dt}v(t) = v(t)\left(\gamma u(t) - \delta\right). \end{cases}$$

Here $u(t)$ stands for the population of prey, $v(t)$ for the population of predators; $r > 0$ is the reproduction rate of prey, $\beta > 0$ is the predation rate of a predator, $\gamma > 0$ is the prey uptake for a predator and $\delta > 0$ is the natural mortality rate of the predator.

In the second volume, we will also consider the equation introduced by Fisher [108] and discovered separately by Kolmogorov, Petrovski and Piskunov [108, 187] in 1937. This equation describes the genetic evolution of a population by using diffusion combined with a logistic equation term, and takes the following form, for $t \geq 0$ and $x \in \mathbb{R}$

$$\partial_t u(t,x) = \partial_x^2 u(t,x) + \lambda u(t,x) \left[1 - \frac{u(t,x)}{\kappa}\right], \text{ with initial value } u(0,x) = u_0(x),$$

where $\lambda > 0$ and $\kappa > 0$.

In 1926–1927 Kermack and McKendrick [176, 177, 178] introduced the first SIR epidemic model, by combining the ideas of Bernoulli and Ross. Kermack and McKendrick's model takes the following form

$$\begin{cases} S'(t) = -\beta S(t)I(t) \\ I'(t) = \beta S(t)I(t) - \gamma I(t) \\ R'(t) = \gamma I(t). \end{cases}$$

Here $S(t)$ is the density of susceptible individuals, $I(t)$ the density of infected individuals, and $R(t)$ the density of reported individuals. The constant $\beta > 0$ is the *transmission rate*, defined as the fraction of all possible contacts between S and I that result in a new infection per unit of time; the constant $\gamma > 0$ is the *recovery rate*, meaning that $1/\gamma$ is the average duration of infection.

As we will see in the second volume, Ricker's model, which was presented in 1954 [290], takes the following form for $t \geq 0$ and $x \in \mathbb{R}$,

$$N(t+1) = \beta N(t) \exp\left(-\alpha N(t)\right), \text{ with } N(0) = N_0 \geq 0,$$

where $\beta > 0$ is the growth rate of the population and the term $\exp(-\alpha N(t))$ (with $\alpha \geq 0$) describes the intra-specific competition. This model was introduced to describe the migration of adult salmon returning back to their natal stream for reproduction.

Ricker's model is known to generate chaos. Such chaos was first described by Sharkovsky [312, 313] in 1964, with his famous order of appearance for periodic orbits. This result was also rediscovered by Li and Yorke [202] in 1975, who proved that the existence of a period three orbit implies the existence of an orbit of any period (a special case of Sharkovsky's theorem), but they prove in addition the existence of ergodic invariant measures.

Age in population dynamics

(i) *Chronological age:* The chronological age is the time since birth. This age is used by all of us to describe life history. It serves, for example, to describe the maturity of individuals, that is, the time at which individuals start to be able to produce newborns. Continuous-time chronological age will be reconsidered by using Volterra's integral equations in Chapter 2.

(ii) *Age as a clock*: Chronological age is nothing but a measure of time determined by a clock which is started at birth. It is very convenient to describe the history of a process by considering other kinds of clocks, such as the time since infection takes place (which is called the age of infection, introduced by Kermack and McKendrick [177]). It is indeed possible to extend this idea to many kinds of clocks to track the history of a process.

Leslie's matrix model was extended by Usher [346] in 1969. An application of Usher matrices to demography is presented in Gaudard et al. [117]. For models with discrete age groups, we refer Caswell [50] and Newman [266] for more results.

For continuous age-structured models, we refer to Cushing [69], Thieme [338], Smith and Thieme [328], Webb [363, 364], Iannelli [166], Inaba [169], and [96, 101, 232, 234, 236] for more results on the subject.

Age and diffusion

Since Gurtin's work [133] in the early 1970s, the interplay between the spatial motion of individuals and age structure has also been widely considered in the literature, for single populations and also for interacting species. Similar types of models (both linear and nonlinear) have been studied. We refer for instance to the papers of Gurtin and MacCamy [134], Di Blasio [82], Garroni and Langlais [116], Langlais [197, 198], and Ducrot and Magal [97].

We also refer to the monograph of Busenberg and Cooke [42], where both diffusive population models with chronological age structure and with age since infection in epidemic problems are presented. We refer to Busenberg and Iannelli [44] for the study of age-structured problems with nonlinear diffusion and to Aniţa [8] and the references cited therein for results on the control of age-structured problems with spatial diffusion. Let us also refer to Di Blasio [83] for epidemic problems coupling age since infection and spatial diffusion and [96, 101, 234] for some studies of the spatial spread of infection with age since infection. Population models taking into account the interplay between age structure and non-local diffusion have also been developed. We refer, for instance, to Kang and Ruan [171] and the references cited therein.

The Kermack and McKendrick model with age of infection

Let $a > 0$ be the time since the first infection of an individual in a population by a pathogen. Then the Kermack and McKendrick model with age of infection can be rewritten as follows. The number of susceptible individuals $S(t)$ satisfies the following equation

$$S'(t) = \lambda - \eta S(t) - v\, S(t) \int_0^\infty \beta(a) i(t, a) da, \text{ for } t \geq 0, \text{ with } S(0) = S_0 \geq 0,$$

and the distribution of population of infected $a \rightarrow i(t, a)$ at time t satisfies

$$i(t, a) = \begin{cases} \dfrac{\Pi(a)}{\Pi(a-t)} i_0(a-t), & \text{if } a > t, \\ \Pi(a)\, v\, S(t-a)\, B(t-a), & \text{if } t > a, \end{cases}$$

where $a \to i_0(a) \in L^1_+(0, \infty)$ is the initial distribution of population of infected.

Here *distribution of population* refers to the number of infected individuals with age of infection in between a_1 and a_2 at time $t = 0$ (respectively at time $t > 0$), that is,

$$\int_{a_1}^{a_2} i_0(a)\mathrm{d}a \quad \left(\text{respectively } \int_{a_1}^{a_2} i(t, a)\mathrm{d}a\right).$$

The function $a \to \beta(a) \in L^\infty_+(0, \infty)$ gives the fraction of infectious (i.e. capable of transmitting the pathogen to the susceptible) for individuals with infection age a, and $a \to \Pi(a)$ gives the probability of remaining infected for individuals with infection age a.

Define

$$B(t) = \int_0^\infty \beta(a) i(t, a)\mathrm{d}a,$$

then we deduce that $t \to B(t) \in C_+([0, \infty), \mathbb{R})$ is the unique solution of the Volterra integral equation for $t \geq 0$,

$$B(t) = \left[\int_t^\infty \beta(a) \frac{\Pi(a)}{\Pi(a-t)} i_0(a-t)\mathrm{d}a + \int_0^t \beta(a)\Pi(a)\, v\, S(t-a)B(t-a)\mathrm{d}a\right],$$

where

$$S'(t) = \lambda - \eta S(t) - v\, S(t)B(t),$$

or equivalently

$$S(t) = \mathrm{e}^{-\int_0^t \eta + vB(\sigma)\mathrm{d}\sigma} S_0 + \int_0^t \mathrm{e}^{-\int_s^t \eta + vB(\sigma)\mathrm{d}\sigma} \lambda \mathrm{d}s.$$

The existence and uniqueness of solutions for Volterra's integral equation will be briefly explained in Chapter 2, where it will also provide one of the motivations to consider several types of methods to prove the existence of solutions. We will reconsider the Kermack–McKendrick model with age of infection in the remarks and notes section of Chapter 8.

The global dynamics of the Kermack and McKendrick model with age of infection was first completely understood by Magal, McCluskey and Webb [230]. We also refer to Magal and McCluskey [229] for a version of this result with two groups. A more elementary presentation of such a result with Liapunov function arguments is presented in Ma and Magal [221].

Movement in space in population dynamics

(i) *Patch models:* Patches can be defined as spatial areas which are sufficiently small so that spatial effects can be neglected. Patch models have been used in population genetics since the 1940s with the introduction by Wright of the so-called "Island models" [371], which he used to study the genetic effects of isolation. Let us also mention the "Stepping stones" model, introduced by Kimura in 1953 [183] and developed in more detail by Kimura and Weiss [184]. Stepping stones are patches on which there exists a one-dimensional structure, meaning that the motion of an individual from a given node is constrained to two neighboring patches (and no other). Patch models are often used in the context of meta-populations, which are populations divided into different spatial locations. In the context of human epidemiology, patch models have been used to describe the spread of epidemics across cities [11, 181].

(ii) *Diffusion processes:* Diffusion processes and the heat equation were originally developed to describe the random motion of microscopic particles. Their use to model the behavior of living bodies can be traced back to the seminal works of Kolmogorov, Petrovski and Piskuov [187] and Fisher [108]. These two studies were published simultaneously in 1937, and are concerned with a population genetics model

$$\partial_t u(t,x) = \partial_{xx} u(t,x) + r u(t,x) \left(1 - u(t,x)\right),$$

where $u(t,x)$ stands for the proportion at time $t \geq 0$ of individuals possessing a genetic advantage measured by the rate $r > 1$, in a population structured by a space variable $x \in \mathbb{R}$. This equation, called the Fisher–KPP equation, can be obtained in some sense as a limit of differential equations on large lattices, which will be presented in Chapter 8 of this book. Skellam [319] may have been the first biologist to use this equation in the context of a biological invasion, the invasion of the muskrat *Ondatra zibethica* L. after its introduction in central Europe in 1910. We refer to the books of Okubo [269] and Cantrell and Cosner [47] for a review of the subject and its historical developments.

(iii) *Lévy flight process:* To understand the laws of human displacement, a comparison between the Lévy flight process and real data was made by Brockmann et al. [39]. Since then the Lévy flight process, which is a mixture between patch model (long-distance) and daily motion (short distance), has been observed in many contexts.

(iv) *Long-short distance dispersal:* Shigesada Kawasaki [316], Bennett and Sherratt [27].

Various classes of practical problems

(i) *Ecology:* Iannelli and Pugliese [167], Murray [263, 264], Turchin [344], Bolker [30], Keyfitz and Caswell [180], Kot [188], Cushing [69, 70] , Tuljapurkar [343], Perthame [276, 277], Thieme [338], Smith and Thieme [328].

(ii) *Demography:* Keyfitz [179].

(iii) *Evolution:* Roff [293], Pianka [278].

(iv) *Epidemics:* Busenberg and Cooke [42], Diekmann and Heesterbeek [87] , Brauer and Castillo-Chávez [32], Brauer, Van den Driessche, Wu [35], Ma, Zhou and Wu [222], Chen, Moulin and Wu [52], Brauer, Castillo-Chavez and Feng [34], Li, Yang and Martcheva [203], Marcheva [247], Murray [263, 264], Keeling and Rohani [174], and Smith and Thieme [328].

(v) *Others:* Hofbauer and Sigmund [157].

1.12 MATLAB codes

Figure 1.1

```
1  t =0:1:10;
2
3  x1=exp(0.15*t )*100;
4  x2=exp(0*t)*100;
5  x3=exp(-0.15*t)*100;
6
7  clf ;
8  hold on;
9
10 plot(t,x1,'k'  , 'LineWidth', 8 );
11 plot(t,x2,'k'  , 'LineWidth', 8 );
12 plot(t,x3,'k'  , 'LineWidth', 8 );
13
14 xlabel('t');
15 ylabel('N( t )');
16
17 set(gca,'YLim',[0 200])
18 set(gca,'XLim',[0 10])
19
20
21 set(gca, 'FontSize', 30);
22 set(gca, 'FontWeight', 'bold');
```

Figure 1.2

```
1   t =0:0.01:3;
2   figure(1)
3
4   plot(t,b(t),'k','LineWidth', 4)
5
6   set(gca, 'FontSize', 20);
7   set(gca, 'FontWeight', 'bold');
8
9
10  figure(2)
11
12  plot(t,m(t),'k','LineWidth', 4)
13
14  set(gca, 'FontSize', 20);
15  set(gca, 'FontWeight', 'bold');
16
17  figure(3)
18  plot(t,r(t),'k','LineWidth', 4)
19
20  set(gca, 'FontSize', 20);
21  set(gca, 'FontWeight', 'bold');
22
23
24  function y=b(t)
25
26  y=2*(cos(2*pi*(t+0.6))+1);
27  end
28  function y=m(t)
29
30  y=cos(2*pi*t)+1;
31  end
32
33
34  function y=r(t)
35
36  y=b(t)-m(t);
37  end
```

Figure 1.3

```
1   t =0:0.01:3;
2
3   n=size(t);
```

```
4   fun = @(t)  2*(cos(2*pi*(t+0.6))+1)-(cos(2*pi*t)+1);
5
6   for i=1:n(2)
7   aux(i) = integral(fun,0,t(i));
8   end
9
10  plot(t,100*exp(aux),'k','LineWidth', 4)
11
12  set(gca, 'FontSize', 20);
13  set(gca, 'FontWeight', 'bold');
```

Figure 1.4

```
1   t=0:0.01:3;
2
3   n=size(t);
4   fun = @(t)  2*(cos(2*pi*(t+0.6))+1)-(cos(2*pi*t)+1);
5
6   for i=1:n(2)
7   aux(i) = integral(fun,0,t(i));
8   end
9
10  plot(t,100*exp(aux),'k','LineWidth', 4)
11
12  set(gca, 'YScale', 'log')
13  set(gca, 'Ylim',[7*10^1,4*10^3])
14  set(gca, 'FontSize', 20);
15  set(gca, 'FontWeight', 'bold');
```

Figure 1.5

```
1   R1=exp(0.15);
2   R2=1;
3   R3=exp(-0.15);
4   t=0:1:10;
5   x1=R1.^t*100;
6   x2=R2.^t*100;
7   x3=R3.^t*100;
8   clf ;
9   hold on;
10  plot( t , x1 ,'o', 'MarkerEdgeColor','k',...
11      'MarkerFaceColor','[ 0.4660 , 0.6740 ,
          0.1880]',...
12      'MarkerSize',20 ) ;
```

```
13
14  plot ( t , x2 ,'o', 'MarkerEdgeColor','k' ,...
15      'MarkerFaceColor','[  0.8500 ,   0.3250  ,
            0.0980]' ,...
16      'MarkerSize',20 ) ;
17
18  plot ( t , x3 ,'o', 'MarkerEdgeColor','k' ,...
19      'MarkerFaceColor','[   0.3010 ,  0.7450  ,
            0.9330]' ,...
20      'MarkerSize',20 ) ;
21
22
23  xlabel('n');
24  ylabel('N(n)');
25
26  set(gca,'YLim',[0  500])
27  set(gca,'XLim',[0  10])
28
29
30  set(gca,  'FontSize',  20);
31  set(gca,  'FontWeight',  'bold');
```

Figures 1.7 and 1.8

```
1   beta1 =0;
2   beta2 =2.5;
3   pi1 =0.5
4
5
6   L=[beta1  beta2;  pi1  0];
7   tmax =6;  % final time
8   t =0:tmax ;
9   X=zeros (2 ,tmax +1);
10
11  X(:,1) =[1;0] % initial distribution
12  for n=1:tmax
13      X(:,n+1)=L*X(:,n);
14  end
15  clf ;
16
17  figure (1)
18  hold on;
19  plot ( X(1 ,:) , X(2 ,:) , 'o', 'MarkerEdgeColor','k'
        ,...
20      'MarkerFaceColor','[   0.3010 ,  0.7450  ,
            0.9330]' ,...
```

```
21        'MarkerSize',20 ) ;
22
23   plot( X(1,:) , X(2,:) , '--','color','[  0.8500 ,
         0.3250  , 0.0980]', 'LineWidth',5 ) ;
24
25   xlabel('N_1(n)');
26   ylabel('N_2(n)');
27
28
29   set(gca, 'FontSize', 20);
30   set(gca, 'FontWeight', 'bold');
31
32   figure(2)
33   hold on;
34   plot( t , X(1,:)+X(2,:) , 'o', 'MarkerEdgeColor','k'
         ,...
35        'MarkerFaceColor','[  0.3010 , 0.7450 ,
            0.9330]' ,...
36        'MarkerSize',20 ) ;
37
38   plot( t , X(1,:)+X(2,:) ,'--','color','[  0.8500 ,
         0.3250  , 0.0980]','LineWidth',5) ;
39
40
41   set(gca, 'FontSize', 20);
42   set(gca, 'FontWeight', 'bold');
43   xlabel('n');
44   ylabel('N(n)');
```

Figure 1.17

```
1              tmax=40;
2              dt=0.5;
3              t=0:dt:tmax
4
5              amax=20;
6              da=dt;
7              a=0:da:amax;
8
9
10             n=size(a)
11             L=zeros(n(2),n(2))
12
13             % birth
14
```

```
15        tau=5 % age of maturity
16        beta=0.2 % reproduction rate
17
18        L(1,:)=beta1(a,tau,beta,da);
19
20        % survival
21        c1=0.01;
22        c2=0.00;
23        c3=0.00;
24        pi1=pi2(a,c1,c2,c3,da)
25        L=diag(pi1)*diag(ones(1,n(2)-1),-1)+L;
26
27
28        % compute the solution
29        m=size(t)
30        U=zeros(n(2),m(2));
31        U(:,1)=ones(n(2),1);
32
33        for i=1:m(2)-1
34        U(:,i+1)=L*U(:,i);
35        end
36
37        % plot the solution
38        p=2;
39        q=2;
40        surf(t(1:q:m(2)),a(1:p:n(2)),U(1:p:n(2),1:q:
             m(2)))
41        xlabel('t');
42        ylabel('a');
43        zlabel('u(t,a)');
44     set(gca,'fontweight','bold','FontSize',30);
```

The above code goes together with the function *pi2.m* (which must be in the same directory as the above code) which contains the following:

```
1   function y=pi2(a,c1,c2,c3,da)
2
3   y=exp(-(c1+(a*c2))).*exp(-c3*a)*da);
4
5   end
```

and the function *beta1.m*

```
1   function y=beta1(x,c1,c2,da)
2   n=size(x);
3   y=zeros(n);
4       for i=1:n(2)
5       y(i)=0;
6       if (x(i)>=c1)
```

```
7        y ( i )=c2*da ;
8        end
9    end
```

Figure 1.23

```
1    tmax =5; % Final  at  which  we  want  to  compute  the
            solution
2    xmin =0;
3    xmax =10;
4    epsilon =2; % diffusion  coefficient
5    dx =0.1; % space  step
6
7    % we  fix  dt  in  order  to  satisfy  the  CFL  condition
8    dt=dx^2/(2*epsilon );
9
10   t =0: dt : tmax ;
11   x=xmin : dx : xmax ;
12
13   U=zeros ( size (x ,2) , size (t ,2))  ;
14   aux1=size (x ,2)
15   p=epsilon*dt /(dx*dx);
16
17   u0=sin (x )+1;
18   % initial  distribution
19   U(  :  ,  1  )  =  u0  ;
20
21   D=diag (ones (aux1 -1 ,1) ,-1)+diag (ones (aux1 -1 ,1) ,1) -2*
            diag (ones (aux1  ,1)));
22   D(1  ,1)=-1;
23
24   D(aux1 , aux1 )=-1;
25
26
27   aux2=size (t ,2)
28   D=sparse (D);
29   for  i =1: aux2 -1;
30   U(:  ,i +1)=U(:  ,i )+p*D*U(: ,i );
31
32   end
33
34   % we  plot  the  distribution
35
36   i1 =1;
37   j1 =1;
```

```
38  x1=zeros (1 ,1); t1=zeros (1 ,1);
39  U1=zeros (1 ,1);
40  for i =1:2: aux1
41  for j =1:25: aux2
42  x1(i1 ,j1)=x(i);
43  t1(i1 ,j1 )=t(j) ;
44  U1(i1 ,j1)=U(i ,j);
45  j1=j1 +1;
46  end
47  j1 =1;
48  i1=i1 +1;
49  end
50  clf ;
51  surf(t1 ,x1 ,U1) ;
52  xlabel('t');
53  ylabel('x') ;
54  zlabel('u( t , x )')
55
56  set(gca,'fontweight','bold','FontSize',30);
```

Figure 1.25

```
1  tmax =4; % Final  at  which  we  want  to  compute  the
      solution
2  xmin =0;
3  xmax=3*pi ;
4  epsilon=2; % diffusion  coefficient
5  dx =0.01; % space  step
6
7  % we  fix  dt  in  order  to  satisfy  the  CFL  condition
8  dt=dx^2/(2*epsilon );
9
10  t =0: dt :tmax ;
11  x=xmin : dx :xmax ;
12
13  U=zeros(size(x,2),size(t,2))  ;
14  aux1=size(x,2)
15  p=epsilon*dt /(dx*dx);
16
17  u0=sin(x+pi)+1;
18  % initial  distribution
19  U( : , 1 ) = u0 ;
20
21  D=diag(ones(aux1 -1,1),-1)+diag(ones(aux1 -1,1),1)-2*
      diag(ones(aux1 ,1));
```

```
22  D( 1    , aux 1 ) = 1 ;
23
24  D( aux 1 , 1 ) = 1 ;
25
26
27  aux 2 = s i z e ( t , 2 )
28  D= s p a r s e (D) ;
29  f o r  i = 1 :  aux 2 − 1 ;
30  U ( :    , i + 1 )=U ( :    , i )+p ∗D∗U ( : , i ) ;
31
32  end
33
34  % we  p l o t  the  d i s t r i b u t i o n
35
36  i 1 = 1 ;
37  j 1 = 1 ;
38  x 1 = z e r o s  ( 1    , 1 ) ;  t 1 = z e r o s  ( 1    , 1 ) ;
39  U1= z e r o s  ( 1    , 1 ) ;
40  f o r  i = 1 : 1 0 ∗ 2 : aux 1
41  f o r  j = 1 : 1 0 0 ∗ 2 5 : aux 2
42  x 1 ( i 1 , j 1 )=x ( i ) ;
43  t 1 ( i 1 , j 1  )= t ( j )  ;
44  U1( i 1 , j 1 )=U( i , j ) ;
45  j 1 = j 1 + 1 ;
46  end
47  j 1 = 1 ;
48  i 1 = i 1 + 1 ;
49  end
50  c l f  ;
51  s u r f ( t 1 , x 1 ,U1)  ;
52  x l a b e l ( ' t ' ) ;
53  y l a b e l ( ' x ' )  ;
54  s e t ( g c a , ' x l i m ' , [ 0  tmax ] , ' y l i m ' , [ 0  xmax ] ) ;
55  z l a b e l ( ' u (  t  ,  x  ) ' )
56
57  s e t ( g c a , ' f o n t w e i g h t ' , ' b o l d ' , ' F o n t S i z e ' , 3 0 ) ;
```

Chapter 2
Existence and Uniqueness of Solutions

2.1 Introduction

We consider the n-dimensional system of ordinary differential equations (a vector-valued Cauchy problem)

$$\frac{\mathrm{d}u(t)}{\mathrm{d}t} = Au(t), \quad \forall t \geq 0 \tag{2.1}$$

with the initial condition (at time $t = 0$)

$$u(0) = u_0 \in \mathbb{R}^n,$$

where the matrix A belongs to $M_n(\mathbb{R})$, the space of n by n real matrices.

Definition 2.1 A continuous function $u \in C([0, \tau], \mathbb{R}^n)$ (for some $\tau > 0$) is a *solution* of (2.1) if u satisfies, for each $t \in [0, \tau]$,

$$u(t) = u_0 + \int_0^t Au(s)\mathrm{d}s. \tag{2.2}$$

Remark 2.2 If u is a solution, then $u \in C^1([0, \tau], \mathbb{R}^n)$ since the right-hand side of (2.2) is C^1 whenever $t \to u(t)$ is continuous. Moreover, by computing the derivative of the right-hand side of (2.2) we deduce that u satisfies (2.1).

Let $I \subset [0, \infty)$ be an interval containing 0 and not reduced to the single point $\{0\}$. Set

$$\tau := \sup I \in (0, \infty].$$

That is, the interval I can take the following forms:

$$I = [0, \tau), \quad \text{if } \tau \leq \infty$$

or

$$I = [0, \tau], \quad \text{if } \tau < \infty.$$

Define the operator $\Psi_A : C(I, \mathbb{R}^n) \to C(I, \mathbb{R}^n)$ as follows

© The Author(s), under exclusive license to Springer Nature Switzerland AG 2022
A. Ducrot et al., *Differential Equations and Population Dynamics I*, Lecture Notes on
Mathematical Modelling in the Life Sciences, https://doi.org/10.1007/978-3-030-98136-5_2

$$\Psi_A(u)(t) = u_0 + \int_0^t Au(s)\mathrm{d}s, \quad \forall t \in I.$$

Then (2.2) is equivalent to

$$u(t) = \Psi_A(u)(t), \quad \forall t \in I \Leftrightarrow u = \Psi_A(u).$$

In other words, $u \in C(I, \mathbb{R}^n)$ is a solution if and only if u is a fixed point of Ψ_A.

2.2 Banach Spaces of Continuous Functions

To use the Banach fixed point theorem, we first need to define the notion of Banach space.

Definition 2.3 A normed vector space $(E, \|\cdot\|)$ is a *Banach space* (or *complete*) if every Cauchy sequence of E converges in E. That is to say, if $\{u_m\}_{m \geq 0} \subset E$ is a sequence such that for each $\eta > 0$ there exists an integer $r = r(\eta) \geq 0$ with the property

$$\|u_k - u_m\| \leq \eta, \quad \forall k, m \geq r,$$

(a *Cauchy sequence*), then there exists a $u_\infty \in E$ such that

$$\lim_{m \to \infty} \|u_m - u_\infty\| = 0.$$

In this section, $I \subset [0, \infty)$ is an interval containing 0 and not reduced to the single point $\{0\}$ and we set $\tau = \sup I$.

Definition 2.4 We define $BC(I, \mathbb{R}^n)$ to be the set of bounded functions of $C(I, \mathbb{R}^n)$. That is,

$$BC(I, \mathbb{R}^n) = \left\{ u \in C(I, \mathbb{R}^n) : \sup_{t \in I} \|u(t)\| < \infty \right\}.$$

Remark 2.5 The space $BC(I, \mathbb{R}^n)$ coincides with $C(I, \mathbb{R}^n)$ if and only if $\tau < \infty$ and the interval I is closed at τ. Otherwise the continuous functions don't have to be bounded around τ.

Lemma 2.6 *The space $BC(I, \mathbb{R}^n)$ is a normed space endowed with the supremum norm*

$$\|u\|_\infty = \sup_{t \in I} \|u(t)\|.$$

Theorem 2.7 *The normed space $(BC(I, \mathbb{R}^n), \|.\|_\infty)$ is a Banach space.*

Proof Let $\{u_m\}_{m \geq 0} \subset BC(I, \mathbb{R}^n)$ be a Cauchy sequence. Then for each $\eta > 0$, we can find an integer $r = r(\eta) \geq 0$ such that

$$\|u_k - u_m\|_\infty \leq \eta, \quad \forall k, m \geq r.$$

Let $t \in I$. We observe that

$$\|u_k(t) - u_m(t)\| \le \|u_k - u_m\|_\infty,$$

hence the sequence $\{u_m(t)\}_{m \ge 0}$ is a Cauchy sequence in $\mathbb{R}^n$, which is complete. Hence for each $t \in I$

$$u(t) = \lim_{m \to \infty} u_m(t)$$

exists.

Uniform convergence of u_m to u: Let $\eta > 0$ be fixed. We can find an integer $r \ge 0$ such that

$$\|u_k - u_m\|_\infty \le \eta, \quad \forall k, m \ge r.$$

This implies

$$\|u_k(t) - u_m(t)\| \le \eta, \quad \forall k, m \ge r \text{ and } \forall t \in I,$$

and when k goes to infinity we obtain

$$\|u(t) - u_m(t)\| \le \eta, \quad \forall m \ge r \text{ and } \forall t \in I.$$

This implies that $t \to u(t)$ is bounded since

$$\|u(t)\| \le \|u(t) - u_m(t)\| + \|u_m(t)\| \le \eta + \|u_m\|_\infty < \infty,$$

and

$$\|u - u_m\|_\infty \le \eta, \quad \forall m \ge r.$$

Therefore

$$\lim_{m \to \infty} \|u - u_m\|_\infty = 0.$$

Proof of the continuity of u: Let $t_0 \in I$ and $\varepsilon > 0$ be fixed. Let $r \ge 0$ be an integer such that

$$\|u - u_m\|_\infty \le \frac{\varepsilon}{3}, \quad \forall m \ge r.$$

Let $m \ge r$ be fixed. Then

$$\|u(t) - u(t_0)\| \le \|u(t) - u_m(t)\| + \|u_m(t) - u_m(t_0)\| + \|u_m(t_0) - u(t_0)\|$$
$$\le \frac{2\varepsilon}{3} + \|u_m(t) - u_m(t_0)\|.$$

Since $t \to u_m(t)$ is continuous we can find an $\eta > 0$ such that

$$\|t - t_0\| \le \eta \implies \|u_m(t) - u_m(t_0)\| \le \frac{\varepsilon}{3},$$

therefore we obtain

$$\|t - t_0\| \le \eta \implies \|u(t) - u(t_0)\| \le \varepsilon,$$

and the proof is complete. $\qquad\qquad\square$

To obtain Banach spaces of continuous functions when $\tau = \infty$, we will consider some weighted spaces of continuous functions.

Definition 2.8 (Weighted space of continuous functions) Let $\rho : I \rightarrow (0, \infty)$ be a continuous function. We define

$$BC_\rho(I, \mathbb{R}^n) = \left\{ u \in C(I, \mathbb{R}^n) : \sup_{t \in I} \rho(t) \|u(t)\| < \infty \right\}.$$

Lemma 2.9 *The space $BC_\rho(I, \mathbb{R}^n)$ is a normed space endowed with the norm*

$$\|u\|_\rho = \sup_{t \in I} \rho(t) \|u(t)\|.$$

By considering the operators

$$J(u)(t) = \rho(t)u(t) \text{ and } J^{-1}(u)(t) = \rho^{-1}(t)u(t),$$

we observe that

$$J(BC_\rho(I, \mathbb{R}^n)) = BC(I, \mathbb{R}^n) \text{ and } J^{-1}(BC(I, \mathbb{R}^n)) = BC_\rho(I, \mathbb{R}^n)$$

and

$$\|J(u)\|_\infty = \|u\|_\rho \text{ and } \left\|J^{-1}(u)\right\|_\rho = \|u\|_\infty.$$

Therefore J is an isometry from $BC_\rho(I, \mathbb{R}^n)$ into $BC(I, \mathbb{R}^n)$ and we obtain the following corollary.

Corollary 2.10 *The normed space $\left(BC_\rho(I, \mathbb{R}^n), \|\cdot\|_\rho \right)$ is a Banach space.*

Proof Let $\{u_m\}_{m \geq 0} \subset BC_\rho(I, \mathbb{R}^n)$ be a Cauchy sequence in $BC_\rho(I, \mathbb{R}^n)$. Then $\{J(u_m)\}_{m \geq 0} \subset BC(I, \mathbb{R}^n)$ is a Cauchy sequence since

$$\|u_k - u_m\|_\rho = \|J(u_k) - J(u_m)\|_\infty, \quad \forall k, m \geq 0.$$

By using Theorem 2.7, there exists a $v_\infty \in BC(I, \mathbb{R}^n)$ such that

$$\lim_{m \to \infty} \|v_\infty - J(u_m)\|_\infty = 0.$$

By setting $u_\infty = J^{-1}(v_\infty) \in BC_\rho(I, \mathbb{R}^n)$ we obtain

$$\lim_{m \to \infty} \|u_\infty - u_m\|_\rho = \lim_{m \to \infty} \|v_\infty - J(u_m)\|_\infty = 0,$$

and the proof is complete. □

2.3 The Banach Fixed Point Theorem

Definition 2.11 Let $\Psi : E \to F$ be a map from a Banach space $(E, \| \cdot \|_E)$ into a Banach space $(F, \| \cdot \|_F)$. A map Ψ is said to be *k-Lipschitz continuous* if

$$\|\Psi(x) - \Psi(y)\|_F \le k\|x - y\|_E, \quad \forall x, y \in E.$$

The map F is called a *contraction* if F is k-Lipschitz continuous for some $k < 1$.

Definition 2.12 Let $\Psi : E \to F$ be a map from a Banach space $(E, \| \cdot \|_E)$ into a Banach space $(F, \| \cdot \|_F)$. The *Lipschitz norm* of Ψ is defined as

$$\|\Psi\|_{\mathrm{Lip}} := \sup_{x,y \in E : x \ne y} \frac{\|\Psi(x) - \Psi(y)\|_F}{\|x - y\|_E}.$$

The function Ψ is *Lipschitzian* or *Lipschitz continuous* if its Lipschitz norm $\|\Psi\|_{\mathrm{Lip}}$ is finite.

Remark 2.13 If Ψ is k-Lipschitz continuous for some real number $k \ge 0$ then

$$\|\Psi\|_{\mathrm{Lip}} \le k.$$

Conversely, if $\|\Psi\|_{\mathrm{Lip}} < +\infty$ then Ψ is k-Lipschitz for each $k \ge \|\Psi\|_{\mathrm{Lip}}$.

Theorem 2.14 (Banach fixed point theorem) *Let $\Psi : E \to E$ be a contraction from a Banach space $(E, \| \cdot \|_E)$ into itself. Then there exists a unique $u \in E$ satisfying $\Psi(u) = u$.*

Proof **Proof of uniqueness:** Assume by contradiction that there exist two fixed points $u, v \in E$ of Ψ. Then

$$\|u - v\| = \|\Psi(u) - \Psi(v)\| \le \|\Psi\|_{\mathrm{Lip}}\|u - v\|.$$

Hence

$$\left(1 - \|\Psi\|_{\mathrm{Lip}}\right) \|u - v\| \le 0.$$

Since $\|\Psi\|_{\mathrm{Lip}} < 1$ and $\|u - v\| \ge 0$, we deduce that $\|u - v\| = 0$. Therefore we must have $u = v$.

Proof of existence: Let $u_0 \in E$ and consider the sequence $\{u_m\}_{m \ge 0}$ recursively defined as

$$u_m = \Psi(u_{m-1}), \quad \forall m \in \mathbb{N}. \tag{2.3}$$

Let us prove that $\{u_m\}_{m \ge 0}$ is a Cauchy sequence. Indeed, we first observe that

$$\|u_{m+1} - u_m\| = \|\Psi(u_m) - \Psi(u_{m-1})\| \le \|\Psi\|_{\mathrm{Lip}}\|u_m - u_{m-1}\|,$$

and we obtain by induction

$$\|u_{m+1} - u_m\| \le \|\Psi\|_{\mathrm{Lip}}^m\|u_1 - u_0\|, \quad \forall m \in \mathbb{N}. \tag{2.4}$$

Next if we consider two integers $k, m \in \mathbb{N}$ with $k \geq m$ we have

$$\|u_k - u_m\| \leq \|u_k - u_{k-1} + u_{k-1} - u_m\| \leq \|u_k - u_{k-1}\| + \|u_{k-1} - u_m\|,$$

and we obtain by induction

$$\|u_k - u_m\| \leq \sum_{j=m}^{k-1} \|u_{j+1} - u_j\|.$$

By using (2.4) we obtain

$$\|u_k - u_m\| \leq \|u_1 - u_0\| \sum_{j=m}^{k-1} \|\Psi\|_{\text{Lip}}^j,$$

and

$$\sum_{j=m}^{k-1} \|\Psi\|_{\text{Lip}}^j = \|\Psi\|_{\text{Lip}}^m \sum_{j=0}^{k-1-m} \|\Psi\|_{\text{Lip}}^j \leq \|\Psi\|_{\text{Lip}}^m \sum_{j=0}^{\infty} \|\Psi\|_{\text{Lip}}^j,$$

and by using the sum of an infinite geometric series we deduce that

$$\|u_k - u_m\| \leq \|u_1 - u_0\| \frac{\|\Psi\|_{\text{Lip}}^m}{1 - \|\Psi\|_{\text{Lip}}}.$$

Let $\eta > 0$. We can find an integer r such that

$$\frac{\|\Psi\|_{\text{Lip}}^m}{1 - \|\Psi\|_{\text{Lip}}} \leq \eta, \quad \forall m \geq r$$

and it follows that $\{u_m\}_{m \geq 0}$ is a Cauchy sequence. Since E is a Banach space, there exists a u_∞ such that

$$\lim_{m \to \infty} \|u_m - u_\infty\| = 0.$$

By taking the limit when m goes to infinity on both sides of the equality

$$u_m = \Psi(u_{m-1}),$$

we deduce by using the continuity of Ψ that

$$u_\infty = \Psi(u_\infty)$$

and the proof is complete. $\square$

The existence of the solution on $[0, 2\varepsilon]$ follows from the first part of the proof. By using a proof by induction, we obtain the existence of a global solution (i.e. a solution defined on $[0, +\infty)$).

2.5.2 Existence and uniqueness on an arbitrary bounded interval $[0, \tau]$ by using the iteration of Ψ_A

We observe that

$$\Psi_A^2(u)(t) - \Psi_A^2(\widehat{u})(t) = \int_0^t \int_0^{s_1} A^2(u(s_2) - \widehat{u}(s_2))\mathrm{d}s_2\mathrm{d}s_1,$$

$$\vdots$$

$$\Psi_A^m(u)(t) - \Psi_A^m(\widehat{u})(t) = \int_0^t \int_0^{s_1} \cdots \int_0^{s_{m-1}} A^m(u(s_m) - \widehat{u}(s_m))\mathrm{d}s_m \ldots \mathrm{d}s_1.$$

Thus

$$\|\Psi_A^m(u) - \Psi_A^m(\widehat{u})\|_\infty \le \|A\|^m \|u - \widehat{u}\|_\infty \int_0^\tau \int_0^{s_1} \cdots \int_0^{s_{m-2}} \int_0^{s_{m-1}} 1\mathrm{d}s_m \ldots \mathrm{d}s_1.$$

One can prove by induction that

$$\int_0^\tau \int_0^{s_1} \cdots \int_0^{s_{m-2}} \int_0^{s_{m-1}} 1\mathrm{d}s_m\mathrm{d}s_{m-1} \ldots \mathrm{d}s_2\mathrm{d}s_1 = \frac{\tau^m}{m!},$$

and we obtain

$$\|\Psi_A^m(u) - \Psi_A^m(\widehat{u})\|_\infty \le \frac{(\tau\|A\|)^m}{m!} \|u - \widehat{u}\|_\infty.$$

By using Stirling's formula (for example), that is,

$$m! \underset{\infty}{\sim} \sqrt{2\pi m} \left(\frac{m}{e}\right)^m,$$

we deduce that

$$\|\Psi_A^m\|_{\mathrm{Lip}} \le \frac{(\tau\|A\|)^m}{m!} \underset{m\to\infty}{\to} 0.$$

Therefore, we can apply Banach's fixed point theorem to Ψ_A^m for each sufficiently large integer m. We deduce that there exists a $u \in C([0, \tau], \mathbb{R}^n)$ satisfying

$$\Psi_A^m(u) = u.$$

Setting

$$u_i = \Psi_A^i(u), \quad i \in \{1, \ldots, m-1\},$$

we have

$$\Psi_A^m(u_1) = \Psi_A^m(\Psi_A(u)) = \Psi_A(\Psi_A^m(u)) = \Psi_A(u) = u_1.$$

By uniqueness of the fixed point for Ψ_A^m, we deduce that $u = u_1$. Similarly, we can prove that $u = u_1 = \cdots = u_{m-1}$. Finally, since $\Psi_A(u) = u_1$ and $u = u_1$, we deduce that u is the unique fixed point of Ψ_A.

2.5.3 Existence and uniqueness by using some weighted spaces of continuous functions

By choosing $\rho(t) = \mathrm{e}^{-\alpha t}$ in Corollary 2.10 we deduce the following lemma.

Lemma 2.17 *The space*

$$BC_\alpha([0, +\infty), \mathbb{R}^n) := \{\varphi \in C([0, +\infty), \mathbb{R}^n) : \sup_{t \geq 0} \mathrm{e}^{-\alpha t} \|\varphi(t)\| < \infty\},$$

endowed with the norm

$$\|\varphi\|_\alpha := \sup_{t \geq 0} \mathrm{e}^{-\alpha t} \|\varphi(t)\|,$$

is a Banach space.

We have

$$
\begin{aligned}
\mathrm{e}^{-\alpha t} \|\Psi_A(u)(t) - \Psi_A(\widehat{u})(t)\| &= \mathrm{e}^{-\alpha t} \left\| \int_0^t A\left(u(s) - \widehat{u}(s)\right) \mathrm{d}s \right\| \\
&\leq \mathrm{e}^{-\alpha t} \left| \int_0^t \|A\left(u(s) - \widehat{u}(s)\right)\| \mathrm{d}s \right| \\
&\leq \|A\|_{\mathcal{L}(\mathbb{R}^n)} \left| \int_0^t \mathrm{e}^{-\alpha t} \|u(s) - \widehat{u}(s)\| \mathrm{d}s \right| \\
&\leq \|A\|_{\mathcal{L}(\mathbb{R}^n)} \left| \int_0^t \mathrm{e}^{-\alpha(t-s)} \mathrm{e}^{-\alpha s} \|u(s) - \widehat{u}(s)\| \mathrm{d}s \right| \\
&\leq \|A\|_{\mathcal{L}(\mathbb{R}^n)} \left| \int_0^t \mathrm{e}^{-\alpha(t-s)} \|u - \widehat{u}\|_\alpha \mathrm{d}s \right| \\
&\overset{l=t-s}{\leq} \|A\|_{\mathcal{L}(\mathbb{R}^n)} \|u - \widehat{u}\|_\alpha \int_0^t \mathrm{e}^{-\alpha l} \mathrm{d}l \\
&\leq \|A\|_{\mathcal{L}(\mathbb{R}^n)} \|u - \widehat{u}\|_\alpha \int_0^{+\infty} \mathrm{e}^{-\alpha l} \mathrm{d}l \\
&\leq \frac{\|A\|_{\mathcal{L}(\mathbb{R}^n)}}{\alpha} \|u - \widehat{u}\|_\alpha, \quad \forall \alpha > 0.
\end{aligned}
$$

Therefore, for each $\alpha > 0$,

$$\|\Psi_A(u) - \Psi_A(\widehat{u})\|_\alpha \leq \frac{\|A\|_{\mathcal{L}(\mathbb{R}^n)}}{\alpha} \|u - \widehat{u}\|_\alpha.$$

Moreover,

$$
\begin{aligned}
\|\Psi_A(u)\|_\alpha &= \|\Psi_A(u) - u_0 + u_0\|_\alpha \\
&= \|\Psi_A(u) - \Psi_A(0) + u_0\|_\alpha \\
&\leq \frac{\|A\|_{\mathcal{L}(\mathbb{R}^n)}}{\alpha} \|u\|_\alpha + \frac{1}{\alpha} \|u_0\|.
\end{aligned}
$$

We obtain for each $\alpha > \|A\|_{\mathcal{L}(\mathbb{R}^n)}$ that

$$\Psi_A\left(BC_\alpha([0, +\infty), \mathbb{R}^n)\right) \subset BC_\alpha([0, +\infty), \mathbb{R}^n),$$

and the map Ψ_A is a contraction on $BC_\alpha([0, +\infty), \mathbb{R}^n)$. Therefore by applying the Banach fixed point theorem we deduce that Ψ_A admits a unique fixed point u in $BC_\alpha([0, +\infty), \mathbb{R}^n)$. Moreover, for each $\varepsilon > 0$, we have

$$\|u(t)\| \leq \frac{(\|A\|_{\mathcal{L}(\mathbb{R}^n)} + \varepsilon)}{\varepsilon} e^{(\|A\|_{\mathcal{L}(\mathbb{R}^n)} + \varepsilon)t} \|u_0\|, \quad \forall t \geq 0,$$

where u is the fixed point. Indeed, let $\varepsilon > 0$ be fixed. Set $\alpha := \|A\|_{\mathcal{L}(\mathbb{R}^n)} + \varepsilon$. We have

$$u = u_0 + \Psi_A(u) - \Psi_A(0).$$

Then

$$\|u\|_\alpha \leq \|u_0\|_\alpha + \|\Psi_A(u) - \Psi_A(0)\|_\alpha \leq \|u_0\| + \frac{\|A\|_{\mathcal{L}(\mathbb{R}^n)}}{\alpha} \|u\|_\alpha.$$

Thus

$$\|u\|_\alpha \leq \frac{\alpha}{\alpha - \|A\|_{\mathcal{L}(\mathbb{R}^n)}} \|u_0\|.$$

By using the definition of the norm $\|\cdot\|_\alpha$, we obtain

$$\|u(t)\| \leq \frac{\alpha}{\alpha - \|A\|_{\mathcal{L}(\mathbb{R}^n)}} \|u_0\| e^{\alpha t}, \quad \forall t \geq 0,$$

and the result follows.

2.5.4 Existence and uniqueness of solution by using the exponential of a matrix

Definition 2.18 Let $A \in M_n(\mathbb{R})$. The *exponential* of A is defined by

$$e^A := \sum_{k=0}^{\infty} \frac{A^k}{k!} = \lim_{m \to +\infty} \sum_{k=0}^{m} \frac{A^k}{k!},$$

where

$$A^0 = I \text{ and } A^k = \underbrace{A \times A \times \ldots \times A}_{k \text{ times}},$$

and

$$0! = 1 \text{ and } k! = k \times (k-1) \times \ldots \times 1.$$

Proposition 2.19 *We have the following properties:*

(i) $e^0 = I$;
(ii) $e^{\lambda I} = e^\lambda I, \quad \forall \lambda \in \mathbb{C}$;
(iii) $\|e^A\|_{\mathcal{L}(\mathbb{R}^n)} \leq e^{\|A\|_{\mathcal{L}(\mathbb{R}^n)}}$, *where* $\|A\|_{\mathcal{L}(\mathbb{R}^n)}$ *is the operator norm of* A;
(iv) $e^A e^B = e^B e^A$ *whenever* $AB = BA$;
(v) $\frac{d}{dt} e^{At} = A e^{At} = e^{At} A, \quad \forall t \in \mathbb{R}$;
(vi) $(e^{At})^{-1} = e^{-At}$;
(vii) $e^{At + As} = e^{At} e^{As}, \quad \forall t, s \in \mathbb{R}$;
(viii) $e^{A+B} = e^A e^B$ *whenever* $AB = BA$.

Proof The properties (i) to (iv) are trivial. Let us prove the last four properties.

Proof of (v): Let $r > 0$ be fixed. Let $t, t + h \in [-r, r]$. Consider

$$E(h) := e^{A(t+h)} - e^{At} - hAe^{At} = \sum_{k=1}^{\infty} \frac{A^k}{k!} \left[(t+h)^k - t^k - ht^{k-1} \frac{k!}{(k-1)!} \right].$$

Then

$$E(h) = \sum_{k=1}^{\infty} \frac{A^k}{(k-1)!} \left[\frac{(t+h)^k - t^k}{k} - ht^{k-1} \right],$$

and we observe that $\frac{(t+h)^k - t^k}{k} - ht^{k-1} = 0$ for $k = 1$. Therefore

$$E(h) = \sum_{k=2}^{\infty} \frac{A^k}{(k-1)!} \left[\frac{(t+h)^k - t^k}{k} - ht^{k-1} \right].$$

Let us evaluate

$$\frac{(t+h)^k - t^k}{k} - ht^{k-1} = \int_t^{t+h} (\sigma^{k-1} - t^{k-1}) d\sigma$$

$$= \int_t^{t+h} (\sigma - t)(\sigma^{k-2} + \sigma^{k-3}t + \sigma^{k-4}t^2 + \cdots + t^{k-2}) d\sigma.$$

We obtain

$$\left| \frac{(t+h)^k - t^k}{k} - ht^{k-1} \right| \le (k-1)r^{k-2} \left| \int_t^{t+h} (\sigma - t) d\sigma \right| \le (k-1)r^{k-2} \frac{h^2}{2}.$$

Hence

$$\|E(h)\| \le \frac{h^2}{2} \sum_{k=2}^{\infty} \frac{\|A\|_{\mathcal{L}(\mathbb{R}^n)}^k}{(k-1)!} (k-1)r^{k-2} = \frac{h^2}{2} \|A\|_{\mathcal{L}(\mathbb{R}^n)}^2 \exp(\|A\|_{\mathcal{L}(\mathbb{R}^n)} r),$$

and (v) follows.

Proof of (vi): We observe that

$$\frac{d}{dt} \left(e^{At} e^{-At} \right) = \frac{d}{dt} \left(e^{At} \right) e^{-At} + e^{At} \frac{d}{dt} \left(e^{-At} \right)$$

$$= Ae^{At} e^{-At} + e^{At} (-A) e^{-At}$$

$$= (A - A) e^{At} e^{-At} = 0.$$

It follows that the function $t \to e^{At} e^{-At}$ is constant and by using $t = 0$, we obtain

$$e^{At} e^{-At} = I, \quad \forall t \in \mathbb{R},$$

and by replacing A by $-A$ we obtain

$$e^{-At}e^{At} = I, \quad \forall t \in \mathbb{R},$$

and the proof is complete.

Proof of (vii) and (viii): We observe that

$$
\begin{aligned}
\frac{d}{dt}\left(e^{-At}e^{-Bt}e^{(A+B)t}\right) &= \frac{d}{dt}\left(e^{-At}\right)e^{-Bt}e^{(A+B)t} + e^{-At}\frac{d}{dt}\left(e^{-Bt}\right)e^{(A+B)t} \\
&\quad + e^{-At}e^{-Bt}\frac{d}{dt}\left(e^{(A+B)t}\right) \\
&= -Ae^{-At}e^{-Bt}e^{(A+B)t} + e^{-At}(-B)e^{-Bt}e^{(A+B)t} \\
&\quad + e^{-At}e^{-Bt}(A+B)e^{(A+B)t}.
\end{aligned}
$$

Since A and B commute we obtain

$$\frac{d}{dt}\left(e^{-At}e^{-Bt}e^{(A+B)t}\right) = 0.$$

Therefore the function $t \to e^{-At}e^{-Bt}e^{(A+B)t}$ is constant and by using $t = 0$ we obtain

$$e^{-At}e^{-Bt}e^{(A+B)t} = I.$$

Therefore

$$e^{(A+B)t} = e^{Bt}e^{At}.$$

This completes the proof since (viii) is a special case of (vii). □

By using Proposition 2.19 (only) we can also prove the existence and the uniqueness of the solutions of (2.1).

Existence of solution: The existence of a solution of (2.1) follows trivially from property (v) of Proposition 2.19. Indeed $t \to e^{At}u_0$ is a solution of (2.1).

Uniqueness of solution: We now prove the uniqueness of the solution by using only Proposition 2.19. Assume that $t \to v(t)$ and $t \to u(t)$ are two continuous functions on $[0, \tau]$ and are solutions of (2.1) with

$$v(0) = u(0) = u_0.$$

Then $w = u - v$ is a continuous function on $[0, \tau]$ and a solution of (2.1). Thus

$$w(t) = A\int_0^t w(s)ds, \quad \forall t \in [0, \tau].$$

Set

$$W(t) = \int_0^t w(s)ds, \quad \forall t \in [0, \tau].$$

We have

$$W'(t) = AW(t), \quad \forall t \in [0, \tau], \text{ and } W(0) = 0.$$

Let $t \in (0, \tau]$. Consider $G : [0, t] \to \mathbb{R}^n$

$$G(s) := e^{A(t-s)} W(s), \quad \forall s \in [0, t].$$

Then for each $s \in [0, t]$,

$$G'(s) = -e^{A(t-s)} AW(s) + e^{A(t-s)} W'(s) = e^{A(t-s)} [-AW(s) + W'(s)] = 0$$

and we deduce that $G(s)$ is constant on $[0, t]$. So

$$W(t) = G(t) = G(0) = e^{At} W(0) = 0.$$

It follows that

$$w(t) = W'(t) = AW(t) = 0, \quad \forall t \in [0, \tau],$$

and the uniqueness of the solution follows.

2.6 An Example of a Continuous-Time Leslie Model

One may consider a continuous-time model to describe the evolution of a population

$$\frac{dn_0(t)}{dt} = \underbrace{\beta_0 n_0(t) + \beta_1 n_1(t) + \beta_2 n_2(t)}_{\text{flux of newborn}} - \underbrace{\mu_0 n_0(t)}_{\text{exit or death}} - \underbrace{\eta_0 n_0(t)}_{\text{flux going to the class 1}}$$

$$\frac{dn_1(t)}{dt} = \underbrace{\eta_0 n_0(t)}_{\text{flux coming from the class 0}} - \underbrace{\mu_1 n_1(t)}_{\text{exit or death}} - \underbrace{\eta_1 n_1(t)}_{\text{flux going to the class 2}}$$

$$\frac{dn_2(t)}{dt} = \eta_1 n_1(t) - \mu_2 n_2(t)$$

with the initial distribution

$$n_i(0) = n_0^i \geq 0, \quad \forall i = 0, 1, 2.$$

The parameters of the system as well as the state variables are defined below

- $n_i(t) \geq 0$ is the number of i-year old individuals at time t;
- $\beta_i \geq 0$ is the birth rate of i-year old individuals;
- $\mu_i \geq 0$ is the mortality rate of i-year old individuals;
- $\eta_i \geq 0$ is the flux rate at which individuals pass from age class i to age class $i + 1$.

The total number of individuals in the population at time t is given by

$$N(t) := n_0(t) + n_1(t) + n_2(t).$$

This model can be rewritten in matrix form as follows

$$\frac{dn(t)}{dt} = Ln(t), \quad \forall t \geq 0, n(0) = \begin{pmatrix} n_0^0 \\ n_0^1 \\ n_0^2 \end{pmatrix},$$

where the matrix L has the following form

$$L := \begin{pmatrix} \beta_0 - (\mu_0 + \eta_0) & \beta_1 & \beta_2 \\ \eta_0 & -(\mu_1 + \eta_1) & 0 \\ 0 & \eta_1 & -\mu_2 \end{pmatrix}.$$

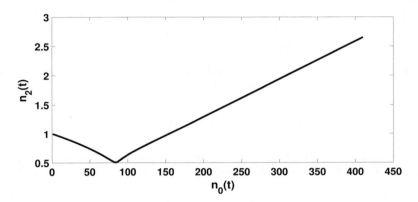

Fig. 2.1: *We plot $(n_0(t), n_2(t))$ for $t = [0, 1000]$. We choose $\beta_0 = \beta_1 = 0$, $\beta_2 = 2$, $\mu_0 = \mu_1 = \mu_2 = 0.01$ and $\eta_0 = \eta_1 = 0.001$. The initial distribution is $n_0^i = 1$, $\forall i = 0, 1, 2$.*

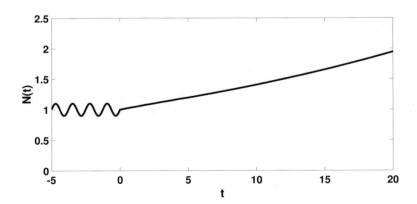

Fig. 2.2: *We plot $(t, N(t))$ for $t = [0, 1000]$. We use the same parameter values as well as the same initial distribution as in Figure 2.1.*

2.7 The Variation of Constant Formula

A *non-homogeneous Cauchy problem* is an ordinary differential equation of the form

$$\frac{du}{dt} = Au(t) + f(t), \forall t \geq t_0 \text{ and } u(t_0) = x \in \mathbb{R}^n, \tag{2.6}$$

where $A \in M_n(\mathbb{R})$ is an n by n real matrix, $t_0 \in \mathbb{R}$ is the time at which we start to compute the solution of (2.6) and f is a continuous function from $\mathbb{R}$ into $\mathbb{R}^n$. The term $f(t)$ is called a *non-homogeneous* (or *non-autonomous*) *perturbation* of the linear ordinary differential equation $u' = Au$.

Definition 2.20 Let $t_0 \in \mathbb{R}$. A continuous function $u \in C([t_0, \tau + t_0], \mathbb{R}^n)$ (for some $\tau > 0$) is a *solution* of (2.6) if u satisfies for each $t \in [t_0, \tau + t_0]$,

$$u(t) = x + \int_{t_0}^t Au(\sigma)\,d\sigma + \int_{t_0}^t f(\sigma)\,d\sigma. \tag{2.7}$$

Proposition 2.21 (Variation of constant formula) *The Cauchy problem (2.6) has a unique solution which is given by the variation of constant formula for each $t \geq t_0$,*

$$u(t) = e^{A(t-t_0)}x + \int_{t_0}^t e^{A(t-\sigma)} f(\sigma)\,d\sigma. \tag{2.8}$$

Proof **Existence of solution:** Let us start by observing that the map $t \to e^{At}$ satisfies for each $t \geq 0$

$$e^{At} = I + A \int_0^t e^{A\sigma}\,d\sigma \Leftrightarrow e^{At} - I = A \int_0^t e^{A\sigma}\,d\sigma.$$

So by using (2.8) and by using Fubini's theorem,

$$\begin{aligned}
A \int_{t_0}^t u(\sigma)d\sigma &= A \int_{t_0}^t e^{A(\sigma-t_0)}x\,d\sigma + A \int_{t_0}^t \int_{t_0}^\sigma e^{A(\sigma-l)} f(l)\,dl\,d\sigma \\
&= A \int_{t_0}^t e^{A(\sigma-t_0)}x\,d\sigma + A \int_{t_0}^t \int_l^t e^{A(\sigma-l)} f(l)\,d\sigma\,dl \\
&= A \int_0^{t-t_0} e^{Ar}x\,dr + \int_{t_0}^t A \int_0^{t-l} e^{Ar}\,dr\,f(l)\,dl \\
&= \left(e^{A(t-t_0)} - I\right)x + \int_{t_0}^t \left(e^{A(t-l)} - I\right) f(l)\,dl \\
&= e^{A(t-t_0)}x + \int_{t_0}^t e^{A(t-l)} f(l)dl - x - \int_{t_0}^t f(l)\,dl \\
&= u(t) - x - \int_{t_0}^t f(l)\,dl.
\end{aligned}$$

So the function $t \to u(t)$ defined by (2.8) is a solution of (2.7).

Uniqueness of solution: Assume that there exist two continuous functions u_1 and u_2 satisfying (2.7). Then by computing the difference, we have

$$u_1(t) - u_2(t) = A \int_{t_0}^t (u_1(\sigma) - u_2(\sigma))\,d\sigma, \forall t \geq t_0,$$

therefore by setting

$$\widehat{u}(t) := (u_1 - u_2)(t + t_0),$$

we have

$$\widehat{u}(t) = A \int_{t_0}^{t+t_0} (u_1 - u_2)(l)dl = A \int_0^t (u_1 - u_2)(r + t_0)dr = A \int_0^t \widehat{u}(r)dr.$$

This implies

$$\widehat{u}(t) = e^{At}0 = 0, \quad \forall t \geq 0.$$

The uniqueness of the solution follows. □

Theorem 2.22 (Perturbation theorem) *Let A and B be two n by n matrices. Then*

$$u(t) = e^{(A+B)t}x,$$

the solution of

$$\frac{du}{dt} = Au(t) + Bu(t), \quad \forall t \geq t_0 \text{ and } u(t_0) = x \in \mathbb{R}^n, \tag{2.9}$$

satisfies the fixed point problem

$$u(t) = e^{A(t-t_0)}x + \int_{t_0}^t e^{A(t-\sigma)}Bu(\sigma)d\sigma, \quad \forall t \geq t_0. \tag{2.10}$$

2.8 The Variation of Constant Formula for Non-Autonomous Systems

By using the fixed point method presented in Section 2.5, we can investigate the existence and uniqueness of solutions for the *non-autonomous linear Cauchy problem*

$$\frac{du(t)}{dt} = A(t)u(t), \quad \forall t \geq t_0, \text{ and } u(t_0) = x \in \mathbb{R}^n, \tag{2.11}$$

where $t_0 \in \mathbb{R}$ and the map $t \to A(t)$ is continuous from $\mathbb{R}$ to the space of n by n real matrices $M_n(\mathbb{R})$.

Definition 2.23 For each $t_0 \in \mathbb{R}$, a continuous function $u \in C([t_0, \infty), \mathbb{R}^n)$ is a *solution* of (2.11) if u satisfies for each $t \in [t_0, +\infty)$,

$$u(t) = x + \int_{t_0}^t A(\sigma)u(\sigma)d\sigma. \tag{2.12}$$

Proposition 2.24 (Non-autonomous linear semiflow) *There exists a unique family of matrices $\{U(t, t_0)\}_{t \geq t_0} \subset M_n(\mathbb{R})$ such that for each $u_0 \in \mathbb{R}^n$ the map $t \to U(t, t_0)x$ is a solution of (2.12). That is, $t \to U(t, t_0)x$ is a continuous map from $[t_0, +\infty)$ into $\mathbb{R}^n$ and satisfies*

$$U(t, t_0)x = x + \int_{t_0}^{t} A(\sigma)U(\sigma, t_0)x \, d\sigma, \quad \forall t \geq t_0, \forall x \in \mathbb{R}^n.$$

Moreover, we have the following properties:

(i) $U(t_0, t_0) = I$;

(ii) $U(t, t_1)U(t_1, t_0) = U(t, t_0), \quad \forall t \geq t_1 \geq t_0$;

(iii) *The map* $(t, t_0, x) \rightarrow U(t, t_0)x$ *is continuous;*

(iv) $\partial_t U(t, t_0) = A(t)U(t, t_0), \quad \forall t \geq t_0$.

Proof We can proceed by using the fixed point method presented in Section 2.5. Let $t_0 \in \mathbb{R}$. We consider the fixed point problem

$$U(t, t_0) = \Psi_{t_0}\left(U(\cdot, t_0)\right)(t),$$

where $\Psi_s : C\left([t_0, t_0 + \tau], M_n(\mathbb{R})\right) \rightarrow C\left([t_0, t_0 + \tau], M_n(\mathbb{R})\right)$ is defined by

$$\Psi_{t_0}\left(U(\cdot, t_0)\right)(t) := I + \int_{t_0}^{t} A(\sigma)U(\sigma, t_0) dl, \quad \forall t \in [t_0, t_0 + \tau].$$

By using the same argument as in Section 2.5, we prove that for $n > 0$ large enough, Ψ^n is a contraction (for the usual supremum topology on $C\left([t_0, t_0 + \tau], M_n(\mathbb{R})\right)$). The existence and the uniqueness follows. We trivially have

$$U(t_0, t_0) = I.$$

Let $t_1 \geq t_0$. If we consider

$$V(t, t_0) := \begin{cases} U(t, t_1)U(t_1, t_0) & \text{for } t \geq t_1, \\ U(t, t_0) & \text{for } t \in [t_0, t_1], \end{cases}$$

it is not difficult to check that $V(t, t_0)$ satisfies the fixed point problem

$$V(t, t_0) = \Psi_{t_0}\left(V(\cdot, t_0)\right)(t),$$

and by uniqueness of the solution we deduce that

$$U(t, t_1)U(t_1, t_0) = U(t, t_0).$$

For the continuity part, we consider

$$U(t, t_0) - U(\widehat{t}, \widehat{t_0}) = \int_{t_0}^{t} A(\sigma)U(\sigma, t_0) \, d\sigma - \int_{\widehat{t_0}}^{\widehat{t}} A(\sigma)U(\sigma, \widehat{t_0}) \, d\sigma.$$

Assume for example that $t_0 \geq \widehat{t_0}$. Then we have

$$U(t, t_0) - U(\widehat{t}, \widehat{t_0}) = \int_{t_0}^{t} A(\sigma) U(\sigma, t_0) \, \mathrm{d}\sigma - \int_{\widehat{t_0}}^{\widehat{t}} A(\sigma) U(\sigma, t_0) U(t_0, \widehat{t_0}) \, \mathrm{d}\sigma$$

$$= \int_{t_0}^{t} A(\sigma) U(\sigma, t_0) \, \mathrm{d}\sigma - \int_{\widehat{t_0}}^{\widehat{t}} A(\sigma) U(\sigma, t_0) \, \mathrm{d}\sigma$$

$$+ \int_{\widehat{t_0}}^{\widehat{t}} A(\sigma) U(\sigma, t_0) \left[I - U(t_0, \widehat{t_0}) \right] \, \mathrm{d}\sigma$$

and the continuity result follows. The last property is immediate. $\qquad \square$

Exercise 2.25 Prove that

$$A(t)A(s) = A(s)A(t), \forall t, s \ge t_0 \Rightarrow U(t, t_0) = \exp\left(\int_{t_0}^{t} A(l) \mathrm{d}l\right), \forall t \ge t_0.$$

Let us now consider the Cauchy problem

$$u'(t) = A(t)u(t) + f(t), \quad \forall t \ge t_0, \text{ with } u(t_0) = x \in \mathbb{R}^n. \tag{2.13}$$

Definition 2.26 Let $t_0 \in \mathbb{R}$. A continuous function $u \in C([t_0, \tau + t_0], \mathbb{R}^n)$ (for some $\tau > 0$) is a *solution* of (2.13) if u satisfies, for each $t \in [t_0, \tau + t_0]$,

$$u(t) = x + \int_{t_0}^{t} A(\sigma) u(\sigma) \, \mathrm{d}\sigma + \int_{t_0}^{t} f(\sigma) \, \mathrm{d}\sigma. \tag{2.14}$$

Proposition 2.27 (Variation of constant formula) *The Cauchy problem* (2.13) *has a unique solution which is given by the variation of constant formula for each $t \ge t_0$,*

$$u(t) = U(t, t_0)x + \int_{t_0}^{t} U(t, l) f(l) \mathrm{d}l, \quad \forall t \ge t_0. \tag{2.15}$$

Proof Let $u(t)$ be defined by (2.15). We have

$$U(t, t_0) - I = \int_{t_0}^{t} A(\sigma) U(\sigma, t_0) \, \mathrm{d}\sigma, \quad \forall t \ge t_0.$$

Therefore

$$\int_{t_0}^{t} A(\sigma) u(\sigma) \mathrm{d}\sigma = \int_{t_0}^{t} A(\sigma) U(\sigma, t_0) x \, \mathrm{d}\sigma + \int_{t_0}^{t} \int_{t_0}^{\sigma} A(\sigma) U(\sigma, l) f(l) \, \mathrm{d}l \, \mathrm{d}\sigma$$

$$= \int_{t_0}^{t} A(\sigma) U(\sigma, t_0) x \, \mathrm{d}\sigma + \int_{t_0}^{t} \int_{l}^{t} A(\sigma) U(\sigma, l) \, \mathrm{d}\sigma \, \mathrm{d}l$$

$$= (U(t, t_0) - I) x + \int_{t_0}^{t} (U(t, l) - I) f(l) \, \mathrm{d}l$$

$$= u(t) - x - \int_{t_0}^{t} f(l) \, \mathrm{d}l.$$

It follows that $t \to u(t)$ satisfies (2.14). The uniqueness part of the proof is similar to the autonomous case. $\qquad \square$

2.9 Convergence of an Implicit Euler Numerical Scheme

Let $\tau \in (0, \infty)$. We consider the *vector-valued* (i.e. *n-dimensional*) *Cauchy problem*

$$\frac{du(t)}{dt} = Au(t), \quad \forall t \in [0, \tau], \tag{2.16}$$

with the initial condition

$$u(0) = u_0 \in \mathbb{R}^n,$$

where A belongs to the space of n by n real matrices $M_n(\mathbb{R})$.

To define an approximation scheme for the above linear ordinary differential equation we will use

$$\Delta t = \frac{\tau}{m + 1}, \tag{2.17}$$

for some integer $m \geq 0$.

The exact solution satisfies

$$u(t + \Delta t) = u(t) + \int_{t-}^{t+\Delta t} Au(\sigma)d\sigma,$$

and the idea of the *Euler implicit scheme* is to use the following approximation formula

$$u(t + \Delta t) = u(t) + \int_{t}^{t+\Delta t} Au(t + \Delta t)d\sigma.$$

Therefore the discrete-time approximated solution y_j is a solution of the implicit Euler numerical scheme

$$y_{j+1} = y_j + \Delta t \, A y_{j+1}, \, \forall j \in \{0, \ldots, m + 1\} \text{ with } y_0 = u_0, \tag{2.18}$$

or equivalently

$$(I - \Delta t A)y_{j+1} = y_j, \, \forall j \in \{0, \ldots, m + 1\} \text{ with } y_0 = u_0.$$

Intuitively, the sequence y_j should approach $u(j\Delta t)$ whenever m is large enough.

To prove such a result, we consider the map

$$u_m(t) = y_j + (t - j\Delta t)A y_{j+1}, \text{ if } t \in [j\Delta t, (j + 1)\,\Delta t). \tag{2.19}$$

By considering the limits (right and left)

$$u_m((j\Delta t)^+) = y_j \text{ and } u_m(((j + 1)\,\Delta t)^-) = y_j + \Delta t A y_{j+1} = y_{j+1},$$

we deduce that $t \to u_m(t)$ is continuous and piecewise affine.

To obtain the existence of the solution for the problem (2.18) we will fix Δt small enough and use the following proposition.

Proposition 2.28 *Let $L \in M_n(\mathbb{R})$ with $\|L\|_{\mathcal{L}(\mathbb{R}^n)} < 1$ (where $\|L\|_{\mathcal{L}(\mathbb{R}^n)}$ is the operator norm of L).*

Then the matrix $I - L$ is invertible and

$$(I - L)^{-1} = \sum_{m=0}^{\infty} L^m,$$

where

$$L^0 = I \text{ and } L^{m+1} = L \times L^m, \quad \forall m \geq 0.$$

Moreover,

$$\left\| (I - L)^{-1} \right\|_{\mathcal{L}(\mathbb{R}^n)} \leq \frac{1}{1 - \|L\|_{\mathcal{L}(\mathbb{R}^n)}}. \tag{2.20}$$

Proof Set

$$B_m = I + L + \cdots + L^m, \quad \forall m \geq 0.$$

By using the fact that $\|L\|_{\mathcal{L}(\mathbb{R}^n)} < 1$ and

$$\|L^m\|_{\mathcal{L}(\mathbb{R}^n)} \leq \|L\|_{\mathcal{L}(\mathbb{R}^n)}^m, \quad \forall m \geq 1,$$

we deduce that the sequence B_m is a Cauchy sequence in $M_n(\mathbb{R})$. Therefore we can define

$$B_\infty = \lim_{m \to \infty} B_m.$$

Moreover, we have for each integer $m \geq 1$

$$(I - L) B_m = B_m (I - L) = I - L^{m+1}.$$

Hence by taking the limit when m goes to infinity we obtain

$$(I - L) B_\infty = B_\infty (I - L) = I.$$

Finally

$$B_\infty = I + L B_\infty.$$

Therefore

$$\|B_\infty\|_{\mathcal{L}(\mathbb{R}^n)} = \|I + L B_\infty\|_{\mathcal{L}(\mathbb{R}^n)} \leq \|I\|_{\mathcal{L}(\mathbb{R}^n)} + \|L B_\infty\|_{\mathcal{L}(\mathbb{R}^n)}.$$

Thus

$$\left(1 - \|L\|_{\mathcal{L}(\mathbb{R}^n)} \right) \|B_\infty\|_{\mathcal{L}(\mathbb{R}^n)} \leq 1$$

and the proof is complete since by definition, $\sum_{m=0}^{\infty} L^m = B_\infty$. □

Assumption 2.29 Assume that the integer $m \in \mathbb{N}$ is chosen large enough such that

$$\Delta t \|A\|_{\mathcal{L}(\mathbb{R}^n)} = \frac{\tau}{m+1} \|A\|_{\mathcal{L}(\mathbb{R}^n)} < 1.$$

Lemma 2.30 *Let Assumption 2.29 be satisfied. Then*

$$\left\| y_j \right\| \le e^{\frac{j}{m+1}\delta} \left\| y_0 \right\| \le e^{\delta} \left\| u_0 \right\|, \quad \forall j \in \{0, \dots, m\}, \tag{2.21}$$

where

$$\delta := \frac{\tau \left\| A \right\|_{\mathcal{L}(\mathbb{R}^n)}}{1 - \Delta t \left\| A \right\|_{\mathcal{L}(\mathbb{R}^n)}}. \tag{2.22}$$

Proof The equation (2.18) can be rewritten as

$$(1 - \Delta t A)\, y_j = y_{j-1} \Leftrightarrow y_j = (1 - \Delta t A)^{-1}\, y_{j-1}$$

and we obtain

$$y_j = (1 - \Delta t A)^{-(j+1)} u_0, \quad \forall j \in \{0, \dots, m\}.$$

We have

$$\left\| y_j \right\| \le \left\| (1 - \Delta t A)^{-1} \right\|_{\mathcal{L}(\mathbb{R}^n)} \left\| y_{j-1} \right\|.$$

Hence

$$\left\| y_j \right\| \le \frac{1}{1 - \Delta t \left\| A \right\|_{\mathcal{L}(\mathbb{R}^n)}} \left\| y_{j-1} \right\| = \left(1 + \frac{\Delta t \left\| A \right\|_{\mathcal{L}(\mathbb{R}^n)}}{1 - \Delta t \left\| A \right\|_{\mathcal{L}(\mathbb{R}^n)}} \right) \left\| y_{j-1} \right\|.$$

We obtain

$$\left\| y_j \right\| \le e^{\frac{\Delta t \left\| A \right\|_{\mathcal{L}(\mathbb{R}^n)}}{1 - \Delta t \left\| A \right\|_{\mathcal{L}(\mathbb{R}^n)}}} \left\| y_{j-1} \right\|, \quad \forall j \in \{0, \dots, m\},$$

and the result follows by using the fact that $\Delta t = \frac{\tau}{m+1}$. $\square$

Estimation of the errors: The error between the approximated solution and the real solution is

$$e(t) = u(t) - u_m(t), \quad \forall t \in [0, \tau].$$

Let $j = 0, \dots, m+1$ and $t \in [j\Delta t, (j+1)\Delta t)$. We have

$$
\begin{aligned}
e(t) &= u(t) - u_m(t) \\
&= u(t) - \left(y_j + (t - j\Delta t)\, A y_{j+1} \right) \\
&= u(j\Delta t) - y_j + \int_{j\Delta t}^{t} A u(\sigma)\mathrm{d}\sigma - (t - j\Delta t)\, A y_{j+1} \\
&= e(j\Delta t) + \int_{j\Delta t}^{t} A e(\sigma)\mathrm{d}\sigma + \int_{j\Delta t}^{t} A \left(y_j + (\sigma - j\Delta t)\, A y_{j+1} \right) \mathrm{d}\sigma \\
&\quad - (t - j\Delta t)\, A y_{j+1} \\
&= e(j\Delta t) + \int_{j\Delta t}^{t} A e(\sigma)\mathrm{d}\sigma + \int_{j\Delta t}^{t} A \left(y_j - y_{j+1} \right) \mathrm{d}\sigma \\
&\quad + \int_{j\Delta t}^{t} (\sigma - j\Delta t)\, A^2 y_{j+1}\mathrm{d}\sigma.
\end{aligned}
$$

Therefore by using the fact that $y_{j-1} - y_j = -\Delta t A y_j$

$$e(t) = e(j\Delta t) + \int_{j\Delta t}^{t} A e(\sigma) d\sigma + \left[\frac{(t - j\Delta t)^2}{2} - \Delta t (t - j\Delta t) \right] A^2 y_j.$$

Moreover, we have

$$\left[\frac{(t - j\Delta t)^2}{2} - \Delta t (t - j\Delta t) \right] = (t - j\Delta t) \left[\frac{(t - j\Delta t)}{2} - \Delta t \right]$$

and for $t \in [j\Delta t, (j + 1)\Delta t)$, we obtain

$$\left| \frac{(t - j\Delta t)^2}{2} - \Delta t (t - j\Delta t) \right| \leq (t - j\Delta t) \left[\Delta t - \frac{\Delta t}{2} \right] \leq \frac{\Delta t^2}{2}.$$

Define

$$E_j = \sup_{t \in [j\Delta t, (j+1)\Delta t)} |u(t) - u_m(t)|.$$

Then we have, for all $j = 1, \ldots, m + 1$,

$$E_j \leq E_{j-1} + \Delta t \|A\|_{\mathcal{L}(\mathbb{R}^n)} E_j + \Delta t^2 \|A\|_{\mathcal{L}(\mathbb{R}^n)}^2 \|y_j\|.$$

Hence by using Lemma 2.30 we obtain the following result.

Lemma 2.31 *We have, for all $j = 1, \ldots, m + 1$,*

$$E_j \leq \alpha E_{j-1} + \beta, \tag{2.23}$$

with

$$\alpha = 1 + \Delta t \frac{\|A\|_{\mathcal{L}(\mathbb{R}^n)}}{1 - \Delta t \|A\|_{\mathcal{L}(\mathbb{R}^n)}} \quad and \quad \beta = \Delta t^2 \frac{\|A\|_{\mathcal{L}(\mathbb{R}^n)}^2}{1 - \Delta t \|A\|_{\mathcal{L}(\mathbb{R}^n)}} e^{\delta} \|u_0\|.$$

We will use the following lemma.

Lemma 2.32 (A discrete-time Gronwall's lemma) *Let $a > 0$ with $a \neq 1$ and $b > 0$. Assume that*

$$v_j \leq a v_{j-1} + b, \quad \forall j = 1, \ldots, m + 1.$$

Then

$$v_j \leq a^j v_0 + \frac{a^j - 1}{a - 1} b, \quad \forall j = 1, \ldots, m + 1.$$

Exercise 2.33 Prove Lemma 2.32.

Next we have

$$\alpha = 1 + \Delta t \frac{\|A\|_{\mathcal{L}(\mathbb{R}^n)}}{1 - \Delta t \|A\|_{\mathcal{L}(\mathbb{R}^n)}} \leq e^{\frac{\Delta t \|A\|_{\mathcal{L}(\mathbb{R}^n)}}{1 - \Delta t \|A\|_{\mathcal{L}(\mathbb{R}^n)}}}.$$

Therefore

$$\alpha^j \leq e^{\frac{j}{m+1} \frac{\tau\|A\|_{\mathcal{L}(\mathbb{R}^n)}}{1-\Delta t\|A\|_{\mathcal{L}(\mathbb{R}^n)}}} \leq e^\delta.$$

Thus by combining equation (2.23) and Lemma 2.32 we obtain

$$E_j \leq e^\delta E_0 + e^\delta \frac{\beta}{\alpha-1} = e^\delta E_0 + \Delta t \|A\|_{\mathcal{L}(\mathbb{R}^n)} e^{2\delta} \|u_0\|.$$

By using the fact that

$$E_0 = \sup_{t\in[0,\Delta t]} \left| u_0 + \int_0^t Au(s)\mathrm{d}s - [u_0 + tAy_1] \right| \to 0 \text{ as } m \to \infty$$

and

$$\delta \to \tau \|A\|_{\mathcal{L}(\mathbb{R}^n)} \text{ as } m \to \infty$$

we deduce that $u_m(t)$ converges to $u(t)$ uniformly on $[0, \tau]$. That is,

$$\lim_{m\to\infty} \sup_{t\in[0,\tau]} |u(t) - u_m(t)| = 0.$$

By considering the specific time $t = j\Delta t$ we deduce the following theorem.

Theorem 2.34 (Convergence result) *Let* $t \to u(t)$ *be the solution of the Cauchy problem*

$$\frac{\mathrm{d}u(t)}{\mathrm{d}t} = Au(t), \quad \forall t \in [0, \tau], \text{ with } u(0) = u_0 \in \mathbb{R}^n.$$

There exists an integer $m_0 \geq 0$ *such that the implicit Euler numerical scheme*

$$y_{j+1}^m = y_j^m + \frac{\tau}{m+1} Ay_{j+1}^m, \quad \forall j \in \{0, \ldots, m+1\} \text{ with } y_0^m = u_0$$

has a unique solution for each $m \geq m_0$. *Moreover, we have the following convergence result (uniform in* $j = 0, \ldots, m+1$)

$$\lim_{m\to\infty} \sup_{j=0,\ldots,m+1} \left| u\left(\frac{j\tau}{m+1}\right) - y_j^m \right| = 0.$$

2.10 A Delay Differential Equation

Let $\beta > 0$, $\mu > 0$ and $N(t)$ be the number of adults in a given population at time t. Then $N(t)$ may satisfy (in some simplified situations) the following *delay differential equation*

$$N'(t) = - \underbrace{\mu N(t)}_{\text{flux of exiting or death}} + \underbrace{\beta N(t - \tau)}_{\text{flux of newborn}}, \quad \forall t \geq 0, \quad (2.24)$$

with initial value

$$N(t) = N_0(t), \quad \forall t \in [-\tau, 0],$$

where

$$N_0 \in C([-\tau, 0], \mathbb{R}).$$

Here $\tau > 0$ is the time needed for a newborn to become an adult, μ is the mortality rate and β is the birth rate.

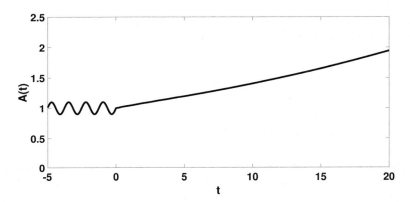

Fig. 2.3: *We run a simulation of the above delay differential equation for $\beta = 0.05$ and $\mu = 0.01$ and with the initial distribution $N_0(t) = 1 + 0.1 \sin(5t)$.*

Definition 2.35 We will say that $N \in C([-\tau, +\infty), \mathbb{R})$ is a *solution* of (2.24) if, for each $t \geq -\tau$,

$$N(t) = \begin{cases} N_0(0) + \int_0^t -\mu N(s) + \beta N(s - \tau) \mathrm{d}s, & \text{if } t \geq 0, \\ N_0(t), & \text{if } t \leq 0. \end{cases}$$

Exercise 2.36 Apply the methods in Section 2.5.1 to prove the global existence and the uniqueness of solutions for this equation.

Hint for Exercise 2.36: For each $t \in [0, \tau]$, we have

$$N(t) = F(t) + \int_0^t -\mu N(s) \mathrm{d}s$$

with

$$F(t) := N_0(0) + \int_0^t \beta N_0(s - \tau) \mathrm{d}s.$$

Then as before we set

$$\Phi(N)(t) := F(t) + \int_0^t -\mu N(s) \mathrm{d}s, \quad \forall t \in [0, \tau],$$

and by using the methods in Sections 2.5.1 and 2.5.2, we deduce the existence of a solution on $[0, \tau]$. Then by induction we prove the existence of a solution on $[\tau, 2\tau]$, $[2\tau, 3\tau]$, etc.

Exercise 2.37 Prove the positivity of solutions starting from a non-negative initial distribution.

Hint for Exercise 2.37: Prove that $N(t)$ is a solution if and only if $N(t)$ satisfies the variation of constant formula for each $t \geq 0$

$$N(t) = e^{-\mu t} N_0(0) + \int_0^t e^{-\mu(t-s)} \beta N(s - \tau) ds.$$

2.11 The Sharpe–Lotka Model

Discrete-time renewal equation: For a discrete-time age-structured model, let $B(n)$ be the flux of newborn at time n, $\beta_i, i = 0, 1$ the reproduction rate for individuals with age i and π_0 the probability for a newborn individual to survive until age 1. By setting

$$B(n) := \beta_0 n_0(n) + \beta_1 n_1(n),$$

one has

$$n_0(n) = B(n - 1)$$

and

$$n_1(n) = \pi_0 n_0(n - 1) = \pi_0 B(n - 2).$$

Thus we obtain the so-called *renewal equation*

$$B(n) = \beta_0 B(n - 1) + \beta_1 \pi_0 B(n - 2), \quad \forall n \in \mathbb{N} \text{ with } n \geq 2.$$

Continuous-time renewal equation: By analogy with the discrete-time case, one can write a continuous-time version of this model. Let $B(t)$ be the flux of newborn at time t. The *Sharpe–Lotka model* [213, 314] (1907–1911) is described by the equation

$$B(t) = F(t) + \int_0^t \beta(a) \pi(a) B(t - a) da, \quad \forall t \geq 0,$$

where $\beta(a)$ is the reproduction rate for individuals with age a and $\pi(a)$ is the probability for a newborn individual to survive until age a. The term $F(t)$ is the production of newborn at time t by the individuals that were already present at time $t = 0$. Therefore

$$F(t) = \int_t^{+\infty} \beta(a) \frac{\pi(a)}{\pi(a - t)} u_0(a - t) da,$$

where $u_0(a)$ is the density of population at time $t = 0$. That is,

$$\int_{a_1}^{a_2} u_0(a) da$$

is the number of individuals with age in between a_1 and a_2 (whenever $a_1 \le a_2$) at time $t = 0$. In particular,

$$\int_0^\infty u_0(a)\mathrm{d}a$$

is the total number of individuals at time $t = 0$. It follows that we must assume that

$$u_0 \in L_+^1((0, \infty), \mathbb{R}).$$

Theorem 2.38 *Assume that $\beta \in L_+^\infty((0, \infty), \mathbb{R})$ and assume that*

$$\pi(a) = \exp\left(-\int_0^a \mu(\sigma)\mathrm{d}\sigma\right), \quad \forall a \ge 0,$$

where

$$\mu \in L_+^\infty((0, \infty), \mathbb{R}).$$

There exists a unique continuous function $t \to B(t)$ satisfying

$$B(t) = F(t) + \int_0^t \beta(a)\pi(a)B(t - a)\mathrm{d}a, \quad \forall t \ge 0.$$

Exercise 2.39 Prove the above Theorem 2.38 by using the fixed point methods in Sections 2.5.1, 2.5.2 and 2.5.3.

Remark 2.40 It is interesting to observe that a Volterra integral equation of the form

$$X(t) = F(t) + \int_0^t G(t - s)X(s)\mathrm{d}s, \quad \forall t \ge 0$$

or equivalently

$$X(t) = F(t) + \int_0^t G(l)X(t - s)\mathrm{d}s$$

coincides with the solution of the linear ordinary differential equation

$$X'(t) = (A + B)X(t), \quad \forall t \ge 0, X(0) = X_0 \in \mathbb{R}^n$$

whenever

$$F(t) = \mathrm{e}^{At}X_0 \text{ and } G(t) = \mathrm{e}^{At}B,$$

and A and B are two n by n real matrices.

Numerical simulations: Assume that

$$u_0(a) = \begin{cases} N_0/(a_2 - a_1), & \text{if } a \in [a_1, a_2], \\ 0, & \text{otherwise,} \end{cases}$$

where N_0 is the number of individuals at time $t = 0$. We assume that

$$\beta(a) = \begin{cases} \beta^*, & \text{if } a \in [a_{\min}, a_{\max}], \\ 0, & \text{otherwise,} \end{cases}$$

and

$$\pi(a) = \exp(-\mu a).$$

Recall that

$$F(t) = \int_t^{+\infty} \beta(a) \frac{\pi(a)}{\pi(a-t)} u_0(a-t) da,$$

so by setting $\sigma = a - t$ we obtain

$$F(t) = \int_0^{+\infty} \beta(\sigma + t) \frac{\pi(\sigma + t)}{\pi(\sigma)} u_0(\sigma) d\sigma.$$

In Figure 2.4, we use Simpson's rule to compute $F(t)$ at each time step.

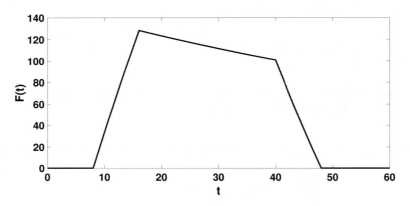

Fig. 2.4: *In this figure we plot the function $t \to F(t)$, which is the flux of newborn produced at time t by the individuals that were present at time 0. We use $N_0 = 50$, $a_1 = 2$, $a_2 = 10$, $\beta^\star = 3$, $a_{min} = 18$, $a_{max} = 50$, and $\mu = 0.01$.*

Recall that

$$B(t) = F(t) + \int_0^t \beta(a)\pi(a)B(t-a)da, \quad \forall t \geq 0.$$

In Figure 2.5, we use Simpson's rule to compute $B(t)$ at each time step.

Derivation of the delay differential equation: Assume for simplicity that

$$\beta(a) = \begin{cases} \overline{\beta}, & \text{if } a \geq \tau, \\ 0, & \text{if } a < \tau \end{cases}$$

and

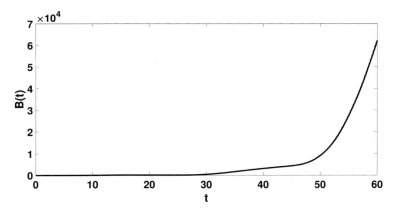

Fig. 2.5: *In this figure we plot the function $t \to B(t)$, which is the flux of newborn produced at time t by the individuals that were present at time 0. We use $N_0 = 50$, $a_1 = 2$, $a_2 = 10$, $\beta^\star = 3$, $a_{min} = 18$, $a_{max} = 50$, and $\mu = 0.01$.*

$$\pi(a) = e^{-\mu a}.$$

Then for $t \geq \tau$ we have

$$F(t) = \begin{cases} e^{-\mu t} \overline{\beta} \int_0^{+\infty} u_0(a)\mathrm{d}a, & \text{if } t \geq \tau \\ e^{-\mu t} \overline{\beta} \int_{\tau-t}^{+\infty} u_0(a)\mathrm{d}a, & \text{if } t \in [0, \tau]. \end{cases}$$

Moreover, set

$$J(t) := \int_0^t \beta(a)\pi(a)B(t-a)\mathrm{d}a, \quad \forall t \geq 0.$$

Then for $t \geq \tau$,

$$J(t) = \overline{\beta} \int_\tau^t e^{-\mu a} B(t-a)\mathrm{d}a$$

$$= \overline{\beta} \int_0^{t-\tau} e^{-\mu(t-s)} B(s)\mathrm{d}s$$

$$= \overline{\beta}e^{-\mu t} \int_0^{t-\tau} e^{\mu s} B(s)\mathrm{d}s$$

and

$$J(t) = 0, \quad \forall t \in [0, \tau].$$

Thus

$$J'(t) = -\mu J(t) + \overline{\beta}e^{-\mu\tau} B(t-\tau), \quad \forall t \geq \tau.$$

Therefore for $t \geq \tau$, the birth flux $B(t) = F(t) + J(t)$ satisfies the delay differential equation

$$B'(t) = -\mu B(t) + \overline{\beta}e^{-\mu\tau} B(t-\tau), \quad \forall t \geq \tau,$$

with the initial condition

$$B(t) = e^{-\mu t}\overline{\beta}\int_{\tau-t}^{+\infty} u_0(a)da, \quad \forall t \in [0, \tau].$$

So we can use a delay differential equation to take into account the fact that reproduction is not taking place immediately after birth.

Exercise 2.41 (Volterra integral equation) Let $F \in C([0, +\infty), \mathbb{R})$. Assume that F is an exponentially bounded function. That is, there exists a real number $\alpha_0 > 0$ such that

$$\sup_{t \geq 0} e^{-\alpha_0 t}|F(t)| < +\infty.$$

Assume that $G \in L^1_{loc}([0, +\infty), \mathbb{R})$. That is, $t \to G(t)$ is Lebesgue measurable, and for each $t > 0$

$$\int_0^t |G(s)|\, ds < +\infty.$$

We assume in addition that

$$\kappa_G(\alpha) := \int_0^t e^{-\alpha s}|G(s)|\, ds \to 0 \text{ as } \alpha \to +\infty.$$

Apply the method in Section 2.5.3 to prove that for all $\alpha > 0$ large enough, there exists a unique solution $B \in C_\alpha([0, +\infty), \mathbb{R})$ of the Volterra integral equation

$$B(t) = F(t) + \int_0^t G(t-s)B(s)ds, \quad \forall t \geq 0.$$

Hint for Exercise 2.41: Consider the fixed point map $: \Phi : C_\alpha([0, +\infty), \mathbb{R}) \to C([0, +\infty), \mathbb{R})$ defined by

$$\Phi(B)(t) = F(t) + \int_0^t G(t-s)B(s)ds, \quad \forall t \geq 0.$$

Then prove that for each $\alpha > 0$ (large enough) and each $B, \overline{B} \in C_\alpha([0, +\infty), \mathbb{R})$,

$$\|\Phi(B)\|_\alpha \leq \|F\|_{\alpha_0} + \kappa_G(\alpha)\|B\|_\alpha$$

and

$$\left\|\Phi(B) - \Phi(\overline{B})\right\|_\alpha \leq \kappa_G(\alpha)\left\|B - \overline{B}\right\|_\alpha.$$

Exercise 2.42 (Matlab simulation of the Kermack and McKendrick model) We reconsider the Kermack and McKendrick model with infection age presented in Chapter 1. We want to compute the unique solution $t \to B(t) \in C_+([0, \infty), \mathbb{R})$ of the Volterra integral equation for $t \geq 0$,

$$B(t) = \left[\int_t^\infty \beta(a)\frac{\Pi(a)}{\Pi(a-t)}i_0(a-t)da + \int_0^t \beta(a)\Pi(a)\, v\, S(t-a)B(t-a)da\right],$$

coupled with $t \to S(t)$, the solution of the ordinary differential equation

$$S'(t) = -\nu S(t)B(t).$$

Based on the Matlab code obtained for Figure 2.5 in Section 2.13 and/or Section 2.13, write a MATLAB code to simulate

$$i_0(a) = \begin{cases} N_0/(a_2 - a_1), & \text{if } a \in [a_1, a_2], \\ 0, & \text{otherwise,} \end{cases}$$

where I_0 is the number of infected individuals at time $t = 0$.

We also assume

$$\beta(a) = \begin{cases} \overline{\beta}, & \text{if } a \geq \tau, \\ 0, & \text{if } a < \tau, \end{cases}$$

and

$$\pi(a) = e^{-\eta a}.$$

2.12 Notes and Remarks

Delay differential equations

Functional differential equations have been extensively studied in the literature. There are some more theory-oriented texts on this subject, see, for example, the books by Hale [137, 138], Mohammed [258], Kolmanovskii and Nosov [186], Gyori and Ladas [135], Arino, Hbid and Dats [12], MacDonald [226], Diekmann, Van Gils, Lunel and Walther [89], Driver [94], Hale and Lunel [141], and some more application-oriented texts by Busenberg and Cooke [43], Kuang [193], Cushing [71], Smith [327], Wu [372], and Gopalsamy [119]. We also refer to Liu [206] and the book of Magal and Ruan [236] (and references therein) for an approach to understanding delay differential equations as non-densely defined Cauchy problems.

Finite delay

Finite delay differential equations were first studied in the 1970s by Hale's group [137, 138, 141]. Since then people have extended the elementary theorems for ordinary differential equations to functional differential equations by using different methods. For example, in the book of Smith [327], the existence and uniqueness of solutions of the following discrete delay differential equations are established by the method of steps:

$$x'(t) = Ax(t) + Bx(t - r), \quad \forall t \geq 0$$

with the initial condition

$$x(t) = \varphi(t) \in \mathbb{R}^n, \quad \forall t \in [-r, 0],$$

where $t \to \varphi(t)$ is assumed to be bounded continuous from $[-r, 0]$ into $\mathbb{R}^n$, the (single) delay $r > 0$, and $A \in M_n(\mathbb{R})$ and $B \in M_n(\mathbb{R})$ are two matrices.

Infinite delay

To illustrate the case of infinite delay, we can consider the following equation (where all the history anterior to t is needed to compute the variation solution at time t)

$$x'(t) = Ax(t) + \int_0^\infty B(r)x(t-r)\mathrm{d}r, \quad \forall t \geq 0,$$

with the initial condition

$$x(t) = \varphi(t), \quad \forall t \in (-\infty, 0],$$

where $t \to \varphi(t)$ is assumed to be bounded continuous from $(-\infty, 0]$ into $\mathbb{R}^n$, and the function $t \to B(t)$ is a continuous map from $[0, \infty)$ into $M_n(\mathbb{R})$ and satisfies the following exponential bound

$$|B(t)| \leq \mathrm{e}^{-\eta t}, \quad \forall t \geq 0,$$

with $\eta > 0$.

For infinite delay differential equations, various classes of semi-normed spaces have been considered, firstly by Hale and Kato [139]. We refer to the book of Hino, Murakami and Naito [153] for more results and a nice survey on this subject. Along these lines a variation of constant formula has been obtained by Hino, Murakami, Naito and Minh [154]. We also refer to Diekmann and Gyllenberg [85] for infinite delay differential equations in weighted L^1 spaces. In a similar fashion, Matsunaga, Murakami, Nagabuchi and Van Minh [251] recently proved a center manifold theorem for difference equations in L^1 spaces. We also mention that a Hopf bifurcation theorem has been obtained by Hassard, Kazarinof and Wan [148, Chapter 4, Section 5] in L^2 space. We also refer to Liu and Magal [205] for more results on infinite delay in a space of exponentially bounded and uniformly continuous functions.

Partial functional differential equations

To illustrate the case of a partial differential equation with delay, we consider the following equation (where all the history anterior to t is needed to compute the variation solution at time t)

$$\partial_t u(t, x) = \varepsilon \partial_x^2 u(t, x) + a(x)u(t, x) + b(x)u(t-r, x), \quad \forall t \geq 0, x \in \mathbb{R},$$

with the initial condition

$$u(t, x) = \varphi(t, x), \quad \forall t \in (-\infty, 0].$$

In the book of Wu [372] the idea is to explore the combined effect of the diffusion and the delay. Such a combination leads to complicated dynamical behaviors and spatio-temporal patterns. We refer to Ducrot, Magal, and Ruan [102] and references therein for more references and results on this subject.

Competition for light in a forest: an example of a state-dependent delay differential equation

Here we recall a model obtained in [242] to describe the dynamics of a population that is structured in size with intra-specific competition for light. The model extends the model proposed by Smith [323, 324].

It models the number of adult trees $t \rightarrow A(t)$ in a forest at time t by the equation

$$A'(t) = e^{-\mu_J \tau(t)} \frac{f(A(t))}{f(A(t - \tau(t)))} \beta A(t - \tau(t)) - \mu_A A(t),$$

where the maturation time $\tau(t)$ is the unique solution of

$$\int_{t-\tau(t)}^{t} f(A(s)) \mathrm{d}s = s^\star - s,$$

for some fixed constant $s^\star - s > 0$ and a decreasing map $x \rightarrow f(x)$ corresponding to the speed of growth of the trees. An example of such a function is

$$f(x) = \frac{\alpha}{1 + \delta x}.$$

We refer to Magal and Zhang [243, 244] for more results about such a system. We refer to Hartung, Krisztin, Walther and Wu [147] for more references and more results on state-dependent delay differential equations.

Linear Volterra integral equations

The theory of Volterra integral and integro-differential equations started in the 1950s [353]. Since then, the theory has been developed in the literature and in applications. The book of Burton [41] gives a systematic treatment of the theory's basic structure and in particular is devoted to the study of stability properties of solutions of integral and integro-differential equations employing Liapunov functionals or Liapunov–Razumikhin functions. We also refer to Gripenberg, Londen and Staffans [128], Lakshmikantham [196], Brunner [40], and Polyanin and Manzhirov [280] for more results on this subject.

As an exercise, one may reconsider the existence and uniqueness problem for the Volterra integral equation

$$u(t) = F(t) + \int_0^t G(t-a)u(a)\mathrm{d}a,$$

whenever the functions $t \to F(t) \in \mathbb{R}^n$, $t \to G(t) \in M_n(\mathbb{R})$ are continuous on $[0, \infty)$.

We can also consider systems of Volterra integro-differential equations

$$u'(t) - H(t)u(t) = v(t)$$

and

$$v(t) = F(t) + \int_0^t G(t-a)u(a)\mathrm{d}a$$

whenever the functions $t \to F(t) \in \mathbb{R}^n$, $t \to G(t) \in M_n(\mathbb{R})$, and $t \to H(t) \in M_n(\mathbb{R})$ are continuous on $[0, \infty)$.

The Hille–Yosida theorem

The basic idea of the Hille–Yosida theorem is to extend the notion of $t \to e^{At}$ whenever A is a linear operator that is possibly unbounded. This corresponds to the theory of semigroups of linear operators and we refer to Pazy [274], Brezis [38], Engel and Nagel [104, 105], Magal and Ruan [236] and references therein for more results on this subject.

Definition 2.43 Let $A : D(A) \subset X \to X$ be a linear operator (possibly unbounded) on a Banach space X. The *resolvent set* of A (denoted $\rho(A))$) is the set of $\lambda \in \mathbb{C}$ such that the map $\lambda I - A$ is invertible from $D(A)$ in X. That is,

(i) For each $y \in X$ there exists a unique $x \in D(A)$ such that $(\lambda I - A)x = y$ and we define
$$x = (\lambda I - A)^{-1}y.$$

(ii) The inverse $y \to (\lambda I - A)^{-1}y$ is continuous or bounded from X into itself.

Assumption 2.44 (Hille–Yosida condition) Let $A : D(A) \subset X \to X$ be a linear operator on a Banach space X. We assume that there exists a real number $\omega_A \in \mathbb{R}$ such that
$$(\omega_A, \infty) \subset \rho(A).$$

Moreover, we assume that there exists a constant $M_A \geq 1$ such that

$$\| (\lambda I - A)^{-n} \|_{\mathcal{L}(X)} \leq \frac{M_A}{(\lambda - \omega_A)^n}, \quad \forall n \in \mathbb{N}, \forall \lambda > \omega_A.$$

Linear semigroup theory started with the Hille–Yosida generation theorem in 1948 (see Hille [152] and Yosida [379]).

Theorem 2.45 (Hille–Yosida) *Let Assumption 2.44 be satisfied. Consider the abstract Cauchy problem*

$$u'(t) = Au(t), \text{ for } t \geq 0, \text{ with } u(0) = x \in X. \tag{2.25}$$

Then, for each $x \in X$ there exists a unique mild solution $t \to u(t)$ of the Cauchy problem (2.25). That is, the map $t \to u(t)$ satisfies

$$\int_0^t u(s)\mathrm{d}s \in D(A), \forall t \geq 0,$$

and

$$u(t) = x + A \int_0^t u(s)\mathrm{d}s, \quad \forall t \geq 0.$$

Moreover, for each $x \in X$, if $t \to u(t)$ is the mild solution satisfying $u(0) = x$, then we can define

$$T(t)x = u(t), \quad \forall t \geq 0.$$

Then we have

$$T(t) \in \mathcal{L}(X),$$

$$\|T(t)\|_{\mathcal{L}(X)} \leq M_A \mathrm{e}^{\omega_A t}, \quad \forall t \geq 0,$$

and

$$T(0) = I \text{ and } T(t + s) = T(s)T(t), \quad \forall t, s \geq 0.$$

2.13 MATLAB Codes

Figure 2.1

```
1   T=1000;
2   deltaT =0.1;
3
4   eta =0.001;
5   mu=0.01;
6   beta =2;
7   A=[-(eta+mu) 0 beta;eta -(eta+mu) 0;0 eta -mu]
8
9   X0=[1  1  1];
10  t0 =0:deltaT :T;
11  [t ,x]=ode45 (@Model1 ,t0 ,X0,[] ,A) ;
12
13  clf ;
14  plot (x(: ,1) ,x (: ,3) ,'k' ,'LineWidth' ,5)
15  xlabel ('n_0(t)');
16  ylabel ('n_2(t)');
```

```
17
18
19  set(gca,'fontweight','bold','FontSize',30);
```

The above code goes together with the function *Model1.m* (which must be in the same directory as the above code), which contains the following:

```
1  function dy=Model1(t,y,A)
2  n=size(A);
3  dy=zeros(n(1),1);
4
5  dy=A*y;
6  end
```

Figure 2.2

```
1   T=1000;
2   deltaT=0.1;
3
4   eta=0.001;
5   mu=0.01;
6   beta=2;
7   A=[-(eta+mu) 0 beta;eta -(eta+mu) 0;0 eta -mu]
8
9   X0=[1 1 1];
10  t0=0:deltaT:T;
11  [t,x]=ode45(@Model1,t0,X0,[],A);
12
13  clf;
14  plot(t,x(:,1)+x(:,2)+x(:,3),'k','LineWidth',5)
15  xlabel('t');
16  ylabel('N(t)');
17
18  set(gca,'fontweight','bold','FontSize',30);
```

Figure 2.3

```
1  mu=0.01;
2  beta=0.05;
3
4  T=20;
5  dt=0.01;
6  tau=5;
7  t0=-tau:dt:0;
8
```

```
9   m= s i z e ( t0 ) ;
10  M=m( 2 ) ;
11  lambda =5;
12  N= p h i ( lambda , t0 ) ;
13  time = t0 ;
14  k=M;
15
16  for  t =0: dt :T
17
18  N( k +1)=N( k ) + dt *( −mu*N( k ) + b e t a *N( k −(M−1) ) ) ;
19  time ( k +1)= time ( k ) + dt ;
20  k=k +1;
21  end
22
23  p l o t ( time ,N, ' k ' , ' L i n e W i d t h ' ,5) ;
24  x l a b e l ( ' t ' ) ;
25  y l a b e l ( 'N( t ) ' ) ;
26  s e t ( gca , 'YLim ' ,[0  2.5 ])
27  s e t ( gca , 'XLim ' ,[ − t a u  T ])
28
29  s e t ( gca , ' f o n t w e i g h t ' , ' b o l d ' , ' F o n t S i z e ' ,30) ;
```

The above code goes together with the function *phi.m* (which must be in the same directory as the above code), which contains the following:

```
1  function  y= p h i ( lambda , t )
2  y =1+0.1* s i n ( lambda * t ) ;
3  end
```

Figure 2.4 and 2.5

```
1   T=60;                 % time until which we compute the
          s o l u t i o n
2
3   deltaT =0.1;          % time step and age step
4
5   amax = 50;            % largest age of reproduction
6   amin = 18;            % smallest age of reproduction ( age
          of maturity )
7   Beta =3;              % reproduction rate
8
9   a1 = 2;               % smallest age of individuals at
          time t =0
10  a2= 10;               % largest age of individuals at time
          t =0
11  N0=50;                % number of individuals at time t =0
```

```
12
13
14
15   mu=0.01;% mortality  rate
16   t=0:deltaT:T;
17
18   a=0:deltaT:amax;
19
20   M=size(t);
21   N=size(a);
22
23   %
24   % computation  of  F(  t  )  by  using  Simpson's  rule
25   %
26
27   F=zeros(1,M(2));
28
29   aux=zeros(1,N(2)+1);
30   for  k = 1:M(2)
31       for  l = 1:N(2)
32       aux(l) = beta(a(l)+t(k),Beta,amax,amin)...
33           *pi(a(l)+t(k),mu)/pi(a(l),mu)...
34           *U0(a(l),a1,a2,N0);
35       end
36       aux(N(2)+1) = beta(a(N(2))+deltaT+t(k),Beta,amax
                 ,amin)...
37       *pi(a(N(2))+deltaT+t(k),mu)/pi(a(N(2))+deltaT,mu
                 )...
38       *U0(a(N(2))+t(k),a1,a2,N0);
39
40
41       S1=0;
42       S2=0;
43
44       for  l  =2:2:N(2)
45           S1 = S1 + aux(l);
46       end
47       for  l  =3:2:N(2)
48           S2 = S2 + aux(l);
49       end
50
51       F(k) = (deltaT/3)*(aux(1) + 4*S1 + 2*S2 + aux(N
                 (2)+1));
52   end
53   figure(1)
54   plot(t,F,'k','LineWidth',4);
```

```matlab
55  xlabel('t')
56  ylabel('F(t)')
57  set(gca,'fontweight','bold','FontSize',30);
58
59  %
60  % computation of B( t ) by using Simpson's rule
61
62  B = zeros(1,M(2));
63  for k=1:M(2)
64      aux=B;
65      s1=0;
66      s2=0;
67
68
69      for l=2:2:M(2)
70          s1 = s1 + beta(t(k)-t(l),Beta,amax,amin)*pi(
              t(k)-t(l),mu)*aux(l);
71      end
72
73      for l=3:2:M(2)
74          s2 = s2 + beta(t(k)-t(l),Beta,amax,amin) ...
75              * pi(t(k)-t(l),mu) * aux(l);
76      end
77
78      B(k) = F(k) +deltaT/3 * ( beta(t(k)-t(1),Beta,
          amax,amin) ...
79              * pi(t(k)-t(1),mu)+ 4*s1+2*s2 ...
80              +beta(t(k)-t(k),Beta,amax,amin)* pi(t(k)
              -t(k),mu));
81  end
82  figure(2)
83  plot(t ,B, 'k','LineWidth',4);
84  xlabel('t')
85  ylabel('B(t)')
86  set(gca,'fontweight','bold','FontSize',30);
87
88  function y=U0(a,a1,a2,N0)
89  y=0;
90  if (a>=a1) && (a<=a2)
91      y = N0/(a2-a1);
92  end
93  end
94
95  function y=pi(a,mu)
96  y = exp(-mu*a);
97  end
```

```
98
99
100
101   function y=beta(a,Beta,amax,amin)
102   y=0;
103   if (a>amin) && (a<amax)
104       y=Beta;
105   end
106   end
```

Alternative code for Figure 2.4 and 2.5

The difference with the previous code is that we use an external function to apply
Simpson's rule. So the code should be more accessible.

```
1   T=60;                % time until which we compute the
                           solution
2
3   deltaT =0.05;        % time step and age step
4
5   amax = 50;           % largest age of reproduction
6   amin = 18;           % smallest age of reproduction (age
                           of maturity)
7   Beta =3;             % reproduction rate
8
9   a1 = 2;              % smallest age of individuals at
                           time t=0
10  a2= 10;              % largest age of individuals at time
                           t=0
11  N0=50;               % number of individuals at time t=0
12
13
14
15  mu=0.01;% mortality rate
16  t =0: deltaT :T;
17
18  a =0: deltaT : amax ;
19
20  M=size(t);
21  N=size(a);
22
23  %
24  % computation of F( t ) by using Simpson's rule
25  %
26
27  F=zeros(1,M(2));
```

```
28
29  aux=zeros(1,N(2)+1);
30  for k = 1:M(2)
31      for l = 1:N(2)
32          aux(l) = beta(a(l)+t(k),Beta,amax,amin)...
33              *pi(a(l)+t(k),mu)/pi(a(l),mu)...
34              *U0(a(l),a1,a2,N0);
35      end
36      aux(N(2)+1) = beta(a(N(2))+deltaT+t(k),Beta,amax
            ,amin)...
37          *pi(a(N(2))+deltaT+t(k),mu)/pi(a(N(2))+deltaT,mu
            )...
38          *U0(a(N(2))+t(k),a1,a2,N0);
39
40
41
42      F(k) =Simp(aux,t);
43  end
44  figure(1)
45  plot(t,F,'k','LineWidth',4);
46  xlabel('t')
47  ylabel('F(t)')
48  set(gca,'fontweight','bold','FontSize',30);
49
50
51  %
52  % computation of B( t ) by using Simpson's rule
53
54  B = zeros(1,M(2));
55  for k=1:M(2)
56
57      aux=zeros(1,M(2));
58      for l=1:k
59          aux(l)=beta(t(k)-t(l),Beta,amax,amin)*pi(t(k)-t(
            l),mu)*B(l);
60      end
61
62      B(k) =F(k)+ Simp(aux,t);
63  end
64  figure(2)
65  plot(t ,B, 'k','LineWidth',4);
66  xlabel('t')
67  ylabel('B(t)')
68  set(gca,'fontweight','bold','FontSize',30);
69
70  function y=U0(a,a1,a2,N0)
```

```
71   y=0;
72   if (a>=a1) && (a<=a2)
73        y = N0/(a2-a1);
74   end
75   end
76
77   function y=pi(a,mu)
78   y = exp(-mu*a);
79   end
80
81
82
83   function y=beta(a,Beta,amax,amin)
84   y=0;
85   if (a>amin) && (a<amax)
86        y=Beta;
87   end
88   end
```

The above code goes together with the function *Simp.m* (which must be in the same directory as the above code), which contains the following:

```
1    function [ I ] = Simp(F,t)
2
3    dt=t(2)-t(1);
4
5    N=length(t);
6
7    % If N-1 is an even number
8    if mod(N-1,2)==0
9
10   % It considers the multiple application of the
         Simpson 1/3 rule
11       I=(dt/3)*(F(1)+F(end)+4* sum(F(2:2:end-1)) + 2*
             sum (F(3:2:end-1)));
12
13   % If N-1 is divisible by 3
14   elseif mod(N-1,3)==0
15       if N-1==3
16   % It considers the simple application of the Simpson
         3/8 rule
17           I=(t(end)-t(1))/8*(fun(X(1))+3*fun(X(2))+3*
             fun(X(3))+fun(X(4)));
18
19   % It considers the multiple application of the
         Simpson 3/8 rule
20       else
21           L=sort([0:N,3:3:N-1]);
```

```
22          B=reshape(L,4,[])+1;
23          B=B';
24          I=3*dt/8*sum(fun(X(B(:,1)))+3*fun(X(B(:,2)))
              +3*fun(X(B(:,3)))+fun(X(B(:,4))));
25       end
26
27  % If none of the previous cases is possible, a
       composed Simpson's rule is done
28  else
29       I1=((X(end-3)-X(1))/(3*(N-3)))*(F(1)+F(end-3)+4*
              sum(F(2:2:end-4)) + 2*sum (F(3:2:end-4)));
30       I2=(X(end)-X(end-3))/8*(fun(X(end-3))+3*fun(X(
              end-2))+3*fun(X(end-1))+fun(X(end)));
31       I=I1+I2;
32  end
33
34  end
```

Chapter 3
Stability and Instability of Linear Systems

3.1 Jordan's Reduction

Definition 3.1 Let $A \in M_n(\mathbb{K})$ (with $\mathbb{K} = \mathbb{R}$ or $\mathbb{C}$) be a square matrix of size n over the field $\mathbb{K}$. The set

$$\sigma(A) := \{\lambda \in \mathbb{C} : \det(\lambda I - A) = 0\}$$

of all eigenvalues of A is called the *spectrum* of A. The *null space* of A (or the *kernel of A*) is the subspace

$$N(A) := \{x \in \mathbb{K}^n : Ax = 0\},$$

and the *range* of A is the subspace

$$R(A) := \{y \in \mathbb{K}^n : y = Ax \text{ for some } x \in \mathbb{K}^n\}.$$

Let $A \in M_n(\mathbb{C})$ and $\lambda_0 \in \sigma(A)$ be an eigenvalue of A. We observe that for each integer $k \geq 1$ we have

$$N(\lambda_0 I - A)^k \subset N(\lambda_0 I - A)^{k+1}$$

as well as

$$R(\lambda_0 I - A)^k \supset R(\lambda_0 I - A)^{k+1}.$$

By using the fact that the dimension of $\mathbb{K}^n$ is finite, we obtain that the series $N(\lambda_0 I - A)^k$ and $R(\lambda_0 I - A)^k$ have to be stationary for k larger than n. The following version of Jordan's theorem is built on this observation.

Theorem 3.2 *Let $A \in \mathbb{M}_n(\mathbb{C})$ be given. For each eigenvalue $\lambda_0 \in \sigma(A)$, there exists a smallest integer $k_0 \in \{1, \ldots, n\}$ such that*

$$N(\lambda_0 I - A)^{k_0} = N(\lambda_0 L - A)^{k_0+1}$$

and

$$R(\lambda_0 I - A)^{k_0} = R(\lambda_0 I - A)^{k_0+1}.$$

A. Ducrot et al., *Differential Equations and Population Dynamics I*, Lecture Notes on Mathematical Modelling in the Life Sciences, https://doi.org/10.1007/978-3-030-98136-5_3

Moreover, the subspaces $N(\lambda_0 I - A)^{k_0}$ *and* $R(\lambda_0 I - A)^{k_0}$ *are positively invariant by* A*, that is,*

$$A(N(\lambda_0 I - A)^{k_0}) \subset N(\lambda_0 I - A)^{k_0} \text{ and } A(R(\lambda_0 I - A)^{k_0}) \subset R(\lambda_0 I - A)^{k_0}.$$

We have the following decomposition of the space $\mathbb{C}^n$

$$\mathbb{C}^n = N(\lambda_0 I - A)^{k_0} \oplus R(\lambda_0 I - A)^{k_0}$$

and, finally, we have the following properties:

(i) *The spectrum of* A *restricted to the subspace* $N(\lambda_0 I - A)^{k_0}$ *is equal to* $\{\lambda_0\}$;

(ii) *The spectrum of* A *restricted to the subspace* $R(\lambda_0 I - A)^{k_0}$ *is equal to* $\sigma(A) \backslash \{\lambda_0\}$.

Remark 3.3 The integer k_0 is necessarily smaller than or equal to n, the dimension of the ambient space $\mathbb{C}^n$. Indeed for each $k < k_0$, the dimension of $N(\lambda_0 I - A)^{k+1}$ must be larger than $\dim N(\lambda_0 I - A)^k + 1$.

Definition 3.4 Let $\lambda_0 \in \sigma(A)$ be given. The space $N(\lambda_0 I - A)$ is the *eigenspace* of A associated with the eigenvalue λ_0. The subspace $N(\lambda_0 I - A)^{k_0}$ is the *generalized eigenspace* of A associated to the eigenvalue λ_0.

By using the above version of Jordan's theorem, we deduce the following result.

Theorem 3.5 (Jordan) *Let* $A \in M_n(\mathbb{C})$ *be a square matrix of size n over the field* $\mathbb{C}$*. There exists an invertible matrix* $P \in M_n(\mathbb{C})$ *such that*

$$P^{-1}AP = J \qquad (\Leftrightarrow A = PJP^{-1})$$

where

$$J = \begin{pmatrix} J_{\lambda_1} & 0 & \cdots & 0 \\ 0 & J_{\lambda_2} & \ddots & \vdots \\ \vdots & \ddots & \ddots & 0 \\ 0 & \cdots & 0 & J_{\lambda_p} \end{pmatrix}$$

is the Jordan reduced form *or* Jordan canonical form *of A and the blocks* $J_{\lambda_i} \in M_{n_i}(\mathbb{C})$ *(called* Jordan blocks*) have the form*

$$J_{\lambda_i} = \begin{pmatrix} \lambda_i & 1 & 0 & \cdots & 0 \\ 0 & \lambda_i & 1 & \ddots & \vdots \\ \vdots & 0 & \ddots & \ddots & 0 \\ \vdots & & \ddots & \ddots & 1 \\ 0 & \cdots & \cdots & 0 & \lambda_i \end{pmatrix}$$

whenever $n_i \geq 2$ *and*

$$J_{\lambda_i} = (\lambda_i)$$

whenever $n_i = 1$.

3.2 Projectors on Generalized Eigenspaces and the Resolvent

The goal of this section is to understand the relationship between the resolvent operator $(\lambda I - A)^{-1}$ and the projectors on the generalized eigenspaces. More precisely, we will describe how to compute the projector on the generalized eigenspace of A from the resolvent. Before going further let us recall the definition of the spectral projector of a generalized eigenspace.

Definition 3.6 Let $\lambda_0 \in \sigma(A)$ be given. The *projector* $\Pi_{\lambda_0} \in M_n(\mathbb{C})$ *on the generalized eigenspace* of A associated to λ_0 is the unique linear projector satisfying

$$\Pi_{\lambda_0}(\mathbb{C}^n) = \text{N}(\lambda_0 I - A)^n$$

and

$$(I - \Pi_{\lambda_0})(\mathbb{C}^n) = \text{R}(\lambda_0 I - A)^n.$$

The computation of such a spectral projector presented below is based on the Jordan decomposition. It is also related to some general properties of the resolvent matrix $\lambda \to (\lambda I - A)^{-1}$ that will be studied in detail later: the resolvent matrix is analytic on $\mathbb{C} \backslash \sigma(A)$ and λ_0 is a pole (singularity) of the resolvent matrix.

To compute the spectral projector, we start with a Jordan reduced form and we consider a single $m_0 \times m_0$ Jordan block (for some $m_0 \leq n$)

$$J_{\lambda_0} = \begin{pmatrix} \lambda_0 & 1 & 0 & \cdots & 0 \\ 0 & \lambda_0 & 1 & \ddots & \vdots \\ \vdots & 0 & \ddots & \ddots & 0 \\ \vdots & & \ddots & \ddots & 1 \\ 0 & \cdots & \cdots & 0 & \lambda_0 \end{pmatrix} \in M_{m_0}(\mathbb{C}).$$

Now let us observe that for all $\lambda \in \mathbb{C}$

$$\lambda I - J_{\lambda_0} = (\lambda - \lambda_0)I - N = (\lambda - \lambda_0)\left[I - (\lambda - \lambda_0)^{-1}N\right],$$

where N is a nilpotent matrix. Since $N^n = N^{m_0}0$, one deduces from a direct computation that the matrix $\lambda I - J_{\lambda_0}$ is invertible whenever $\lambda \neq \lambda_0$ and its inverse is given by the (truncated) Neumann series

$$(\lambda I - J_{\lambda_0})^{-1} = (\lambda - \lambda_0)^{-1} \sum_{k=0}^{n} \left((\lambda - \lambda_0)^{-1}N\right)^k.$$

Set for $\lambda \neq \lambda_0$

$$G_0(\lambda) := (\lambda - \lambda_0)^n (\lambda I - J_{\lambda_0})^{-1},$$

which can be rewritten for all $\lambda \neq \lambda_0$ as

$$G_0(\lambda) = (\lambda - \lambda_0)^{n-1}I + (\lambda - \lambda_0)^{n-2} + \cdots + (\lambda - \lambda_0)^{n-2} + N^{n-1},$$

and it follows that

$$\frac{1}{(n-1)!} \frac{d^{n-1} G_0(\lambda)}{d\lambda^{n-1}} = I.$$

Next we let $\lambda_1 \in \sigma(A)$ be another eigenvalue $\lambda_1 \neq \lambda_0$. Consider the following Jordan block with size $m_1 \leq n$

$$J_{\lambda_1} = \begin{pmatrix} \lambda_1 & 1 & 0 & \cdots & 0 \\ 0 & \lambda_1 & 1 & \ddots & \vdots \\ \vdots & 0 & \ddots & \ddots & 0 \\ \vdots & & \ddots & \ddots & 1 \\ 0 & \cdots & \cdots & 0 & \lambda_1 \end{pmatrix} \in M_{m_1}(\mathbb{C}).$$

As above, we have for each $\lambda \neq \lambda_1$,

$$(\lambda I - J_{\lambda_1})^{-1} = (\lambda - \lambda_1)^{-1} \sum_{k=0}^{n} \left((\lambda - \lambda_1)^{-1} N \right)^k.$$

Set

$$G_1(\lambda) := (\lambda - \lambda_0)^n (\lambda I - J_{\lambda_1})^{-1},$$

then we infer from Leibniz's formula that

$$\frac{d^{n-1} G_1(\lambda)}{d\lambda^{n-1}} = (\lambda - \lambda_0)^n \frac{d^{n-1}(\lambda I - J_{\lambda_1})^{-1}}{d\lambda^{n-1}} + \binom{1}{n} n (\lambda - \lambda_0)^{n-1} \frac{d^{n-2}(\lambda I - J_{\lambda_1})^{-1}}{d\lambda^{n-2}} + \cdots.$$

Since the map $\lambda \to (\lambda I - J_{\lambda_1})^{-1}$ has no singularity in a neighborhood of λ_0, we end-up with

$$\lim_{\lambda \to \lambda_0} \frac{1}{(n-1)!} \frac{d^{n-1} G_1(\lambda)}{d\lambda^{n-1}} = 0.$$

As a consequence of Jordan's theorem combined with the above idea, we obtain the following lemma.

Lemma 3.7 *Let $A \in M_n(\mathbb{C})$ and $\lambda_0 \in \sigma(A)$ be given. Let Π_{λ_0} be the projector on the generalized eigenspace associated to λ_0, that is, satisfying (see Definition 3.6)*

$$\Pi_{\lambda_0}(\mathbb{C}^n) = \mathrm{N}(\lambda_0 I - A)^n \text{ and } (I - \Pi_{\lambda_0})(\mathbb{C}^n) = \mathrm{R}(\lambda_0 I - A)^n.$$

Then the following properties are satisfied

(i) *The linear maps A and Π_{λ_0} commute, that is,*

$$\Pi_{\lambda_0} A = A \Pi_{\lambda_0}.$$

(ii) *The projector Π_{λ_0} can be obtained from the resolvent of A by using the formula*

$$\Pi_{\lambda_0} = \lim_{\lambda \to \lambda_0} \frac{1}{(n-1)!} \frac{d^{n-1} G(\lambda)}{d\lambda^{n-1}},$$

where $G : \mathbb{C}\backslash\sigma(A) \to M_n(\mathbb{C})$ is the map given by

$$G(\lambda) := (\lambda - \lambda_0)^n (\lambda I - A)^{-1}.$$

(iii) *The projector Π_{λ_0} can be obtained from the resolvent of A by using the formula*

$$\Pi_{\lambda_0} = \frac{1}{2i\pi} \int_C (\lambda I - A)^{-1} \mathrm{d}\lambda,$$

wherein C denotes a positively oriented circle of the complex plane chosen so that λ_0 is the unique eigenvalue of A which lies in the interior of C.

Remark 3.8 In item (iii) of Lemma 3.7, we could have chosen the closed curve C differently. Actually, C could be any closed curve such that the index of all eigenvalues of A is 0, except λ_0, which has index 1.

Remark 3.9 More results can be found in the book of Yosida [380, p. 228] concerning in particular the Laurent series expansion of the resolvent operator. We also refer to the book of Kato [172] for more results on this topic.

3.3 Change of Variable

Let $A \in M_n(\mathbb{C})$ be a square matrix of size n over the field $\mathbb{C}$. Let $P \in M_n(\mathbb{C})$ be an invertible matrix such that

$$P^{-1}AP = J,$$

where J is the Jordan canonical form of A. Then on the one hand we have

$$P^{-1}e^{At}P = \sum_{n=0}^{+\infty} \frac{P^{-1}A^n P t^n}{n!} = \sum_{n=0}^{+\infty} \frac{(P^{-1}AP)^n t^n}{n!} = \sum_{n=0}^{+\infty} \frac{(Jt)^n}{n!} = e^{Jt}, \ \forall t \geq 0.$$

On the other hand, if $u(t)$ is the solution of the ODE

$$\begin{cases} \dfrac{\mathrm{d}u(t)}{\mathrm{d}t} = Au(t), & t \geq 0, \\ u(0) = u_0 \in \mathbb{C}^n, \end{cases}$$

then we have

$$\frac{\mathrm{d}}{\mathrm{d}t}(P^{-1}u(t)) = P^{-1}\frac{\mathrm{d}u(t)}{\mathrm{d}t} = P^{-1}Au(t) = P^{-1}APP^{-1}u(t).$$

Therefore by setting $v(t) := P^{-1}u(t)$ and $v_0 := P^{-1}u_0$ we deduce that $v(t)$ is a solution to the equation

$$\frac{\mathrm{d}v(t)}{\mathrm{d}t} = Jv(t) \text{ and } v(0) = v_0 \in \mathbb{C}^n.$$

3.4 Computation of the Solution for a Jordan Block

Consider for some $p \geq 1$ the matrix

$$
N := \begin{pmatrix}
0 & 1 & 0 & \cdots & 0 \\
0 & 0 & 1 & \ddots & \vdots \\
\vdots & \ddots & \ddots & \ddots & 0 \\
\vdots & & \ddots & 0 & 1 \\
0 & \cdots & \cdots & 0 & 0
\end{pmatrix} \in M_p(\mathbb{R}).
$$

Then N is a nilpotent matrix (here we have $N^p = 0$) and the infinite series e^{tN} reduces to a finite sum

$$
e^{Nt} = I + tN + \frac{t^2}{2!}N^2 + \frac{t^3}{3!}N^3 + \cdots + \frac{t^{p-1}}{(p-1)!}N^{p-1} = \sum_{k=0}^{p-1} \frac{t^k}{k!}N^k.
$$

As a consequence we obtain

$$
e^{Nt} = \begin{pmatrix}
1 & t & \frac{t^2}{2!} & \cdots & \frac{t^{p-1}}{(p-1)!} \\
0 & 1 & t & \ddots & \vdots \\
\vdots & \ddots & \ddots & \ddots & \frac{t^2}{2!} \\
\vdots & & \ddots & \ddots & t \\
0 & \cdots & \cdots & 0 & 1
\end{pmatrix} \in M_p(\mathbb{R}).
$$

Now since, for all $\lambda \in \mathbb{C}$, we have

$$
J_\lambda = \lambda I + N,
$$

one obtains for all $t \geq 0$

$$
e^{J_\lambda t} = e^{\lambda t} e^{Nt} = \begin{pmatrix}
e^{\lambda t} & te^{\lambda t} & \frac{t^2}{2!}e^{\lambda t} & \cdots & \frac{t^{p-1}}{(p-1)!}e^{\lambda t} \\
& \ddots & \ddots & \ddots & \vdots \\
& & \ddots & \ddots & \frac{t^2}{2!}e^{\lambda t} \\
& 0 & & \ddots & te^{\lambda t} \\
& & & & e^{\lambda t}
\end{pmatrix}.
$$

3.5 Equilibrium

Definition 3.10 An *equilibrium solution* is a solution which is constant in time.

Lemma 3.11 *All the equilibrium solutions of the ordinary differential equation*

$$\begin{cases} u'(t) = Au(t), \quad t \geq 0, \\ u(0) = u_0, \end{cases} \tag{3.1}$$

are solutions of the form

$$u(t) = \bar{u} \in \mathbb{R} \text{ for all } t \geq 0,$$

where $\bar{u}$ belongs to the null space of A

$$A\bar{u} = 0.$$

Conversely, any element $\bar{u} \in \mathrm{N}(A)$ of the null space of A is an equilibrium solution to (3.1).

Remark 3.12 Let $\tau > 0$ be given and consider the delay differential equation

$$u'(t) = -\mu u(t) + \beta u(t - \tau) \text{ for all } t \geq 0,$$

with initial value
$$u(t) = \psi(t) \text{ for all } t \in [-\tau, 0]$$

with $\psi \in C([-\tau, 0], \mathbb{R})$. Then the equilibrium solutions (or constant solutions) have the form
$$u(t) = \bar{u} \text{ for all } t \geq -\tau,$$

and $\bar{u}$ must satisfy
$$0 = -\mu\bar{u} + \beta\bar{u}.$$

So in this case, we need to return back to the notion of constant solution to determine the equilibria.

We also have the following properties.

Lemma 3.13 *Consider the linear differential equation*

$$\begin{cases} u'(t) = Au(t), \quad \text{for all } t \geq 0, \\ u(0) = u_0. \end{cases}$$

Then we have the following properties

(i) *If A is invertible, then the only equilibrium is $\bar{u} = 0$.*
(ii) *If A is not invertible, every distribution $\bar{u} \in \mathrm{N}(A)$ is an equilibrium.*

Example 3.14 Consider the linear system

$$\begin{cases} \dfrac{dx(t)}{dt} = y(t), \\[2mm] \dfrac{dy(t)}{dt} = 0. \end{cases}$$

Setting $u(t) = \begin{pmatrix} x(t) \\ y(t) \end{pmatrix}$, we can rewrite this system in matrix form

$$\frac{du(t)}{dt} = Au(t)$$

with

$$A = \begin{pmatrix} 0 & 1 \\ 0 & 0 \end{pmatrix}.$$

The set

$$\left\{ \begin{pmatrix} \bar{x} \\ 0 \end{pmatrix} : \bar{x} \in \mathbb{R} \right\}$$

is the set of all equilibria of this system. In other words, any solution starting with this distribution remains constant in time.

3.6 Exponential Asymptotic Stability of Linear Systems

3.6.1 The case of continuous time

Definition 3.15 We will say that the equilibrium 0 of the linear ordinary differential equation

$$\begin{cases} u'(t) = Au(t), \forall t \geq 0, \\ u(0) = u_0 \end{cases}$$

is *exponentially asymptotically stable* if we can find two constants $M \geq 1$ and $\alpha > 0$ such that for each initial distribution $u_0 \in \mathbb{R}^n$ the corresponding solution $u(t)$ satisfies

$$\|u(t)\| \leq Me^{-\alpha t}\|u_0\|, \text{ for all } t \geq 0,$$

or equivalently (since $u(t) = e^{At}u_0$)

$$\|e^{At}u_0\| \leq Me^{-\alpha t}\|u_0\|, \text{ for all } t \geq 0.$$

Consider the example of Malthus's model

$$\begin{cases} N'(t) = rN(t), & t \geq 0 \\ N(0) = N_0. \end{cases}$$

Since

$$|N(t)| = e^{rt}|N_0|,$$

the equilibrium 0 is exponentially asymptotically stable whenever $r < 0$. The notion of stability of 0 can be regarded here as a notion corresponding to the extinction of the population. The converse notion of instability will correspond to the case $r > 0$. In that case, the instability corresponds to an expanding population.

Definition 3.16 Recall the definition of the spectrum of A (first defined in Definition 3.1):

$$\sigma(A) = \{\lambda \in \mathbb{C} : \det(\lambda I - A) = 0\}.$$

The number

$$s(A) := \sup\{\mathrm{Re}(\lambda) : \lambda \in \sigma(A)\}$$

is called the *spectral radius* or *spectral bound* of A.

Theorem 3.17 (Exponential stability) *If $s(A) < 0$ (i.e. if all the eigenvalues have a strictly negative real part), then 0 is exponentially asymptotically stable. More precisely for each $\alpha \in (0, -s(A))$ we can find $M = M(\alpha) \geq 1$ such that*

$$\|e^{At}u\| \leq Me^{-\alpha t}\|u\| \text{ for all } t \geq 0, u \in \mathbb{R}^n. \tag{3.2}$$

Remark 3.18 In the next chapter (see Lemma 4.4) we will prove the converse of this theorem, namely that if 0 is exponentially asymptotically stable, then $s(A) < 0$.

Proof Let $\alpha \in (0, -s(A))$ be given. We first prove the result for each Jordan block of A, then deduce the estimate for A.

Let $\sigma(A) = \{\lambda_1, \ldots, \lambda_m\}$ for some $m \leq n$ and fix $i \in \{1, \ldots, m\}$. Let J_{λ_i} be the Jordan block of size p_i associated with λ_i. We have for all $t \geq 0$

$$e^{J_{\lambda_i}t} = e^{\lambda_i t}\begin{pmatrix} 1 & t & \frac{t^2}{2!} & \cdots & \frac{t^{p_i-1}}{(p_i-1)!} \\ 0 & 1 & t & \ddots & \vdots \\ \vdots & \ddots & \ddots & \ddots & \frac{t^2}{2!} \\ \vdots & & \ddots & \ddots & t \\ 0 & \cdots & \cdots & 0 & 1 \end{pmatrix}$$

and therefore there exists some constant $C(p_i) > 0$ such that for all $t \geq 0$

$$\|e^{J_{\lambda_i}t}\| \leq C(p_i)e^{\mathrm{Re}(\lambda_i)t}(1+t)^{p_i}$$
$$\leq C(p_i)e^{(\mathrm{Re}(\lambda_i)+\alpha)t}(1+t)^{p_i}e^{-\alpha t},$$

thus

$$\|e^{J_{\lambda_i}t}\| \leq C(p_i)e^{(s(A)+\alpha)t}(1+t)^{p_i}e^{-\alpha t}.$$

Next, since $s(A) + \alpha < 0$ the function $t \to e^{(s(A)+\alpha)t}(1+t)^{p_i}$ is bounded on $[0, \infty)$. Hence setting $M_i := C(p_i)\sup_{t \geq 0} s^{(s(A)+\alpha)t}(1+t)^{p_i}$ yields

$$\|e^{J_{\lambda_i}t}\| \leq M_i e^{-\alpha t}, \ \forall t \geq 0.$$

By Jordan's theorem (see Theorem 3.5), there exists a matrix $P \in M_n(\mathbb{C})$ such that

$$A = PJP^{-1},$$

where

$$J = \begin{pmatrix} J_{\lambda_1} & 0 & \cdots & 0 \\ 0 & J_{\lambda_2} & \ddots & \vdots \\ \vdots & \ddots & \ddots & 0 \\ 0 & \cdots & 0 & J_{\lambda_p} \end{pmatrix}$$

and therefore

$$\|e^{At}\| = \|Pe^{Jt}P^{-1}\| \leq \|P\|\|P^{-1}\|\|e^{Jt}\| \leq \|P\|\|P^{-1}\| \left(\sup_{1 \leq i \leq m} M_i \right) e^{-\alpha t}$$

$$\leq Me^{-\alpha t},$$

where $M := \|P\|\|P^{-1}\| \left(\sup_{1 \leq i \leq m} M_i \right)$. Theorem 3.17 is proved.   □

Consider for example

$$\begin{cases} x'(t) = -cx(t) + y(t) \\ y'(t) = -cy(t) \end{cases} \tag{3.3}$$

with initial value

$$x(0) = 0.1 \text{ and } y(0) = 0.9.$$

Then the matrix of the linear system (3.3) is

$$A = \begin{pmatrix} -c & 1 \\ 0 & c \end{pmatrix}$$

and the spectrum of A is $\sigma(A) = \{-c\}$. Therefore the system (3.3) is exponentially asymptotically stable as soon as $c > 0$. The solution of (3.3) can be computed explicitly as

$$\begin{cases} x(t) = (x_0 + y_0 t)e^{-ct} \\ y(t) = y_0 e^{-ct} \end{cases}$$

Remark 3.19 In practice, we can use different criteria (depending on the form of a given matrix) to prove that all the eigenvalues have a strictly negative real part. The most general criterion for stability is called the *Routh–Hurwitz criterion* (see Section 3.7) which provides a method to compute the stability of a linear system. We will also see that the Perron–Frobenius theorem provides a criterion for stability for matrices with non-negative off-diagonal coefficients.

That a system is linearly stable doesn't necessarily mean that the unit ball is left invariant by e^{At} (for a given norm). The following lemma shows that we can always choose the norm (in a way that depends on A) to ensure the invariance of the balls.

Lemma 3.20 *Let $A \in M_n(\mathbb{C})$ be a square matrix of size n over the field $\mathbb{R}$. Assume that $s(A) < 0$. Let $\alpha \in (0, -s(A))$. The map $\| \cdot \|_1 : \mathbb{R}^n \to [0, +\infty)$ defined by*

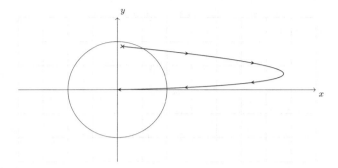

Fig. 3.1: *In this figure we plot the solution $(x(t), y(t))$ of equation (3.3) with $c = 0.1$ when t varies between 0 and 100. We consider the solution starting from the initial distribution $(0.1, 0.9)$ at time $t = 0$ and we observe that the solution leaves the ball of radius 1 during a period of time before converging to $(0, 0)$. This example shows why in general, a constant $M > 1$ may be needed in (3.2). In the case of the example we need a constant M which is bigger than 3.*

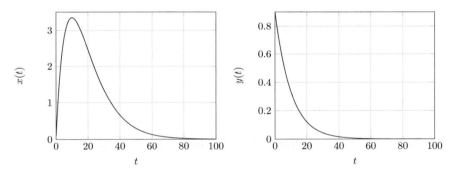

Fig. 3.2: *In this figure we plot the solution $(x(t), y(t))$ of equation (3.3) with $c = 0.1$ when t varies from 0 to 100. On the left we plot $(t, x(t))$ and on the right side we plot $(t, y(t))$. We observe that the x component first increases above the value 3 before converging to 0, while $y(t)$ only decreases.*

$$\|x\|_1 := \sup_{t \geq 0} e^{\alpha t} \|e^{At} x\|$$

is a norm equivalent to $\| \cdot \|$, and we have

$$\|e^{At} x\|_1 \leq e^{-\alpha t} \|x\|_1 \text{ for all } t \geq 0.$$

Proof We have

$$\|e^{At} x\|_1 = \sup_{s \geq 0} e^{\alpha s} \|e^{As} e^{At} x\| = \sup_{l \geq t} e^{\alpha(l-t)} \|e^{Al} x\| = e^{-\alpha t} \sup_{l \geq t} e^{\alpha l} \|e^{Al} x\|$$

and the result follows. □

Lemma 3.21 *Let A be a square real matrix of size 2. Then $s(A) < 0$ if and only if* $\mathrm{tr}(A) < 0$ *and* $\det(A) > 0$.

Proof Let

$$A = \begin{pmatrix} a & b \\ c & d \end{pmatrix}.$$

A direct computation of $\det(\lambda I - A)$ gives

$$\det(\lambda I - A) = 0 \Leftrightarrow \lambda^2 - \mathrm{tr}(A)\lambda + \det(A) = 0$$

where

$$\mathrm{tr}(A) = a + d \text{ and } \det(A) = ad - bc.$$

Consider the discriminant

$$\Delta := \mathrm{tr}(A)^2 - 4\det(A).$$

We have the following alternative

- if $\Delta \leq 0$ then $s(A) < 0 \Leftrightarrow \mathrm{tr}(A) < 0$,
- if $\Delta > 0$ then $s(A) < 0 \Leftrightarrow \mathrm{tr}(A) + \sqrt{\Delta} < 0$,

and the lemma follows.   □

3.6.2 The discrete time case

Definition 3.22 We will say that the equilibrium 0 of the recursion equation

$$\begin{cases} u(t+1) = Au(t), & t = 0, 1, 2, \ldots \\ u(0) = u_0 \end{cases}$$

is *exponentially asymptotically stable* if we can find two constants $M \geq 1$ and $\alpha \geq 0$ such that for each initial distribution $u_0 \in \mathbb{R}^n$ the corresponding solution $u(t)$ satisfies

$$\|u(t)\| \leq Me^{-\alpha t}\|u_0\| \text{ for all } t \geq 0,$$

or equivalently (since $u(t) = A^t u_0$)

$$\|A^t u_0\| \leq Me^{-\alpha t}\|u_0\| \text{ for all } t \geq 0.$$

If we reconsider Malthus's model

$$\begin{cases} N(t+1) = RN(t), & t = 0, 1, 2, \ldots \\ N(0) = N_0, \end{cases}$$

then since

$$|N(t)| = R^t |N_0|$$

the equilibrium 0 is exponentially asymptotically stable whenever $R < 1$. As in the continuous time case, the notion of stability of 0 can be regarded here as a notion corresponding to the extinction of the population. Conversely, the notion of instability corresponds to the case $R > 1$ and therefore to an expanding population.

Theorem 3.23 (Stability) *Define* $r(A) := \max\{|\lambda| : \lambda \in \sigma(A)\}$. *If* $r(A) < 1$ *then the equilibrium* 0 *of the discrete-time system*

$$\begin{cases} u(t+1) = Au(t), \forall t \in \mathbb{N}, \\ u(0) = u_0 \end{cases}$$

is asymptotically exponentially stable.

Exercise 3.24 In order to prove the above result, it is again sufficient to consider the Jordan blocks of the matrix. Consider a Jordan block of the form

$$J_\lambda = \lambda I + N \in M_p(\mathbb{C})$$

for some $\lambda \in \mathbb{C}$ and $p \geq 1$. Prove that if $|\lambda| < 1$ then for each $\delta \in (|\lambda|, 1)$ we can find $M \geq 1$ satisfying

$$\|J_\lambda^t\| \leq M\delta^t \text{ for all } t \in \mathbb{N}.$$

Definition 3.25 The equilibrium 0 is *hyperbolic* if the spectrum $\sigma(A)$ of A contains no eigenvalue of modulus 1.

3.7 The Routh–Hurwitz Criterion

Let P be a polynomial with real coefficients

$$P(\lambda) = p_0\lambda^n + p_1\lambda^{n-1} + \cdots + p_{n-1}\lambda + p_n$$

with $p_0 \neq 0$ and $p_i \in \mathbb{R}, i = 0, \ldots, n$.

Definition 3.26 $P(\lambda)$ is said to be *stable* if and only if all its roots have a strictly negative real part.

For each integer $k \in \mathbb{N}$, we define

$$\hat{p}_k := \begin{cases} p_k, & \text{if } k \leq n, \\ 0, & \text{if } k \geq n+1. \end{cases} \tag{3.4}$$

Then,

$$P(\lambda) = \sum_{k=0}^{+\infty} \hat{p}_k \lambda^{n-k}.$$

We first construct the *Routh table* of $P(\lambda)$ as follows

$$
\begin{array}{llllll}
\lambda^n & r_{1,1} & r_{1,2} & r_{1,3} & r_{1,4} & \cdots \\
\lambda^{n-1} & r_{2,1} & r_{2,2} & r_{2,3} & r_{2,4} & \cdots \\
\lambda^{n-2} & r_{3,1} & r_{3,2} & r_{3,3} & \cdots \\
\lambda^{n-3} & r_{4,1} & r_{4,2} & \cdots \\
\vdots & \vdots & \vdots & \vdots \\
\lambda^1 & r_{n,1} & r_{n,2} & 0 & \cdots \\
\lambda^0 & r_{n+1,1} & 0 & 0 & \cdots
\end{array}
\tag{3.5}
$$

where

$$
(r_{1,1}, r_{1,2}, r_{1,3}, r_{1,4}, \ldots) = (\hat{p}_0, \hat{p}_2, \hat{p}_4, \hat{p}_6, \ldots)
$$

and

$$
(r_{2,1}, r_{2,2}, r_{2,3}, r_{2,4}, \ldots) = (\hat{p}_1, \hat{p}_3, \hat{p}_5, \hat{p}_7, \ldots).
$$

Then for each $i \geq 3$,

$$
(r_{i,1}, r_{i,2}, r_{i,3}, \ldots) = (r_{i-2,2}, r_{i-2,3}, \ldots) - \frac{r_{i-2,1}}{r_{i-1,1}} (r_{i-1,2}, r_{i-1,3}, \ldots).
\tag{3.6}
$$

For example, the Routh table of $P(\lambda) = p_0\lambda^2 + p_1\lambda + p_2$ is

$$
\begin{array}{llllll}
\lambda^2 & p_0 & p_2 & 0 & 0 & \cdots \\
\lambda^1 & p_1 & 0 & 0 & \cdots \\
\lambda^0 & p_2 & 0 & \cdots
\end{array}
$$

and the Routh table of $P(\lambda) = p_0\lambda^3 + p_1\lambda^2 + p_2\lambda + p_3$ is

$$
\begin{array}{llllll}
\lambda^3 & p_0 & p_2 & 0 & 0 & \cdots \\
\lambda^2 & p_1 & p_3 & 0 & 0 & \cdots \\
\lambda^1 & p_2 - \frac{p_0}{p_1}p_3 & 0 & 0 & \cdots \\
\lambda^0 & p_3 & 0 & 0 & \cdots
\end{array}
$$

We state now the Routh–Hurwitz criterion [114, 160]. Here we will prove this result by using an approach due to Meinsma [254]. Another proof can be found in the book of Gantmacher [114].

Theorem 3.27 (Routh–Hurwitz criterion) *A real polynomial $P(\lambda) = p_0\lambda^n + p_1\lambda^{n-1} + \cdots + p_{n-1}\lambda + p_n$ (with $p_0 \neq 0$ and $p_i \in \mathbb{R}$ for all $i = 0, 1, \ldots, n$) is stable if, and only if, all the elements of the first column of the Routh table of (3.5) are non-zero and have the same sign. That is,*

$$
r_{j,1} \times p_0 > 0 \text{ for all } j = 1, \ldots, n + 1.
$$

We prove this result by induction. The key observation to prove Theorem 3.27 is that, when we remove the first line of the Routh table of P, we obtain the Routh table of a polynomial Q whose degree is strictly less than that of P. Moreover, Q can be constructed by a continuous deformation P_η ($\eta \in [0, 1]$) of the polynomial P (i.e. $\eta \to P_\eta$ is continuous, $P_0 = P$ and $P_1 = Q$) which is chosen so that the values taken by P_η on the imaginary axis are non-zero. That is, P_η does not have a purely imaginary root for any $\eta \in [0, 1]$. By Rouché's theorem, the zeros of P_η cannot cross the imaginary axis when η moves from 0 to 1. Therefore P and Q have the same number of zeros on each side of the imaginary axis, except one of the zeros of P, which goes to ∞ when $\eta \to 1^-$ (due to the change of degree). It turns out that the sign of the real part of this exploding root is exactly the opposite sign of $\frac{p_1}{p_0}$. The theorem follows by induction. We make this observation rigorous in the next lemma.

Lemma 3.28 (Meinsma [254]) *The polynomial* $P(\lambda) = p_0\lambda^n + p_1\lambda^{n-1} + \cdots + p_n$ *is stable if, and only if,* p_1 *is non-zero,* p_0 *and* p_1 *have the same sign, and the polynomial of degree* $n - 1$

$$Q(\lambda) := P(\lambda) - \frac{p_0}{p_1}(p_1\lambda^n + p_3\lambda^{n-2} + \cdots)$$

is stable.

Proof Let us assume that p_1 is non-zero, p_0 and p_1 have the same sign, and Q is stable. For any $\eta \in [0, 1]$, let us define the polynomial

$$P_\eta(\lambda) := P(\lambda) - \eta\frac{p_0}{p_1}(p_1\lambda^n + p_3\lambda^{n-2} + \cdots) \tag{3.7}$$

$$= P(\lambda) - \eta\frac{p_0}{p_1}\sum_{k=0}^{+\infty}\hat{p}_{2k+1}\lambda^{n-2k},$$

where $\hat{p}_k$ is defined in (3.4).

We observe that $P_0(\lambda) = P(\lambda)$, $P_1(\lambda) = Q(\lambda)$, and the polynomials $P_\eta(\lambda)$ have exactly the same zeros on the imaginary axis. Indeed, let $\omega \in \mathbb{R}$ and be such that $P_{\eta_0}(i\omega) = 0$ for some $\eta_0 \in [0, 1]$, where i is the imaginary unit $i^2 = -1$. Then we have for all $\eta \in [0, 1]$

$$P_\eta(i\omega) = \sum_{k=0}^{+\infty}\hat{p}_k i^{n-k}\omega^{n-k} - \eta\frac{p_0}{p_1}\sum_{k=0}^{+\infty}\hat{p}_{2k+1}i^{n-2k}\omega^{n-2k}$$

$$= i^n\left(\sum_{k=0}^{+\infty}(-1)^k\hat{p}_{2k}\omega^{n-2k} + \omega\eta\frac{p_0}{p_1}\sum_{k=0}^{+\infty}(-1)^{k+1}\hat{p}_{2k+1}\omega^{n-(2k+1)}\right)$$

$$+ i^{n+1}\sum_{k=0}^{+\infty}(-1)^{k+1}\hat{p}_{2k+1}\omega^{n-(2k+1)}. \tag{3.8}$$

Therefore since $P_{\eta_0}(i\omega) = 0$, by taking the real and imaginary parts of (3.8) with $\eta = \eta_0$ yields

$$\sum_{k=0}^{+\infty}(-1)^{k+1}\hat{p}_{2k+1}\omega^{n-(2k+1)} = 0 \text{ and } \sum_{k=0}^{+\infty}(-1)^k\hat{p}_{2k}\omega^{n-2k} = 0. \tag{3.9}$$

Plugging the above two equalities into (3.8) we obtain that $P_\eta(i\omega) = 0$ for all $\eta \in [0, 1]$. We have proven that all the polynomials $(P_\eta)_{\eta \in [0,1]}$ have exactly the same imaginary zeros. Since Q is stable, there cannot exist a zero of P_η on the imaginary axis for any $\eta \in [0, 1]$.

Claim: *Let $\lambda_1^\eta, \ldots, \lambda_n^\eta$ be an enumeration of the roots of the polynomial P_η, counted with their multiplicities. Since the degree of Q equals $n - 1$ and the map $\eta \to P_\eta$ is continuous for $\eta \in [0, 1]$, there is exactly one root of P_η that becomes unbounded when $\eta \to 1^-$, and the other roots remain bounded when $\eta \to 1$.*

This claim will be justified later, in Lemma 3.30. Up to rearranging the roots, we can therefore assume that the maps $\eta \in [0, 1] \to \lambda_j^\eta$ for $j = 2, \ldots, n$ are all continuous, and

$$\lim_{\eta \to 1^-} |\lambda_1^\eta| = +\infty.$$

Therefore we can write

$$P_\eta(\lambda) = p_0(1 - \eta) \cdot (\lambda - \lambda_1^\eta) \times (\lambda - \lambda_2^\eta) \times \cdots \times (\lambda - \lambda_n^\eta), \tag{3.10}$$

and by expanding the product we obtain

$$P_\eta(\lambda) = p_0(1 - \eta) \left[\lambda^n - \left(\sum_{k=0}^n \lambda_k^\eta \right) \lambda^{n-1} + \cdots \right], \tag{3.11}$$

so that, identifying the coefficients of P_η, we find that

$$-p_0(1 - \eta) \sum_{k=1}^n \lambda_k^\eta = p_1,$$

$$\lambda_1^\eta = -\frac{p_1}{p_0} \cdot \frac{1}{(1 - \eta)\left(1 + \frac{1}{\lambda_1^\eta} \sum_{k=2}^n \lambda_k^\eta\right)} = -\frac{p_1}{p_0} \cdot \frac{1 + \frac{1}{\lambda_1^\eta} \sum_{k=2}^n \lambda_k^\eta}{(1 - \eta)\left|1 + \frac{1}{\lambda_1^\eta} \sum_{k=2}^n \lambda_k^\eta\right|^2}.$$

Since λ_k^η is bounded for $k = 2, \ldots, n$ and $|\lambda_1^\eta| \to +\infty$ when $\eta \to 1^-$, the above equation shows that the real part of λ_1^η has the same sign as $-\frac{p_1}{p_0}$ when $\eta \to 1^-$. Therefore, λ_1^η has a negative real part for all $\eta \in [0, 1)$. Since Q is stable and

$$\lim_{\eta \to 1^-} \lambda_k^\eta = \lambda_k^1 \text{ for all } k = 2, \ldots, n,$$

we conclude that $\lambda_2^\eta, \ldots, \lambda_n^\eta$ all have a negative real part for all $\eta \in [0, 1]$. This shows that P is stable.

Conversely, assume that P is stable. Then P has n roots $\lambda_1, \ldots, \lambda_n$ whose real part is negative. By using the factorized expression (3.10) and developing the product, we obtain (3.11) and therefore

$$p_1 = -p_0 \sum_{k=1}^n \lambda_k,$$

and since p_1 is real we conclude that

$$p_1 = \mathrm{Re}(p_1) = -p_0 \sum_{k=1}^{n} \mathrm{Re}(\lambda_k).$$

In particular p_1 is non-zero and has the same sign as p_0. Next we define $P_\eta(\lambda)$ as in (3.7) and observe that, since (3.8) and (3.9) still hold, P_η cannot have a root on the imaginary axis for any $\eta \in [0, 1]$. By the continuity of the roots of P_η with respect to η, we conclude that Q is stable. This completes the proof of Lemma 3.28. □

It remains to prove the property claimed in the proof of Lemma 3.28. We first recall Rouché's Theorem, as given in the book of Rudin [304].

Theorem 3.29 (Rouché) *Let $\Omega \subset \mathbb{C}$ be an open domain, and $f, g : \Omega \to \mathbb{C}$ be two holomorphic functions. Let $B(a, r) = \{z : |z - a| \leq r\} \subset \Omega$ and assume that*

$$|f(z) - g(z)| < |f(z)| \qquad \text{for all } z \in \Omega \text{ with } |z - a| = r.$$

Then f and g have the same number of zeros in $B(a, r)$ (counting multiplicities).

Lemma 3.30 *Let $n \geq 1$ be given and $P^\eta(z)$ be a family of polynomials of degree n for $\eta \in [0, 1)$, continuous in the sense that*

$$P^\eta(z) = p_0^\eta z^n + p_1^\eta z^{n-1} + \ldots + p_n^\eta,$$

where each of the functions $\eta \mapsto p_i^\eta$ is continuous, for $i = 1, \ldots, n$, with

$$p_0^\eta \neq 0, \forall \eta \in [0, 1).$$

Then the roots of P^η are locally bounded. That is to say, for any $\xi \in (0, 1)$, there exists $R > 0$, such that $|\lambda| \leq R$ for any root λ of P^η with $\eta \in [0, \xi]$.

If we assume in addition that all the coefficient of $P^\eta(z)$ are continuous with respect to η on $[0, 1]$, and

$$\lim_{\eta \to 1} p_0^\eta = 0, \text{ and } \lim_{\eta \to 1} p_1^\eta \neq 0.$$

That is to say that, there exists a polynomial $Q(z)$ of degree $n - 1$ such that $P^\eta(z) \to Q(z)$ as $\eta \to 1$ uniformly on every ball $B(0, R)$ with $R > 0$. Then there exists a reordering of the λ_i^η and $M > 0$ such that

$$\sup_{\eta \in [0,1)} |\lambda_2(\eta)| \leq M, \ldots, \sup_{\eta \in [0,1)} \lambda_{n-1}(\eta) \leq M, \text{ and } \lim_{\eta \to 1^-} |\lambda_1(\eta)| = +\infty.$$

Proof We first prove that the roots of P^η are locally bounded. Suppose by contradiction that there exists $\eta_0 \in [0, 1)$ and a sequence $\eta_k \to \eta_0$ such that at least one root of P^{η_k} is unbounded. Choose $R > 0$ sufficiently large, so that all roots $\lambda_1^0, \ldots, \lambda_n^0$ of P^{η_0} are in the ball of radius R, that is to say, $|\lambda_i| < R$ for all $i = 1, \ldots, n$. Define

$$\inf_{|z|=R} |P^{\eta_0}(z)| =: \delta > 0.$$

For η_k sufficiently close to η_0, by our assumption, P^{η_k} has at least one root λ^{η_k} with $|\lambda^{\eta_k}| > R$, and at the same time

$$\sup_{|z|=R} |P^{\eta_k}(z) - P^{\eta_0}(z)| < \delta,$$

since P^{η_k} converges to P^{η_0}. Applying Rouché's Theorem, P^{η_k} has the same number of roots as P^{η_0} in the ball of radius R, that is to say, n roots. This is a contradiction because P^{η_k} has degree n and one root of modulus strictly larger than R. The contradiction proves our claim.

Suppose now that $P^{\eta}(z) \to Q(z)$ as $\eta \to 1$ uniformly on every ball $B(0, R)$, with Q as in the statement of the Lemma. Let R be sufficiently large, so that all $n - 1$ roots of Q have modulus less than R, and define

$$\inf_{|z|=R} |Q(z)| =: \delta > 0.$$

Then for η_0 sufficiently close to 1, we have

$$\sup_{|z|=R} |P^{\eta}(z) - Q(z)| < \delta \text{ for all } \eta \geq \eta_0.$$

Therefore, applying Rouché's Theorem, P^{η} has exactly $n - 1$ roots of modulus less than R and exactly one of modulus strictly larger than R for all $\eta \in [\eta_0, 1)$. In particular, $(n - 1)$ roots of P^{η} are bounded when $\eta \to 1^-$. Since $R > 0$ can be made arbitrarily large when $\eta_0 \to 1^-$, the root λ^{η} of P^{η} with modulus larger than R satisfies

$$\lim_{\eta \to 1^-} |\lambda^{\eta}| = +\infty.$$

This concludes the proof of Lemma 3.30.   □

Remark 3.31 The continuity of the roots of a polynomial with respect to its coefficients is a classical problem. By using Rouché's Theorem it is possible to prove the continuity of the roots for the Hausdorff metric on sets. But a stronger result holds, namely that the roots are given by continuous functions of the parameter η. We refer to [143, 144] for an elegant proof based on the inversion of symmetric polynomials giving the coefficients as a function of the roots.

Remark 3.32 Even when P is not stable, the Routh table of P can still provide some useful information on the roots of P. By using the same idea as in the proof of Lemma 3.28, we can deduce the number of roots with positive and negative real parts from the Routh table provided the algorithm converges. We refer to the paper of Meinsma [254] for more details on this principle.

Remark 3.33 In practice, given a real matrix $A = (a_{ij}) \in M_n(\mathbb{R})$, we will apply the above theorem to the characteristic polynomial

$$P(\lambda) = \det(\lambda I - A) = \lambda^n + p_1 \lambda^{n-1} + \cdots + p_{n-1}\lambda + p_n,$$

where $(-1)^k p_k$ is the sum of the principal minors of order k of A, that is,

$$p_0 = 1,$$

$$p_1 = -\operatorname{tr}(A) = -\sum_{i=1}^{n} a_{ii},$$

$$\cdots$$

$$p_n = (-1)^n \det(A).$$

To conclude the section we have the following consequence of Lemma 3.28.

Theorem 3.34 *If the polynomial* $P(\lambda) = p_0\lambda^n + p_1\lambda^{n-1} + \cdots + p_n$ *is stable then,*

$$\operatorname{sign}(p_0) = \operatorname{sign}(p_1) = \ldots = \operatorname{sign}(p_n),$$

where

$$\operatorname{sign}(x) = \begin{cases} 1, & \text{if } x > 0, \\ 0, & \text{if } x = 0, \\ -1, & \text{if } x < 0. \end{cases}$$

Proof Assume for simplicity that $p_0 > 0$. We prove this theorem by induction on n. The result is clear for $n = 1$, $n = 2$ and $n = 3$. Assume that the result is true for $n = m - 1$. Then by Lemma 3.28, $P(\lambda)$ is sable if and only if

$$Q(\lambda) := P(\lambda) - \frac{p_0}{p_1}(p_1\lambda^m + p_3\lambda^{m-2} + \cdots)$$

is stable. Then

$$Q(\lambda) := p_1\lambda^{m-1} + \left(p_2 - \frac{p_0}{p_1}p_3\right)\lambda^{m-2} + p_3\lambda^{m-3} + \left(p_4 - \frac{p_0}{p_1}p_5\right)\lambda^{m-4} + \cdots$$

Since the degree of Q is $m - 1$, the induction assumption implies that

$$\operatorname{sign}(p_1) = \operatorname{sign}(p_3) = \ldots > 0,$$

and

$$\operatorname{sign}\left(p_2 - \frac{p_0}{p_1}p_3\right) = \operatorname{sign}\left(p_4 - \frac{p_0}{p_1}p_5\right) = \ldots > 0,$$

and since $\dfrac{p_0}{p_1} > 0$, the result follows. $\qquad\square$

3.8 Stable, Central, Unstable, and Hyperbolic Spaces

Definition 3.35 Let $A \in M_n(\mathbb{C})$ be a given complex square matrix of size n. We can decompose the spectrum of A into the *central spectrum*

$$\sigma_c(A) := \{\lambda \in \sigma(A) : \operatorname{Re}(\lambda) = 0\},$$

the *unstable spectrum*

$$\sigma_u(A) := \{\lambda \in \sigma(A) \,:\, \mathrm{Re}(\lambda) > 0\},$$

and the *stable spectrum*

$$\sigma_s(A) := \{\lambda \in \sigma(A) \,:\, \mathrm{Re}(\lambda) < 0\}.$$

Define

$$\beta_+ := \min_{\lambda \in \sigma_u(A)} \mathrm{Re}(\lambda) > 0,$$

$$\beta_- := \max_{\lambda \in \sigma_s(A)} \mathrm{Re}(\lambda) < 0,$$

and

$$\beta := \min(\beta_+, -\beta_-),$$

with $\beta_+ = +\infty$ if $\sigma_u(A) = \varnothing$ and $\beta_- = -\infty$ if $\sigma_s(A) = \varnothing$.

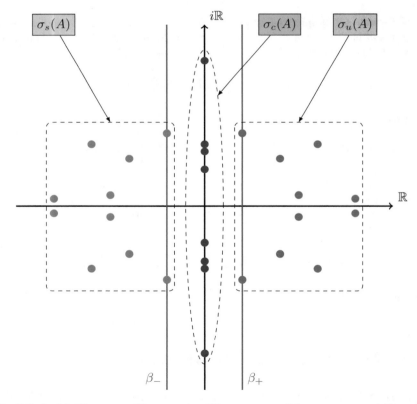

Fig. 3.3: *In this Figure, we illustrate the different parts of the spectrum $\sigma_s(A)$, $\sigma_c(A)$ and $\sigma_u(A)$ as well as β_- and β_+.*

Definition 3.36 Let $\eta \in (0, \beta)$ be given. The *stable subspace* $X_s \subset \mathbb{C}^n$ is defined as

$$X_s = \left\{ x \in \mathbb{C}^n \ : \ \sup_{t \geq 0} e^{\eta t} \|e^{At} x\| < +\infty \right\},$$

the *unstable subspace* $X_u \subset \mathbb{R}^n$ is defined as

$$X_u = \left\{ x \in \mathbb{C}^n \ : \ \sup_{t \leq 0} e^{\eta t} \|e^{At} x\| < +\infty \right\},$$

and the *central subspace* $X_c \subset \mathbb{C}^n$ is defined as

$$X_c = \left\{ x \in \mathbb{C}^n \ : \ \sup_{t \in \mathbb{R}} e^{\eta t} \|e^{At} x\| < +\infty \right\}.$$

The stable subspace X_s corresponds to the subspace on which $t \to e^{At} x$ decays exponentially fast as t goes to $+\infty$. The unstable subspace X_u corresponds to the subspace on which $e^{At} x$ decays exponentially fast as $t \to -\infty$. The central subspace corresponds to the subspace on which $t \to e^{At}$ may grow exponentially fast when $t \to \pm\infty$, but less fast than $M e^{\eta |t|}$.

By using the Jordan reduced form of the matrix A we deduce the following result.

Theorem 3.37 *Let $A \in M_n(\mathbb{C})$. For each $k = s, c, u$, the subspace X_k is the direct sum of the generalized eigenspaces associated to each eigenvalue in $\sigma_k(A)$. That is,*

$$X_k = \bigoplus_{\lambda \in \sigma_k(A)} N\big((\lambda I - A)^n\big).$$

Consequently, each subspace X_k is invariant by e^{At}, that is,

$$e^{At} X_k = X_k, \text{ for all } t \in \mathbb{R} \text{ and } k = s, c, u.$$

For $k = s, c, u$ we define the projector Π_k on the direct sum of the generalized eigenspaces associated to the eigenvalues in $\sigma_k(A)$. That is,

$$\Pi_k = \sum_{\lambda \in \sigma_k(A)} \Pi_\lambda,$$

where Π_λ is the projector on the generalized eigenspace of A associated to the eigenvalue λ. Then one has

$$X_k = R(\Pi_k)$$

and

$$\bigoplus_{m \neq k} X_m = N(\Pi_k).$$

From the previous theorem we deduce the following decomposition

$$\mathbb{C}^n = X_s \oplus X_c \oplus X_u.$$

Lemma 3.38 *For each $\varepsilon > 0$, we can find a constant $M(\varepsilon) > 0$ such that*

$$\|e^{At}x\| \leq M(\varepsilon)e^{[\beta_- + \varepsilon]t}\|x\|, \text{ for all } t \geq 0 \text{ and } x \in X_s,$$

$$\|e^{At}x\| \leq M(\varepsilon)e^{[\beta_x - \varepsilon]t}\|x\|, \text{ for all } t \leq 0 \text{ and } x \in X_u$$

and

$$\|e^{At}x\| \leq M(\varepsilon)e^{|\varepsilon|t}\|x\|, \text{ for all } t \in \mathbb{R} \text{ and } x \in X_c.$$

Proof In order to prove the first inequality, we can assume without loss of generality that $\sigma(A) = \sigma_s(A)$. Then

$$e^{-(\varepsilon + \beta_-)t}e^{At} = e^{[A - (\varepsilon + \beta_-)I]t}$$

and $s(A - (\varepsilon + \beta_-)I) = -\varepsilon$, therefore by using the same arguments as in the proof of stability in Theorem 3.17, the first inequality follows. The second and third inequalities are similar.   □

Definition 3.39 The space $X_{cu} = X_c \oplus X_u$ is called the *center-unstable space*.

The center-unstable space can be characterized as follows.

Lemma 3.40 *Let $\eta \in (0, \beta)$ be given. Then we have*

$$X_{cu} = \left\{ x \in \mathbb{C}^n \ : \ \sup_{t \leq 0} e^{\eta t}\|e^{At}x\| < +\infty \right\}.$$

Proof Let Π_s be the linear projector on X_s along $X_c \oplus X_u$. Then one has

$$\Pi_s(\mathbb{C}^n) = X_s \text{ and } (I - \Pi_s)(\mathbb{C}^n) = X_c \oplus X_u.$$

Let us consider the norm on $\mathbb{C}^n$

$$\|x\|_s = \|\Pi_s x\| + \|(I - \Pi_s)x\|.$$

Then by using the triangle inequality

$$\|x\| = \|\Pi_s x + (I - \Pi_s)x\| \leq \|\Pi_s x\| + \|(I - \Pi_x)x\|$$

and since both Π_s and $I - \Pi_s$ are bounded linear operators we have

$$\|x\|_s \leq \left[\|\Pi_s\| + \|(I - \Pi_s)\| \right] \|x\|.$$

In particular, the norms $\| \cdot \|$ and $\| \cdot \|_s$ are equivalent.

Let $x \in \mathbb{C}^n$ be such that

$$\sup_{t \leq 0} e^{\eta t}\|e^{At}x\| < +\infty,$$

and let us show that $\Pi_s x = 0$, that is $x \in X_{cu}$. First, due to the equivalence of the norms $\| \cdot \|$ and $\| \cdot \|_s$, this is equivalent to

$$\sup_{t \leq 0} e^{\eta t} \|e^{At} x\|_s < +\infty.$$

Assume by contradiction that $\Pi_s x \neq 0$. Then by considering again the Jordan reduced form of the matrix A we deduce that for each $\varepsilon > 0$ we can find a positive constant $M = M(x, \varepsilon) > 0$ such that

$$\|e^{At} \Pi_s x\| \geq M e^{(\beta - \varepsilon)|t|} \text{ for all } t \leq 0.$$

Then by choosing $\varepsilon > 0$ such that $\beta - \varepsilon > \eta$ we obtain a contradiction. This contradiction implies that $\Pi_s x = 0$. □

Definition 3.41 The equilibrium 0 is said to *hyperbolic* if the spectrum $\sigma(A)$ of A contains no purely imaginary eigenvalue (i.e. $\sigma_c(A) = \varnothing$). The equilibrium 0 is said to be *non-hyperbolic* otherwise.

Inspired by the above definition we sometimes make use of the following notion.

Definition 3.42 The *hyperbolic space* $X_h := X_s \oplus X_u$ is defined as the direct sum of the stable and unstable spaces.

Exercise 3.43 Prove that the spectrum $\sigma(A)$ of a real 2×2 matrix $A \in M_2(\mathbb{R})$ contains a purely imaginary eigenvalue if, and only if, one of the following conditions is satisfied

(i) $\det(A) = 0$ (in which case $0 \in \sigma(A)$),
(ii) $\operatorname{tr}(A) = 0$ and $\det(A) > 0$ (in which case $\pm 2i\sqrt{\det(A)} \in \sigma(A)$).

3.9 Planar Linear Differential Equations

In this section, we describe the behavior of linear ordinary differential equations in the plane. We refer to Hirsch, Smale and Devaney [155] for more results on this subject.

3.9.1 Introduction

Consider a linear system

$$\begin{cases} \dfrac{dX(t)}{dt} = AX(t), \text{ for all } t \geq 0, \\ X(0) = X_0 \in \mathbb{R}^2 \end{cases}$$

with

$$A = \begin{bmatrix} a & b \\ c & d \end{bmatrix} \in M_2(\mathbb{R}).$$

The eigenvalues of A satisfy the so-called *characteristic equation* given by

$$\lambda^2 - \text{tr}(A) + \det(A) = 0,$$

where $\text{tr}(A) = a + d$ and $\det(A) = ad - bc$. The eigenvalues satisfy

$$\lambda_\pm = \frac{1}{2}\left(\text{tr}(A) \pm \sqrt{\Delta}\right),$$

where $\Delta := \text{tr}(A)^2 - 4\det(A)$.

For linear systems in the plane, we have the following classification.

Definition 3.44 Assume that 0 is a hyperbolic equilibrium. Then we say that 0 is

- a *node* when both eigenvalues are real and have the same sign (i.e. $0 > \lambda_+ \geq \lambda_-$ or $\lambda_+ \geq \lambda_- > 0$). A node is stable when both eigenvalues are negative and unstable when both eigenvalues are positive.
- a *saddle* when the eigenvalues are real and have opposite signs (i.e. $\lambda_+ > 0 > \lambda_-$). A saddle is always unstable.
- a *focus* (sometimes called a *spiral point*) when the eigenvalues are complex-conjugate (i.e. $\lambda_+ = a + ib$ and $\lambda_- = a - ib$ with $a \neq 0$ and $b \neq 0$). The focus is stable when the eigenvalues have negative real part (i.e. $a < 0$) and unstable when they have positive real part (i.e. $a > 0$).

3.9.2 Case with two real eigenvalues

We fix for example

$$A = \begin{bmatrix} 0.1 & 0.1 \\ 0.1 & 0.1 \end{bmatrix} + cI.$$

We have

$$\lambda_+ = 0.2 + c > \lambda_- = c.$$

The eigenspace associated to the eigenvalue λ_+ is

$$E_{\lambda_+} = \mathbb{R}\begin{pmatrix} 1 \\ 1 \end{pmatrix}.$$

The eigenspace associated to the eigenvalue λ_- is

$$E_{\lambda_-} = \mathbb{R}\begin{pmatrix} 1 \\ -1 \end{pmatrix}.$$

Case 1: We fix

$$c = -0.301$$

and we have

$$\lambda_- < \lambda_+ < 0.$$

Then 0 is a stable node. In this case the *equilibrium is exponentially asymptotically stable*, and in Figure 3.4 we plot the solutions in the phase plane.

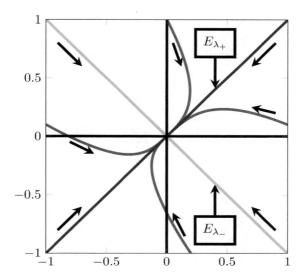

Fig. 3.4: *The blue line (respectively the green line) corresponds to the eigenspace associated with the eigenvalue λ_+ (respectively λ_-). We observe that the solutions are converging to 0 by approaching the blue line.*

Case 2: We fix
$$c = -0.1$$
so that
$$\lambda_- < 0 < \lambda_+.$$

This equilibrium is a saddle. The name "hyperbolic equilibrium" is inspired by such an example, since the red solutions represented in Figure 3.5 look like hyperbolas. In Figure 3.5 we plot the solutions in the phase plane $(x(t), y(t))$.

Case 3: We fix
$$c = 0.2$$
and therefore
$$0 < \lambda_- < \lambda_+.$$

Then 0 is an unstable node and in Figure 3.6 we plot the solutions in the phase plane.

Case 4: Assume that the only eigenvalue of A is 0. That is, $\sigma(A) = \{0\}$, or with the above notation,
$$\lambda_+ = \lambda_- = 0.$$

Then 0 is not hyperbolic anymore. In this case the algebraic multiplicity of the eigenvalue 0 is equal to 2, and we have

$$p_A(\lambda) = \det(\lambda I - A) = \lambda^2.$$

If $\dim(N(A)) = 2$ then we have

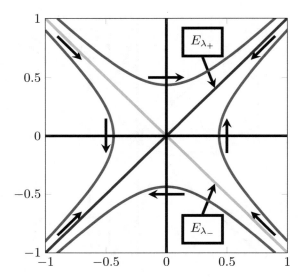

Fig. 3.5: *The blue line (respectively the green line) corresponds to the eigenspace associated with the eigenvalue λ_+ (respectively λ_-). Solutions starting on the green line approach 0. All the other solutions approach the blue line and explode (or blow up) when the time t goes to $+\infty$.*

$$A = 0.$$

There is nothing particular to say since every point in $\mathbb{R}^2$ is an equilibrium.

If $\dim(N(A)) = 1$, then

$$\dim(N(A^2)) = 2.$$

In this case the matrix A is not diagonalizable, but according to Jordan's theorem there exists an invertible matrix P such that

$$P^{-1}AP = \begin{pmatrix} 0 & 1 \\ 0 & 0 \end{pmatrix},$$

the Jordan reduced form of A. We can find this matrix by looking for $V_- \neq 0$ and $V_+ \neq 0$ such that

$$AV_- = 0 \text{ and } AV_+ = V_-.$$

In the basis $\{V_-, V_+\}$ the system has the form

$$\begin{cases} \dfrac{dx(t)}{dt} = y(t) \\ \dfrac{dy(t)}{dt} = 0, \end{cases}$$

with the initial condition

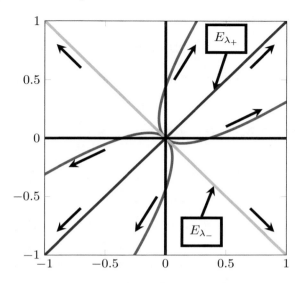

Fig. 3.6: *The blue line (respectively the green line) corresponds to the eigenspace associated with the eigenvalue λ_+ (respectively λ_-). Solutions starting on the green line (respectively, on the blue line) stay on the green line (respectively, on the blue line). For all other solutions, the distance to the green line increases faster than the distance to the blue line.*

$$x(0) = x_0 \text{ and } y(0) = y_0.$$

This system has an explicit solution given by

$$y(t) = y_0,$$
$$x(t) = x_0 + \int_0^t y(s)\mathrm{d}s = x_0 + ty_0.$$

3.9.3 Case with two complex conjugate eigenvalues

Consider the Poincaré normal form (see for example the book of Hassard, Kazarinoff and Wan [148])

$$A = \begin{bmatrix} 0 & -b \\ b & 0 \end{bmatrix} + aI.$$

Then

$$\det(\lambda I - A) = (\lambda - \lambda_+)(\lambda - \lambda_-)$$

with

$$\lambda_+ = a + ib \text{ and } \lambda_- = a - ib.$$

Case 1: Let us fix for instance

$$a = -0.01 \text{ and } b = 0.1.$$

In this case the equilibrium 0 is exponentially asymptotically stable (or a stable focus), since

$$a < 0.$$

In Figure 3.7 we plot the solutions in the phase plane.

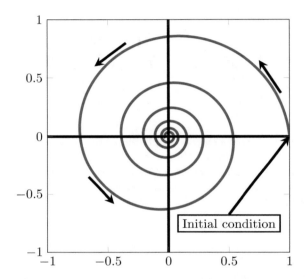

Fig. 3.7: *Stable focus or stable equilibrium with two complex conjugate eigenvalues.*

Remark 3.45 If we change the sign of b we will change the sense of rotation around 0 from the counter-clockwise to the clockwise sense of rotation.

Case 2: We fix

$$a = 0.01 \text{ and } b = 0.1.$$

In this case the equilibrium is *unstable*, since

$$a > 0.$$

In Figure 3.8 we plot the solutions in the phase plane.

Case 3: We fix

$$a = 0 \text{ and } b = 0.1.$$

In this case the equilibrium 0 is called a *center equilibrium*, and all the points of the plane lie in a ω-periodic orbit (i.e. a periodic orbit with period ω). Moreover, the period ω is given by

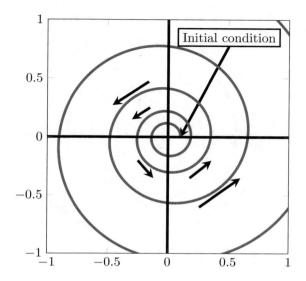

Fig. 3.8: *Unstable focus or unstable equilibrium with two complex conjugate eigenvalues.*

$$\omega = \frac{2\pi}{b} \ (\Leftrightarrow e^{ib\omega} = 1).$$

In Figure 3.9 we plot the solutions in the phase plane.

In the case when we have two complex conjugate purely imaginary eigenvalues, by using a change of basis we can always write the system in the following form

$$\begin{cases} \dfrac{dx(t)}{dt} = ibx(t) \\ \dfrac{dy(t)}{dt} = -iby(t). \end{cases}$$

In this case we have

$$\begin{cases} x(t) = e^{ibt}x(0) \\ y(t) = e^{-ibt}y(0). \end{cases}$$

The functions $x(t)$ and $y(t)$ are ω-periodic, and if we assume in addition that

$$x(0) = \bar{y}(0),$$

then we obtain

$$x(t) = \bar{y}(t) \text{ for each } t \geq 0.$$

We deduce that

$$\begin{cases} x(t) = x_R(t) + ix_I(t) \\ y(t) = x_R(t) - ix_I(t) \end{cases} \Leftrightarrow \begin{cases} x_R(t) = \frac{1}{2}(x(t) + y(t)) \\ x_I(t) = \frac{i}{2}(x(t) - y(t)), \end{cases}$$

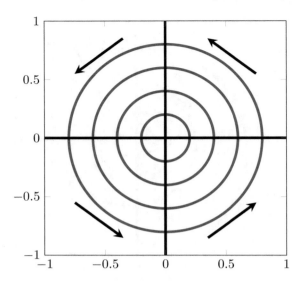

Fig. 3.9: *When the system has only two complex conjugate purely imaginary eigen-values, the system admits an infinite number of periodic orbits with the same period* $\omega = \frac{2\pi}{b}$.

wherein we have set

$$x_R(t) = \mathrm{Re}(x(t)) \text{ and } x_I(t) = \mathrm{Im}(x(t)).$$

Then we get

$$
\begin{aligned}
x(t) &= \mathrm{e}^{ibt} x(0) \\
&= [\cos(bt) + i \sin(bt)][x_R(0) + i x_I(0)] \\
&= [\cos(bt) x_R(0) - \sin(bt) x_I(0)] + i[\sin(bt) x_R(0) + \cos(br) x_I(0)].
\end{aligned}
$$

Thus we obtain the system from which we started, namely

$$\frac{\mathrm{d}}{\mathrm{d}t} \begin{pmatrix} x_R(t) \\ x_I(t) \end{pmatrix} = \begin{pmatrix} 0 & -b \\ b & 0 \end{pmatrix} \begin{pmatrix} x_R(t) \\ x_I(t) \end{pmatrix}$$

and we have for each $t \geq 0$:

$$x_R(t) + i x_I(t) = \mathrm{e}^{ibt}[x_R(0) + i x_I(0)].$$

3.10 Notes and Remarks

Infinite-dimensional Jordan's theorem

Let $(X, \| \cdot \|)$ be a Banach space. Let $A, B, C \in \mathcal{L}(X)$ be three linear operators such that

$$A = B + C,$$

where $C \in \mathcal{L}(X)$ is compact. That is, $\overline{C\,(B_X(0,1))}$ is compact (where $B_X(0,1) = \{x \in X : \|x\| < 1\}$ is the unit ball in X).

Recall that the spectral radius of B is

$$r(B) = \lim_{n \to \infty} \|B^n\|_{\mathcal{L}(X)}^{1/n}.$$

Compactness is the key argument to extend Jordan's theorem from finite to infinite dimensions. The following theorem is a special case of Theorem 4.3.27, p. 199 in the book of Magal and Ruan [236].

Theorem 3.46 *With the preceding notation, let* $\gamma > r(B)$. *Then*

$$\sigma(A) \cap \{\lambda \in \mathbb{C} : |\lambda| \geq \gamma\}$$

is a finite. Furthermore, for each $\lambda_0 \in \sigma(A) \cap \{\lambda \in \mathbb{C} : |\lambda| \geq \gamma\}$, *there exists an integer* $k_0 \geq 1$ *such that*

$$X = R((\lambda_0 I - A)^{k_0}) \oplus N((\lambda_0 I - A)^{k_0}),$$

$$A\left(R((\lambda_0 I - A)^{k_0})\right) \subset R((\lambda_0 I - A)^{k_0}), \text{ and}$$

$$A\left(N((\lambda_0 I - A)^{k_0})\right) \subset N((\lambda_0 I - A)^{k_0}).$$

Moreover, the following properties are satisfied

(i) $A_{R((\lambda_0 I - A)^{k_0})}$ *(the restriction of A to the summand* $R((\lambda_0 I - A)^{k_0})$*) is invertible. In other words,*

$$\lambda_0 \notin \sigma(A_{R((\lambda_0 I - A)^{k_0})}).$$

(ii) *The dimension of* $N((\lambda_0 I - A)^{k_0})$ *(the generalized eigenspace associated to λ_0) is finite.*

(iii) *The spectrum of* $A_{N((\lambda_0 I - A)^{k_0})}$ *(the restriction of A to the summand* $N((\lambda_0 I - A)^{k_0})$*) is equal to* $\{\lambda_0\}$.

Example 3.47 Let $X = C([0, 1], \mathbb{R})$. Define the linear operator $B \in \mathcal{L}(C([0, 1], \mathbb{R}))$ by

$$B(u) = \exp(-\beta(x))u(x),$$

where $\beta \in C([0, 1], \mathbb{R})$ satisfies

$$\beta(x) > \eta > 0, \forall x \in [0, 1],$$

Let $C \in \mathcal{L}(C([0,1], \mathbb{R}))$ be a compact linear operator defined by

$$C(u)(x) = \int_0^1 \gamma(x, y)u(y)dy,$$

where

$$\gamma \in C([0,1] \times [0,1], \mathbb{R}).$$

So a typical example of a linear operator $A \in \mathcal{L}(C([0,1], \mathbb{R}))$ is the following

$$A(u)(x) = \exp(-\beta(x))u(x) + \int_0^1 \gamma(x, y)u(y)dy.$$

For an infinite-dimensional Banach space, the spectrum of A does not coincide with the set of eigenvalues $\lambda \in \mathbb{C}$ such that

$$N(\lambda I - A) \neq \{0\}.$$

By using Theorem 3.46 and the compactness of C one deduces that

$$r(A) = \max\left(\{|\lambda| : \lambda \in \mathbb{C} \text{ such that } N(\lambda I - A) \neq \{0\}\}, r(B)\right).$$

Now one can investigate the sign of $r(A) - 1$ (i.e. the stability of the difference equation $u_{n+1} = Au_n$), by using the fact that $r(B) < 1$ and by considering the eigenvalues of A with modulus strictly larger than $r(B)$.

For finite-dimensional ordinary differential equations, Jordan's theorem leads to stability results, as does Theorem 3.46 for infinite-dimensional systems. Moreover, some continuous-time versions of Theorem 3.46 exist (see Magal and Ruan [236, Theorem 4.5.8, p. 210] for more information).

Stability of ω-periodic non-autonomous systems

The results presented in this chapter can be generalized to non-autonomous (or time-dependent) systems. Let us consider a differential equation of the form

$$u'(t) = A(t)u(t), \ t \geq s \text{ with } u(s) = x \in \mathbb{R}^n, \tag{3.12}$$

where $A : \mathbb{R} \to \mathcal{M}_n(\mathbb{R})$ is assumed to be a continuous map.

Both stability and hyperbolicity have been studied for non-autonomous ordinary differential equations. We refer the reader to the books of Coppel [65], and Barreira and Valls [25], and the references therein.

Definition 3.48 The *principal fundamental matrix* $t \to X(t) \in M_n(\mathbb{R})$ is the unique solution of the problem

$$X'(t) = A(t)X(t), \forall t \in \mathbb{R}, \text{ with } X(0) = I \in M_n(\mathbb{R}).$$

Definition 3.49 The *non-autonomous flow* associated to (3.12) is the two-parameter matrix given by the formula

$$U(t, s) = X(t)X(s)^{-1}, \forall (t, s) \in \mathbb{R}^2.$$

Proposition 3.50 *The flow* $U = U(t, s)$ *satisfies the following properties:*

(i) $U(t, t) = I \in M_n(\mathbb{R})$, *for all* $t \in \mathbb{R}$.

(ii) *The equation*

$$U(t, s) = U(t, r)U(r, s), \ \forall (t, r, s) \in \mathbb{R}^3, \qquad \text{(flow property)}.$$

(iii) *For all* $(t, s) \in \mathbb{R}^2$:

$$\partial_t U(t, s) = A(t)U(t, s),$$

and

$$\partial_s U(t, s) = -U(t, s)A(s).$$

Moreover, if $t \to f(t)$ *is a continuous function from* $\mathbb{R}$ *into* $\mathbb{R}^n$ *and*

$$u(t) = U(t, s)x + \int_s^t U(t, \sigma)f(\sigma)d\sigma, \ \forall t \geq s,$$

then $t \to u(t)$ *is the unique solution of*

$$u'(t) = A(t)u(t) + f(t), \ t \geq s \text{ with } u(s) = x \in \mathbb{R}^n.$$

Remark 3.51 As a consequence of (i) and (ii), for each $(t, s) \in \mathbb{R}^2$ the matrix $U(t, s)$ is invertible and one has

$$U(t, s)^{-1} = U(s, t), \forall (t, s) \in \mathbb{R}^2.$$

The specific case where the map $t \to A(t)$ is ω-periodic for some $\omega > 0$ turns out to be of particular importance and has been widely studied. The analysis of such a periodic system enters into the so-called Floquet theory, based on the so-called Floquet decomposition of the principal fundamental matrix $X = X(t)$, as described below. We refer to the original article of Floquet [109] and to the more recent books of Chicone [53] and Hale [140] for more results. In what follows, $X(t)$ denotes the principal fundamental matrix and $\{U(t, s)\}_{(t,s) \in \mathbb{R}^2}$ denotes the associated flow.

Theorem 3.52 *Assume that* $A : \mathbb{R} \to M_n(\mathbb{R})$ *is continuous and* ω-*periodic with* $\omega > 0$. *Then there exist a matrix* $B \in M_n(\mathbb{R})$ *and a continuous and* ω-*periodic function* $P : \mathbb{R} \to M_n(\mathbb{R})$ *such that*

$$X(t) = P(t)e^{tB}, \ \forall t \in \mathbb{R}.$$

Moreover, for each $t \in \mathbb{R}$ *the matrix* $P(t)$ *is invertible.*

Note that using the above decomposition, the flow $U = U(t, s)$ can be rewritten as follows

$$U(t, s) = P(t)e^{(t-s)B}P(s)^{-1}, \ \forall (t, s) \in \mathbb{R}^2.$$

Let us observe that since P is ω-periodic, $U = U(t, s)$ is an *ω-periodic flow* in the sense that

$$U(t, s) = U(\omega + t, \omega + s), \quad \forall t, s \in \mathbb{R}^2.$$

The matrix $e^{\omega B}$ is usually referred to as the *monodromy matrix*. The eigenvalues of $e^{\omega B}$, denoted by $\varrho_1, \dots, \varrho_n$, are called the *characteristic multipliers* (or sometimes *Floquet multipliers*) while $\lambda_1, \dots, \lambda_n$, the complex numbers such that

$$\varrho_i = e^{\omega \lambda_i},$$

are referred to as the *characteristic exponents* (or the *Floquet exponents*). Note that the imaginary part of each of the characteristic exponents is not uniquely determined uniquely, but up to an additional multiple of $2\pi i / \omega$).

Lemma 3.53 *Let $\{U(t, s)\}_{t \geq s} \subset M_n(\mathbb{R})$ be the ω-periodic flow on $\mathbb{R}^n$ generated by $t \rightarrow A(t)$, a continuous and ω-periodic matrix. Then the spectral radius of $U(\omega + s, s)$ is independent of s. That is,*

$$r\left(U(\omega + s, s)\right) = r\left(U(\omega, 0)\right) = r\left(e^{\omega B}\right), \forall s \in \mathbb{R}.$$

Proof The above lemma is a direct consequence of the Floquet decomposition. Indeed one has

$$U(t, s) = X(t)X(s)^{-1} = P(t)e^{(t-s)B}P(s)^{-1}.$$

Hence we get for all $s \in \mathbb{R}$,

$$U(t + \omega, t) = P(t + \omega)e^{\omega B}P(t)^{-1} = P(t)e^{\omega B}P(t)^{-1}.$$

so that for all $t \in \mathbb{R}$, the Poincaré map $U(t + \omega, t)$ is conjugated to the monodromy matrix $e^{\omega B}$ and the result follows.   □

Using this vocabulary, one can state the following stability result, which is a direct extension of Theorem 3.17.

Corollary 3.54 *Assume that $A : \mathbb{R} \rightarrow M_n(\mathbb{R})$ is continuous and ω-periodic with $\omega > 0$, and assume that the characteristic multipliers have modulus strictly less than one. Then the equilibrium $0 \in \mathbb{R}^n$ of (3.12) is exponentially stable. In other words, there exist $M \geq 1$ and $\alpha > 0$ such that the evolution flow $U = U(t, s)$ satisfies*

$$\|U(t, s)\| \leq Me^{-\alpha(t-s)}, \quad \forall t \geq s.$$

Remark 3.55 Floquet theory has been extended by Sell [310] to almost periodic linear differential equations. The idea is to take advantage of the compactness property of the shift of an almost periodic function.

The spectral theory for ω-periodic linear systems has been used in population dynamics and more particularly in epidemiology to define the basic reproduction number in a periodic environment. We refer to Bacaer [19, 20, 21] and Wang and Zhao [360] for some stability results in the context of time periodic epidemic models.

We also refer to Thieme [339] and Inaba [168] for abstract results concerning general time heterogeneous media.

To explain some of the ideas behind such computations, we consider a linear problem for infection, of the form

$$u'(t) = (F(t) - V(t)) u(t), \tag{3.13}$$

wherein F and V are both continuous and ω-periodic functions from $\mathbb{R}$ into $\mathcal{M}_n(\mathbb{R})$.

Assumption 3.56 We assume in addition that:

(i) $F(t)$ is non-negative for all $t \in \mathbb{R}$;
(ii) $-V(t)$ is cooperative (i.e. all the off-diagonal elements are non-negative) for all $t \in \mathbb{R}$.

Remark 3.57 In this case, $F(t)$ typically describes the rate of new infected while $V(t)$ stands for the rates of transfer of individuals out of compartments such as, for example, deaths, recovery, and emigration.

Define $U(t, s)$ to be the periodic flow associated to the ω-periodic matrix $-V(t)$ and assume that

$$r\left(U(\omega, 0)\right) < 1, \tag{3.14}$$

so that Corollary 3.54 ensures that there exist $M \geq 1$ and $\alpha > 0$ such that

$$\|U(t, s)\| \leq M e^{-\alpha(t-s)}, \ \forall (t, s) \in \mathbb{R}^2.$$

Let us also observe that Assumption 3.56-(ii) implies that

$$U(t, s)\mathbb{R}_+^n \subset \mathbb{R}_+^n, \quad \forall t > s,$$

where

$$\mathbb{R}_+^n = \{(x_1, \cdots, x_n) \in \mathbb{R}^n, \ x_i \geq 0, \ \forall i = 1, \ldots, n\}.$$

We refer to Lemma 8.21 in Chapter 8 for more details.

Now let $s \to \varphi(s) \in \mathbb{R}^n$ be an ω-periodic function that corresponds to the initial distribution of infectious individuals. Next the quantity $F(s)\varphi(s)$ stands for the distribution of new infections produced by the infected individuals who were introduced at time s. Now for $t \geq s$, the quantity $U(t, s)F(s)\varphi(s)$ gives the distribution of those infected individuals who were newly infected at time s and remain in the infected compartments at time t. Hence integrating from $(-\infty, t)$, the quantity $\psi(t)$ given by

$$\psi(t) := \int_{-\infty}^{t} U(t, s)F(s)\varphi(s)\mathrm{d}s = \int_0^{\infty} U(t, t - a)F(t - a)\varphi(t - a)\mathrm{d}a$$

corresponds to the distribution of new infections at time t produced by all those infected individuals $\varphi(s)$ introduced before time t.

To define the basic reproduction number, one considers the Banach space $C_\omega(\mathbb{R}; \mathbb{R}^n)$ of continuous and ω-periodic functions from $\mathbb{R}$ into $\mathbb{R}^n$ endowed with uniform norm topology as well as the linear bounded operator $L \in \mathcal{L}(C_\omega(\mathbb{R};\mathbb{R}^n))$ given for $\varphi \in C_\omega(\mathbb{R};\mathbb{R}^n)$ by

$$L\varphi(t) = \int_0^\infty U(t, t-a)F(t-a)\varphi(t-a)da, \ \forall t \in \mathbb{R}.$$

In [360], this linear (positive and bounded) operator L is referred to as the next infection operator and the basic reproduction number R_0 is defined as the spectral radius of L

$$R_0 = r(L).$$

This quantity R_0 characterizes the stability of the solution 0 of equation (3.13). Indeed, according to Theorem 2.2 in [360], one has

Theorem 3.58 *Let Assumption 3.56 be satisfied. Let* $e^{\omega B}$ *be the monodromy operator of equation* (3.13). *Then one has*

(i) $R_0 = 1$ *if and only if* $r(e^{\omega B}) = 1$;
(ii) $R_0 > 1$ *if and only if* $r(e^{\omega B}) > 1$;
(iii) $R_0 < 1$ *if and only if* $r(e^{\omega B}) < 1$.

Remark 3.59 This quantity can be explicitly computed typically when the matrices F and V are both time independent. In that case the above expression coincides with the usual definition of the basic reproduction number

$$R_0 = r(FV^{-1}),$$

see for instance [88, 93].

This quantity can also be computed when both matrices $F(t)$ and $V(t)$ are diagonal, namely

$$F(t) = \mathrm{diag}\,(F_1(t), \ldots, F_n(t))\,, \ V(t) = \mathrm{diag}\,(V_1(t), \ldots, V_n(t))\,.$$

In that case, one has

$$R_0 = \max_{i=1,\ldots,n} \left(\frac{\int_0^\omega F_i(s)ds}{\int_0^\omega V_i(s)ds} \right).$$

We refer to Bacaer [19, 20, 21], Thieme [339], Inaba [168] and the references therein for more results.

3.11 MATLAB Codes

Figure 3.5

```
1  cla; clf;
2  T=100;
3  deltaT =0.1;
```

```
4   c =0.301;
5   A=[0.1−c   0.1;   0.1   0.1−c];
6
7   X0=[0   1];
8   t0 =0: deltaT :T;
9   [ t1 ,   x1 ] = ode45 (@Model1,   t0 ,   X0,   [],   A);
10
11  clf ;
12  hold  on ;
13  plot ( x1 (: ,   1) ,   x1 (: ,   2) ,   ' r ' ,   ' LineWidth ' ,   2) ;
14  X0 = [0.2   −1];
15  [ t1 ,   x2 ] = ode45 (@Model1,   t0 ,   X0,   [],   A);
16  plot ( x2 (: ,   1) ,   x2 (: ,   2) ,   ' r ' ,   ' LineWidth ' ,   2) ;
17
18  X0 = [−1   0.1];
19  [ t1 ,   x3 ] = ode45 (@Model1,   t0 ,   X0,   [],   A);
20  plot ( x3 (: ,   1) ,   x3 (: ,   2) ,   ' r ' ,   ' LineWidth ' ,   2) ;
21
22  X0 = [1   0.1];
23  [ t1 ,   x4 ] = ode45 (@Model1,   t0 ,   X0,   [],   A);
24  plot ( x4 (: ,   1) ,   x4 (: ,   2) ,   ' r ' ,   ' LineWidth ' ,   2) ;
25
26  aux = −2:0.1:2;
27  plot ( aux ,   aux ,   ' b ' ,   aux ,   −aux ,   ' g ' ,   ' LineWidth ' ,   2) ;
28  plot ( aux ,   0∗aux ,   ' k ' ,   0∗aux ,   −aux ,   ' k ' ,   ' LineWidth ' ,
        2) ;
29
30  xlabel ( ' x ' ) ;
31  ylabel ( ' y ' ) ;
32  set ( gca ,   ' YLim ' ,   [−1,   1]) ;
33  set ( gca ,   ' XLim ' ,   [−1,   1]) ;
34
35  T = table ( t1 ,   x1 (: ,   1) ,   x1 (: ,2) ,   x2 (: ,   1) ,   x2 (: ,2) ,
        x3 (: ,   1) ,   x3 (: ,2) ,   x4 (: ,   1) ,   x4 (: ,2) ,   '
        VariableName ' ,   { ' t ' ,   ' x1 ' ,   ' y1 ' ,   ' x2 ' ,   ' y2 ' ,   ' x3 '
        ,   ' y3 ' ,   ' x4 ' ,   ' y4 ' }) ;
36  writetable (T,   ' Fig3_4 . csv ' )
37
38
39
40  function  dy=Model1 ( t ,   y ,   A)
41          n= size (A) ;
42          dy=zeros (n(1) ,   1) ;
43          dy=A∗y ;
44  end
```

Chapter 4
Positivity and the Perron–Frobenius Theorem

4.1 The Resolvent Formula

Let $A \in M_n(\mathbb{R})$ be an n by n matrix with real elements. Then the following lemma holds.

Lemma 4.1 *For each $\lambda > s(A)$, the matrix $(\lambda I - A)$ is invertible and we have the following formula*

$$(\lambda I - A)^{-1} = \int_0^\infty e^{-\lambda t} e^{At} \, dt,$$

where $(\lambda I - A)^{-1}$ is called the resolvent *of A.*

Remark 4.2 The integral in the resolvent formula is called the *Laplace transform* of $t \to e^{At}$. Note that this integral converges since $s(A - \lambda I) = s(A) - \lambda < 0$ and the convergence follows from the stability theorem.

Remark 4.3 The above formula remains true for any $\lambda \in \mathbb{C}$ such that

$$\mathrm{Re}(\lambda) > s(A).$$

Proof Let $\lambda > s(A)$ be given. We have

$$(\lambda I - A) \int_0^\infty e^{-\lambda t} e^{At} \, dt = -\int_0^\infty (-\lambda I + A) e^{(-\lambda I + A)t} \, dt = -\left[e^{(-\lambda I + A)t} \right]_0^\infty,$$

which yields

$$(\lambda I - A) \int_0^\infty e^{-\lambda t} e^{At} \, dt = \int_0^\infty e^{-\lambda t} e^{At} \, dt \, (\lambda I - A) = I.$$

This ends the proof of the lemma. □

By using the Laplace transform we also prove the following lemma.

© The Author(s), under exclusive license to Springer Nature Switzerland AG 2022
A. Ducrot et al., *Differential Equations and Population Dynamics I*, Lecture Notes on Mathematical Modelling in the Life Sciences, https://doi.org/10.1007/978-3-030-98136-5_4

Lemma 4.4 *Assume that* 0 *is exponentially asymptotically stable for the system*

$$X'(t) = AX(t).$$

Then $s(A) < 0$.

Proof Let $\delta > 0$ and $M > 1$ be such that

$$\|\mathrm{e}^{At}\| \le M\mathrm{e}^{-\delta t}, \ \forall t \ge 0.$$

Let $\lambda \in \mathbb{C}$ with $\mathrm{Re}(\lambda) > -\delta$. Then the integral

$$\int_0^\infty \mathrm{e}^{-\lambda t}\mathrm{e}^{At}\,\mathrm{d}t$$

converges and

$$(\lambda I - A)\int_0^\infty \mathrm{e}^{-\lambda t}\mathrm{e}^{At}\,\mathrm{d}t = \int_0^\infty \mathrm{e}^{-\lambda t}\mathrm{e}^{At}\,\mathrm{d}t(\lambda I - A) = I.$$

Therefore the matrix $(\lambda I - A)$ is invertible and $\lambda \notin \sigma(A)$. $\qquad\qquad\square$

4.2 A Partial Order on $\mathbb{R}^n$

In this section, we introduce partial orders on $\mathbb{R}^n$ and $M_n(\mathbb{R})$.

Definition 4.5 Let $x, y \in \mathbb{R}^n$ be given. We will use the following notations

$$
\begin{aligned}
&x \ge y \iff x_i \ge y_i \text{ for all } i = 1, \cdots, n,\\
&x > y \iff x \ge y \text{ and } x_{i_0} > y_{i_0} \text{ for some } i_0 \in \{1, \cdots, n\},\\
&x \gg y \iff x_i > y_i \text{ for all } i = 1, \cdots, n.
\end{aligned}
$$

Remark 4.6 We can reformulate the above definitions by considering the difference $x - y$ as follows. We have

$$
\begin{aligned}
&x \ge y \iff x - y \ge 0 \iff x - y \in \mathbb{R}^n_+,\\
&x > y \iff x - y > 0 \iff x - y \in \mathbb{R}^n_+ \setminus \{0\},\\
&x \gg y \iff x - y \gg 0 \iff x - y \in \mathrm{Int}\left(\mathbb{R}^n_+\right) = (0, \infty)^n.
\end{aligned}
$$

Remark 4.7 We can generalize the above notion of partial order by replacing $\mathbb{R}^n_+$ by $K \subset \mathbb{R}^n$, a *positive cone*, that is, K is a subset with the following properties:

  (i) K is closed and convex;
 (ii) $\mathbb{R}_+ K \subset K$,   where $\mathbb{R}_+ K := \{\lambda x : \lambda \in \mathbb{R}_+ \text{ and } x \in K\}$;
(iii) $K \cap (-K) = \{0\}$.

Then one can define the partial order $\le_K$ by

$$x \le_K y \iff y - x \in K.$$

Similarly to the elements of $\mathbb{R}^n$ we can define a partial order on the space of real matrices $M_n(\mathbb{R})$ as follows: for $A = (a_{i,j})_{i,j=1,\cdots,n} \in M_n(\mathbb{R})$, we set

$$A \geq 0 \iff a_{ij} \geq 0, \ \forall i, j = 1, \cdots, n,$$
$$A > 0 \iff A \geq 0 \text{ and } A \neq 0,$$
$$A \gg 0 \iff a_{ij} > 0, \ \forall i, j = 1, \cdots, n.$$

Definition 4.8 Let $x \in \mathbb{C}^n$ and $A \in M_n(\mathbb{C})$ be given. We define the *modulus* of x and A respectively by

$$|x| = \begin{pmatrix} |x_1| \\ |x_2| \\ \vdots \\ |x_n| \end{pmatrix} \in \mathbb{R}^n_+ \text{ and } |A| = \begin{pmatrix} |a_{11}| & \cdots & |a_{1n}| \\ \vdots & & \vdots \\ |a_{n1}| & \cdots & |a_{nn}| \end{pmatrix} \in M_n(\mathbb{R}_+).$$

4.3 Positivity of the Solution

Consider the linear Cauchy problem

$$u'(t) = Au(t), \ \forall t \geq 0 \text{ and } u(0) = u_0 \in \mathbb{R}^n.$$

Definition 4.9 We will say that the system is *positivity-preserving* if for any non-negative initial distribution $u_0 \geq 0$ the corresponding solution $t \to u(t)$ stays positive for all time $t \geq 0$. That is,

$$u_0 \geq 0 \implies u(t) \geq 0, \ \forall t \geq 0.$$

Remark 4.10 It is clear that the system is positivity-preserving if and only if

$$e^{At} \geq 0, \quad \forall t \geq 0.$$

The main result of this section is the following theorem.

Theorem 4.11 *The two following properties are equivalent*

(i) *The system is positivity-preserving.*
(ii) *The off-diagonal elements of A are all non-negative. That is,*

$$a_{ij} \geq 0, \ \text{whenever } i, j = 1, \cdots, n \text{ and } i \neq j.$$

Remark 4.12 The above property (ii) is equivalent to the existence of a real number $\lambda \geq 0$ such that

$$(A + \lambda I) \geq 0.$$

Proof $(\Rightarrow)$ Assume that

$$e^{At} \geq 0, \ \forall t \geq 0.$$

Then for all $\lambda \in \mathbb{R}$ we also have

$$e^{-\lambda t} e^{At} = e^{(A - \lambda I)t} \geq 0, \ \forall t \geq 0.$$

Next, using the resolvent formula stated in Lemma 4.1, we deduce that

$$(\lambda I - A)^{-1} = \int_0^\infty e^{(A - \lambda I)t} dt \geq 0, \ \forall \lambda > s(A).$$

Furthermore, for all $\lambda > \max\big(s(A), \|A\|_{\mathcal{L}(\mathbb{R}^n)}\big)$ one has

$$(\lambda I - A)^{-1} = \lambda^{-1} \left(I - \lambda^{-1} A \right)^{-1}$$

$$= \lambda^{-1} \sum_{k=0}^\infty \frac{A^k}{\lambda^k} = \lambda^{-1} \left(I + \frac{A}{\lambda} + \cdots + \frac{A^k}{\lambda^k} + \cdots \right).$$

Hence we get

$$\lambda^2 (\lambda I - A)^{-1} = \left(\lambda I + A + \frac{\lambda A^2}{\lambda^2} \left(I - \frac{A}{\lambda} \right)^{-1} \right).$$

Let $\{e_1, \cdots, e_n\}$ denote the canonical basis of $\mathbb{R}^n$. Let $i, j \in \{1, \ldots, n\}$ with $i \neq j$. Then we have $\langle e_i, e_j \rangle = 0$ and it follows that

$$0 \leq \langle e_i, \lambda^2 (\lambda I - A)^{-1} e_j \rangle = \langle e_i, A e_j \rangle + \left\langle e_i, \frac{\lambda A^2}{\lambda^2} \left(I - \frac{A}{\lambda} \right)^{-1} e_j \right\rangle,$$

and

$$\left\langle e_i, \frac{A^2}{\lambda} \left(I - \frac{A}{\lambda} \right)^{-1} e_j \right\rangle = O\left(\frac{1}{\lambda} \right) \to 0, \text{ as } \lambda \to \infty.$$

Therefore

$$a_{ij} = \langle e_i, A e_j \rangle \geq 0,$$

and the first implication follows.

($\Leftarrow$) Conversely, assume that all the off-diagonal elements of A are non-negative. Let $\delta > 0$ such that

$$(A + \delta I) \geq 0.$$

Then one has

$$e^{\delta t} e^{At} = \sum_{k=0}^\infty \frac{(A + \delta I)^k t^k}{k!} \geq 0, \ \forall t \geq 0,$$

and the result follows.   □

4.4 The Perron–Frobenius Theorem

The theorem presented in this chapter was proved by Perron [275] and Frobenius [111, 112]. This is a classical result in matrix analysis. We refer to the books of Gantmacher [114], Seneta [311], Minc [256] and Horn and Johnson [161] for more results on non-negative matrices.

4.4.1 Definitions and notations for matrices

Recall that the linear operator norm of an n by n matrix A with real elements, denoted by $\|A\|_{\mathcal{L}(\mathbb{R}^n)}$, is defined as

$$\|A\|_{\mathcal{L}(\mathbb{R}^n)} := \sup_{\|x\| \leq 1} \|Ax\|.$$

By using this norm we have the following result.

Lemma 4.13 *Let $A \in M_n(\mathbb{R})$ be given. The sequence $\left(\|A^p\|_{\mathcal{L}(\mathbb{R}^n)}^{1/p} \right)_{p \geq 1}$ converges as $p \to \infty$.*

The proof of this result given below is taken from the book of Kato [172, pp. 27–28].

Proof Set $a_p := \ln(\|A^p\|_{\mathcal{L}(\mathbb{R}^n)})$ for $p \geq 0$. Here $A^0 := I$, which implies that $\|A^0\| = 1$, so that $a_0 = 0$. Let us prove that

$$\lim_{p \to +\infty} \frac{a_p}{p} = \inf_{m > 0} \frac{a_m}{m}.$$

Since we have

$$\|A^{p+q}\|_{\mathcal{L}(\mathbb{R}^n)} \leq \|A^p\|_{\mathcal{L}(\mathbb{R}^n)} \|A^q\|_{\mathcal{L}(\mathbb{R}^n)}, \ \forall p, q \in \mathbb{N},$$

we deduce that the sequence $(a_p)_{p \geq 0}$ is sub-additive, namely it satisfies

$$a_{p+q} \leq a_p + a_q \ \forall p, q \in \mathbb{N}.$$

Let $m > 0$ be a fixed integer. Applying this last inequality to $p = m \times q + r$, for some $q \in \mathbb{N}$ and $r \in \{0, ..., m - 1\}$, we have

$$a_p \leq a_{mq} + a_r \leq q a_m + a_r.$$

Hence for all p large enough (such that $q > 0$) we have

$$\frac{a_p}{p} \leq \frac{q}{p} a_m + \frac{1}{p} a_r \leq \frac{1}{m + \dfrac{r}{q}} a_m + \frac{1}{p} a_r$$

and since $q \to +\infty$ whenever $p \to +\infty$, we obtain

$$\limsup_{p \to +\infty} \frac{a_p}{p} \le \frac{a_m}{m}.$$

Now since this inequality must be true for all $m > 0$ we deduce that

$$\limsup_{p \to +\infty} \frac{a_p}{p} \le \inf_{m>0} \frac{a_m}{m}.$$

Now for each integer $p > 0$ we have

$$\frac{a_p}{p} \ge \inf_{m>0} \frac{a_m}{m},$$

so that we get

$$\liminf_{p \to +\infty} \frac{a_p}{p} \ge \inf_{m>0} \frac{a_m}{m} \ge \limsup_{p \to +\infty} \frac{a_p}{p}.$$

The result follows. $\qquad\qquad\qquad\qquad\qquad\qquad\qquad\qquad\qquad\qquad\qquad\quad$ $\square$

Definition 4.14 The *spectral radius* $r(A)$ of a matrix $A \in M_n(\mathbb{R})$ is defined by

$$r(A) := \lim_{p \to +\infty} \|A^p\|_{\mathcal{L}(\mathbb{R}^n)}^{\frac{1}{p}}.$$

By using the Jordan normal form of A we deduce the following result.

Lemma 4.15 *The following equality holds*

$$r(A) = \sup\{|\lambda| : \lambda \in \sigma(A)\}.$$

Exercise 4.16 Prove the above lemma (Hint: Use Jordan's reduction of A).

By using the same arguments as for the above discrete time case we have the following result.

Lemma 4.17 *Let $A \in M_n(\mathbb{R})$ be given. The limit $\lim_{t \to +\infty} \frac{1}{t} \ln \|e^{tA}\|_{\mathcal{L}(\mathbb{R}^n)}$ exists.*

Definition 4.18 The growth rate of the semigroup $\{e^{At}\}_{t \ge 0}$ is defined as

$$\mathrm{Gr}(A) := \lim_{t \to +\infty} \frac{1}{t} \ln \|e^{tA}\|_{\mathcal{L}(\mathbb{R}^n)}.$$

By using the Jordan normal form of A again we also deduce the following result.

Lemma 4.19 *The growth rate and the growth bound coincide. That is,*

$$\mathrm{Gr}(A) = \sup\{\mathrm{Re}(\lambda) : \lambda \in \sigma(A)\} =: s(A).$$

Figure 4.1 summarizes the above notions for the spectrum.

Definition 4.20 The *peripheral spectrum* of A is defined as

$$\sigma_{\mathrm{per}}(A) = \{\lambda \in \sigma(A) : |\lambda| = r(A)\}.$$

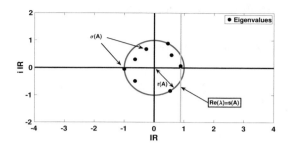

Fig. 4.1: *In this figure the black dots represent the point of the spectrum in the complex plane. In general, the spectral radius does not belong to the spectrum of A. The growth bound $s(A)$ corresponds to the green line. The peripheral spectrum is the spectrum of A (i.e. the black dots) belonging to the red circle. Observe that, in general, the growth bound (green line) is strictly smaller than the spectral radius $r(A)$. The Perron–Frobenius theorem implies that the growth bound and the spectral radius are equal for non-negative matrices (because for non-negative matrices $r(A)$ belongs to the spectrum of A).*

Definition 4.21 The *algebraic multiplicity* of an eigenvalue λ_0 of A is the dimension of the generalized eigenspace of A associated to the eigenvalue λ_0 and is also its multiplicity as a root of the characteristic polynomial of A, i.e. the algebraic multiplicity of λ_0 is the integer $n_0 \geq 1$ satisfying

$$\det(\lambda I - A) = (\lambda - \lambda_0)^{n_0} g(\lambda),$$

where $\lambda \to g(\lambda)$ is a polynomial satisfying $g(\lambda_0) \neq 0$. The *geometric multiplicity* of an eigenvalue λ_0 of A is the dimension of the eigenspace $N(\lambda_0 I - A)$.

Remark 4.22 By considering the Jordan normal form of a given matrix we can prove that the algebraic multiplicity is always greater than or equal to the geometric multiplicity. More precisely, the geometric multiplicity is equal to the number of Jordan blocks, while the algebraic multiplicity is the number of times that the eigenvalue appears on the diagonal of the Jordan reduction.

Definition 4.23 We will say that an eigenvalue of A is *simple* if its algebraic multiplicity is 1.

Remark 4.24 An eigenvalue λ_0 is simple if and only if

$$\dim(N(\lambda_0 I - A)) = 1$$

and

$$N(\lambda_0 I - A) = N(\lambda_0 I - A)^2.$$

4.4.2 The Perron–Frobenius theorem for strictly positive matrices

We start by stating and proving the Perron–Frobenius theorem for strictly positive matrices.

Theorem 4.25 *Let $A \in M_n(\mathbb{R})$ be a strictly positive matrix (i.e. $A \gg 0$). Then A satisfies the following properties*

(i) $r(A) > 0$.

(ii) $r(A)$ *is an eigenvalue of A.*

(iii) $r(A)$ *is the unique eigenvalue of A with modulus $r(A)$ or equivalently $\sigma_{per}(A) = \{r(A)\}$.*

(iv) *There exists a $v_r \gg 0$ (a right eigenvector of A) and there exists a $v_l \gg 0$ (a left eigenvector of A) such that*

$$Av_r = r(A)v_r \text{ and } v_l^T A = r(A)v_l^T .$$

(v) $r(A)$ *is a simple eigenvalue of A.*

Example 4.26 In order to illustrate this theorem we consider the transition matrix of a *homogeneous Markov chain* (see Seneta [311] for more results on this topic). Namely consider a random variable with a finite number of states $1, \ldots, n$. Assume that the system is in the ith state at time t and the next jump will take it to the jth state (at time $t + 1$) with probability m_{ij}. Therefore

$$P[X = j | X = i] = m_{ij}.$$

Then it holds that

$$\sum_{j=1}^{n} m_{ij} = 1, \quad \forall i = 1, \cdots, n.$$

Define

$$M = (m_{ij})_{i,j=1,\ldots,n}.$$

Then, one has

$$M \begin{pmatrix} 1 \\ \vdots \\ 1 \end{pmatrix} = \begin{pmatrix} 1 \\ \vdots \\ 1 \end{pmatrix}.$$

As an example with $n = 4$ we consider the following matrix

$$M = \frac{1}{10} \begin{pmatrix} 1 & 2 & 3 & 4 \\ 4 & 1 & 2 & 3 \\ 3 & 4 & 1 & 2 \\ 2 & 3 & 4 & 1 \end{pmatrix}.$$

The matrix M is said to be *Markovian* because

$$M \begin{pmatrix} 1 \\ 1 \\ 1 \\ 1 \end{pmatrix} = \begin{pmatrix} 1 \\ 1 \\ 1 \\ 1 \end{pmatrix}.$$

Now by the Perron–Frobenius theorem for strictly positive matrices, there exists a vector $V \gg 0$ such that

$$V^T M = r(M) V^T.$$

So we obtain

$$V^T \begin{pmatrix} 1 \\ 1 \\ 1 \\ 1 \end{pmatrix} = V^T M \begin{pmatrix} 1 \\ 1 \\ 1 \\ 1 \end{pmatrix} = r(M) V^T \begin{pmatrix} 1 \\ 1 \\ 1 \\ 1 \end{pmatrix}.$$

This yields

$$V^T \begin{pmatrix} 1 \\ 1 \\ 1 \\ 1 \end{pmatrix} = r(M) V^T \begin{pmatrix} 1 \\ 1 \\ 1 \\ 1 \end{pmatrix},$$

and since $V \gg 0$, one deduces that $r(M) = 1$.

Let Π^t denote the row vector of the probability distribution of X_t at time t. Then it satisfies

$$\Pi^{t+1} = \Pi^t M, \quad \forall t \geq 0.$$

Then whenever M is primitive we have

$$\lim_{t \to \infty} \frac{1}{\Pi_1^t + \cdots + \Pi_n^t} \Pi^t = \frac{1}{V_1 + \cdots + V_n} V,$$

and since $\Pi_1^t + \cdots + \Pi_n^t = 1$ this is also equivalent to

$$\lim_{t \to \infty} \Pi^t = \frac{1}{V_1 + \cdots + V_n} V.$$

Remark 4.27 For the example $M = \frac{1}{10} \begin{pmatrix} 1 & 2 & 3 & 4 \\ 4 & 1 & 2 & 3 \\ 3 & 4 & 1 & 2 \\ 2 & 3 & 4 & 1 \end{pmatrix}$ the left eigenvector is also $V = (1, 1, 1, 1)^T$.

In Figure 4.2 we plot the eigenvalues of the matrix M in the complex plane.

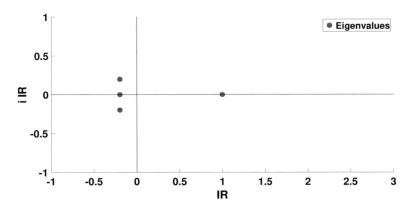

Fig. 4.2: *In the figure we plot the eigenvalues of M in the complex plane. We observe that two eigenvalues are real (the spectral radius 1 and a negative eigenvalue −0.2) and the two last eigenvalues are complex conjugates −0.2 ± 0.2i.*

Lemma 4.28 *Let $z_1, z_2, \ldots, z_n \in \mathbb{C} \setminus \{0\}$ be given, for some $n \geq 2$. Then*

$$\left| \sum_{k=1}^{n} z_k \right| = \sum_{k=1}^{n} |z_k|$$

if and only if for each $j \in \{2, \ldots, n\}$, there exists an $\alpha_j > 0$ such that

$$z_j = \alpha_j z_1.$$

Proof The proof of the above lemma is based on an induction argument.
For $n = 2$, note that using polar coordinates one can rewrite z_1 and z_2 as $z_1 = r_1 e^{i\theta_1}$ and $z_2 = r_2 e^{i\theta_2}$. Hence we get

$$
\begin{aligned}
& |z_1 + z_2| = |z_1| + |z_2| \\
\Leftrightarrow\ & |r_1 e^{i\theta_1} + r_2 e^{i\theta_2}| = r_1 + r_2 \\
\Leftrightarrow\ & |r_1 + r_2 e^{i(\theta_2 - \theta_1)}| = r_1 + r_2 \\
\Leftrightarrow\ & |r_1 + r_2 \cos((\theta_2 - \theta_1)) + i r_2 \sin((\theta_2 - \theta_1))| = r_1 + r_2 \\
\Leftrightarrow\ & (r_1 + r_2 \cos((\theta_2 - \theta_1)))^2 + (r_2 \sin((\theta_2 - \theta_1)))^2 = (r_1 + r_2)^2
\end{aligned}
$$

and after simplification this leads us to

$$2 r_1 r_2 \cos((\theta_2 - \theta_1)) = 2 r_1 r_2.$$

Now since by assumption we have $z_1 \neq 0$ and $z_2 \neq 0$, we end up with $\cos((\theta_2 - \theta_1)) = 1$, that is $(\theta_2 - \theta_1) = 2k\pi$, for some integer $k \in \mathbb{Z}$. Hence we deduce that the result holds true for $n = 2$.

Assume that the result holds true for each integer $2 \leq n \leq n_0$, for some integer $n_0 \geq 2$ and let us prove that the property also holds true for $n_0 + 1$. So assume that

$$|z_1 + z_2 + \cdots + z_{n_0+1}| = |z_1| + |z_2| + \cdots + |z_{n_0+1}|. \tag{4.1}$$

By using the triangle inequality we have

$$|z_1 + \cdots + z_{n_0} + z_{n_0+1}| \leq |z_1 + \cdots + z_{n_0}| + |z_{n_0+1}|.$$

Next by using (4.1) and again the triangle inequality we deduce that

$$|z_1| + \cdots + |z_{n_0}| \leq |z_1 + \cdots + z_{n_0}| \leq |z_1| + \cdots + |z_{n_0}|.$$

This implies that

$$|z_1| + \cdots + |z_{n_0}| = |z_1 + \cdots + z_{n_0}|.$$

By using our induction assumption we obtain that for each $j \in \{2, \ldots, n_0\}$, there exists an $\alpha_j > 0$ such that

$$z_j = \alpha_j z_1,$$

and setting $C := 1 + \alpha_2 + \ldots + \alpha_{n_0} > 0$ the equality (4.1) becomes

$$|Cz_1 + z_{n_0+1}| = |Cz_1| + |z_{n_0+1}|.$$

The result follows by using the case $n = 2$. This completes the proof of the lemma.□

Proof (of Theorem 4.25) *Proof of (i).* The trace of A is given by $\text{tr}(A) = \sum_{i=1}^{n} a_{ii} = \sum_{i=1}^{n} \lambda_i$, where the $\lambda_i \in \mathbb{C}$ are eigenvalues of A. Since $a_{ii} > 0$ for all $i = 1, \cdots, n$ we obtain that $\text{tr}(A) > 0$, which implies that $r(A) > 0$. Indeed if $r(A) = 0$ then $\lambda_i = 0$ for all $i = 1, \cdots, n$ and $\text{tr}(A) = 0$, which is a contradiction.

Proof of (ii). Since $r(A) > 0$ by the previous step, multiplying A by $r(A)^{-1}$ we can assume that

$$r(A) = 1.$$

Moreover, due to Lemma 4.15, there exists at least one eigenvalue $\lambda \in \mathbb{C}$ of A such that

$$|\lambda| = r(A) = 1.$$

Let $x \neq 0$ be an eigenvector associated to λ. Recall that we have defined the modulus of a matrix $|M|$ as the matrix with elements $|m_{ij}|$. With this notation we have

$$|x| = |\lambda||x| = |\lambda x| = |Ax| \leq |A||x|.$$

Since the matrix A is positive, we have $A = |A|$ and we obtain

$$|x| \leq A|x|.$$

Let us prove that $A|x| = |x|$. To see this, assume that

$$A|x| > |x| \Leftrightarrow A|x| - |x| > 0.$$

Since $A \gg 0$, we deduce that

$$A(A|x| - |x|) = A^2|x| - A|x| \gg 0.$$

So there exists an $\varepsilon > 0$ such that

$$A^2|x| - A|x| > \varepsilon A|x| \Leftrightarrow \frac{1}{1+\varepsilon}A^2|x| > A|x|.$$

By setting

$$B := \frac{1}{1+\varepsilon}A,$$

the above inequality can be rewritten as

$$BA|x| > A|x|.$$

By applying the positive matrix B on both sides of this inequality we obtain

$$B^2A|x| > BA|x| > A|x|,$$

and by induction we obtain for each integer $k > 1$,

$$B^k A|x| > B^{k-1}A|x| > \cdots > BA|x| > A|x|.$$

Hence for each $k > 1$ one has

$$B^k A|x| > A|x|. \tag{4.2}$$

On the other hand we also have

$$r(B) = \frac{1}{1+\varepsilon}r(A) = \frac{1}{1+\varepsilon} < 1,$$

which implies that

$$\lim_{k \to \infty} B^k = 0.$$

Taking the limit as k goes to $+\infty$ in (4.2), we obtain

$$0 \geq A|x|,$$

which is impossible since $A \gg 0$ and $|x| > 0$ imply that $A|x| \gg 0$. Therefore we deduce that

$$A|x| = |x|,$$

and 1 is an eigenvalue of A.

Proof of (iii). We still assume that $r(A) = 1$. Let λ be an eigenvalue with modulus 1. Let $x \in \mathbb{C}^n \setminus \{0\}$ be an eigenvector of A associated to λ. Then from the previous part of the proof we have

$$A|x| = |x|. \tag{4.3}$$

This equality implies first that $|x| \gg 0$ (since $A \gg 0$ and $|x| > 0$). Therefore

$$x_j \neq 0, \quad \forall j \in \{1, \ldots, n\}.$$

By using (4.3) again, we have for each $j \in \{1, \ldots, n\}$

$$|x_j| = \sum_{k=1}^{n} a_{jk}|x_k| = \sum_{k=1}^{n} |a_{jk}x_k|$$

and since $Ax = \lambda x$ we also have

$$|x_j| = |\lambda||x_j| = |(\lambda x)_j| = |(Ax)_j| = \left|\sum_{k=1}^{n} a_{jk}x_k\right|.$$

Coupling the above two equalities we obtain, for each $j \in \{1, \ldots, n\}$,

$$\sum_{k=1}^{n} |a_{jk}x_k| = \left|\sum_{k=1}^{n} a_{jk}x_k\right|.$$

Let $j \in \{1, \ldots, n\}$ be fixed and set

$$z_k := a_{jk}x_k \in \mathbb{C}, \quad \forall k \in \{1, \ldots, n\}.$$

Then the above equality can be rewritten as

$$\left|\sum_{k=1}^{n} z_k\right| = \sum_{k=1}^{n} |z_k|.$$

Next Lemma 4.28 applies and ensures that for each $k \in \{2, \ldots, n\}$, there exists an $\alpha_k > 0$ such that

$$z_j = \alpha_j z_1.$$

Hence we can find positive real numbers $\alpha_2 > 0, \ldots, \alpha_n > 0$ such that for each $k \in \{2, \ldots, n\}$,

$$a_{jk}x_k = \alpha_k a_{j1}x_1,$$

so that the vector x can be rewritten as

$$x = x_1 \begin{pmatrix} 1 \\ \alpha_2 \dfrac{a_{j1}}{a_{j2}} \\ \vdots \\ \alpha_n \dfrac{a_{j1}}{a_{jn}} \end{pmatrix}.$$

But since $Ax = \lambda x$, by dividing both sides of this equality by x_1 we obtain

$$\lambda \begin{pmatrix} 1 \\ \alpha_2 \dfrac{a_{j1}}{a_{j2}} \\ \vdots \\ \alpha_n \dfrac{a_{j1}}{a_{jn}} \end{pmatrix} = A \begin{pmatrix} 1 \\ \alpha_2 \dfrac{a_{j1}}{a_{j2}} \\ \vdots \\ \alpha_n \dfrac{a_{j1}}{a_{jn}} \end{pmatrix}.$$

Thus $\lambda \in (0, \infty)$ and since $|\lambda| = 1$, one obtains $\lambda = 1$. As a consequence 1 is the only eigenvalue with modulus 1.

Proof of (iv). Here we still assume that $r(A) = 1$. Let $x \in \mathbb{C}^n \setminus \{0\}$ be an eigenvector of A associated to the eigenvalue 1. Then from the proof of (ii) we have $A|x| = |x|$ and $|x| \gg 0$ (since $A \gg 0$ and $|x| > 0$). Therefore one can choose $v_r = |x|$. Similarly since $r(A) = r(A^T)$ we can apply the same argument to the transposed matrix A^T and we can find $v_l \gg 0$ such that $A^T v_l = v_l$.

Proof of (v). Let us first prove that the geometric multiplicity of $r(A) = 1$ is 1. Assume by contradiction that $\dim(\mathrm{N}(A - r(A)I)) > 1$. Then we can find two linearly independent (non-null) vectors $u \in \mathbb{R}^n \setminus \{0\}$ and $v \in \mathbb{R}^n \setminus \{0\}$ such that

$$Au = u \text{ and } Av = v.$$

From part (ii), we have $A|u| = |u|$ and $A|v| = |v|$, which implies that $|u| \gg 0$ ($\Leftrightarrow u_i \neq 0, \forall i = 1, \ldots, n$) and $|v| \gg 0$ ($\Leftrightarrow v_i \neq 0, \forall i = 1, \ldots, n$) .

Define $w := v_1 u - u_1 v$. Then by construction $w_1 = 0$. Moreover, since $u_1 \neq 0$ and $v_1 \neq 0$ and u and v are linearly independent, we must have $w \neq 0$, and since u and v are two eigenvectors associated to $r(A) = 1$, we must have $Aw = w$. We deduce that

$$A|w| = |w| \gg 0,$$

and we obtain a contradiction with the fact that $w_1 = 0$. We deduce that the geometric multiplicity of $r(A) = 1$ is 1, that is,

$$\dim(\mathrm{N}(A - I)) = 1.$$

Next, assume by contradiction that the algebraic multiplicity of $r(A) = 1$ is not 1. This implies that

$$\mathrm{N}(A - I)^2 \neq \mathrm{N}(A - I).$$

Remember that $\mathrm{N}(A - I) \subset \mathrm{N}(A - I)^2$. It follows that we can find $x \in \mathrm{N}(A - I)^2$ such that

$$x \notin \mathrm{N}(A - I).$$

Therefore we can find

$$Ax = x + y \text{ with } Ay = y \text{ and } y \gg 0.$$

But we also have for each integer $k \in \mathbb{N}$

$$A(x + ky) = (x + ky) + y.$$

Choosing k large enough, one can assume that $z := x + ky \gg 0$ and

$$Az = z + y.$$

We obtain $z \ll Az$ and $z \gg 0$, which is impossible from the proof of part (ii). This completes the proof of the theorem. $\square$

Consider the linear operator $\Pi : \mathbb{R}^n \to \mathbb{R}^n$ defined by

$$\Pi x := \frac{\langle v_l, x \rangle}{\langle v_l, v_r \rangle} v_r.$$

Then Π is a projector, that is,

$$\Pi^2 = \Pi.$$

Moreover, Π commutes with A and we have

$$A\Pi = \Pi A = r(A)\Pi.$$

We deduce that

$$A(I - \Pi) = (I - \Pi)A,$$

and we obtain a state space decomposition

$$\mathbb{R}^n = \mathrm{R}(\Pi) \oplus \mathrm{R}(I - \Pi),$$

where $\mathrm{R}(\Pi)$ (respectively $\mathrm{R}(I - \Pi)$) is the range of Π (respectively $I - \Pi$). Moreover, we have

$$A(\mathrm{R}(\Pi)) \subset \mathrm{R}(\Pi) \text{ and } A(\mathrm{R}(I - \Pi)) \subset \mathrm{R}(I - \Pi).$$

From the Perron–Frobenius theorem we know that $r(A)$ is an eigenvalue of A with algebraic multiplicity 1, so we have

$$\sigma(A|_{\mathrm{R}(I-\Pi)}) = \sigma(A)\backslash\{r(A)\}.$$

Furthermore, since $r(A)$ is the only eigenvalue in the peripheral spectrum of A, we deduce that

$$r(A|_{\mathrm{R}(I-\Pi)}) < r(A).$$

Therefore by choosing $\delta \in \left(\frac{r(A|_{\mathrm{R}(I-\Pi)})}{r(A)}, 1 \right)$, one can find a constant $M = M(\delta) \geq 1$ such that

$$\left\| \frac{1}{r(A)^k} A^k (I - \Pi) \right\| \leq M\delta^k, \forall k \in \mathbb{N}.$$

As a consequence of the Perron–Frobenius theorem, we obtain the following result.

Corollary 4.29 *Let $A \in M_n(\mathbb{R})$ be a strictly positive matrix (i.e. $A \gg 0$). Then the rank 1 projector $\Pi \in M_n(\mathbb{R})$ defined by*

$$\Pi x := \frac{\langle v_l, x \rangle}{\langle v_l, v_r \rangle} v_r$$

satisfies

$$A\Pi = \Pi A = r(A)\Pi$$

and

$$\lim_{k \to +\infty} \frac{1}{r(A)^k} A^k = \Pi.$$

More precisely, we can find two constants $M > 1$ and $\delta \in (0, 1)$ such that for any $x \in \mathbb{R}^n$ one has

$$\left\| \Pi x - \frac{1}{r(A)^k} A^k x \right\| = \left\| \frac{1}{r(A)^k} A^k (I - \Pi) x \right\| \leq M \delta^k \| (I - \Pi) x \|.$$

Remark 4.30 The above property is also called the *asynchronous exponential growth* property. This means that the normalized distribution converges to a distribution that is independent of the initial distribution.

Remark 4.31 Let $A \in M_n(\mathbb{R})$ be a strictly positive matrix (i.e. $A \gg 0$). Assume that the dynamical distribution of population is described by the difference equation in $\mathbb{R}^n$

$$N(t + 1) = AN(t), \quad \forall t \in \mathbb{N} \text{ and } N(0) = N_0 \geq 0.$$

Consider a left eigenvector $v_l \gg 0$ associated to the spectral radius $r(A)$. Then one has

$$\langle v_l, N(t + 1) \rangle = \langle v_l, AN(t) \rangle = r(A) \langle v_l, N(t) \rangle$$

and by induction we get

$$\langle v_l, N(t) \rangle = r(A)^t \langle v_l, X_0 \rangle, \ \forall t \in \mathbb{N}.$$

In addition, observe that the map

$$\| x \|_1 := \langle v_l, |x| \rangle, \ \forall x \in \mathbb{R}^n$$

is a norm on $\mathbb{R}^n$.

As a consequence, when a population density is described by such a discrete-time model, the Perron–Frobenius theorem provides an equivalent indicator of the Malthusian growth. Namely, we have

$$\| N(t) \|_1 = r(A)^t \| N_0 \|_1, \quad \forall t \in \mathbb{N}.$$

Moreover, for $N_0 > 0$ in $\mathbb{R}^n$, the asynchronous exponential growth as stated in Corollary 4.29 means the following convergence for the normalized distribution

$$\lim_{t \to +\infty} \frac{N(t)}{\| N(t) \|_1} = \frac{\Pi N_0}{\langle v_l, N_0 \rangle} = \frac{v_r}{\langle v_l, v_r \rangle}.$$

Herein $v_r \gg 0$ denotes a right eigenvector associated to the spectral radius $r(A)$.

4.4.3 Primitive and irreducible matrices

In this section, we extend the Perron–Frobenius theorem to a larger class of matrices, the class of so-called primitive and irreducible matrices.

Definition 4.32 Let $A \in M_n(\mathbb{R})$ be a non-negative matrix. We will say that A is *primitive* if there exists an integer $m \geq 1$ such that

$$A^m \gg 0.$$

We will say that a matrix $A \in M_n(\mathbb{R})$ is *irreducible* if there exists an integer $m \geq 1$ such that

$$I + A + A^2 + \cdots + A^m \gg 0.$$

Remark 4.33 A matrix is *reducible* if it is not irreducible. For a reducible matrix A, one can find that a permutation of the elements of the basis, such that the matrix of A expressed in the permuted basis is block lower triangular

$$B = \begin{bmatrix} B_{11} & 0 \\ B_{21} & B_{22} \end{bmatrix},$$

where B_{11} and B_{22} are both square blocks.

Definition 4.34 Let $A = (a_{ij})$ be an $n \times n$ non-negative matrix. Consider n distinct points $P_1, P_2, \ldots, P_n$ in the plane, which we call *nodes*. If $a_{ij} > 0$, we connect node P_j to P_i by means of a directed path. The graph obtained is called the *graph $G(A)$ associated with the matrix A.*

Definition 4.35 A directed graph $G(A)$ is *strongly connected* if for any pair of nodes P_i and P_j there exists a directed path connecting P_i to P_j (such a direct path can eventually be composed by several single paths joining some intermediate nodes).

Proposition 4.36 *The following properties are equivalent*

(i) *A is irreducible.*
(ii) *The matrix $\varepsilon I + A$ is primitive for all $\varepsilon > 0$.*
(iii) *For each $i, j \in 1, \ldots, n$, there exists an integer $m = m(i, j) > 0$ such that*

$$\langle e_j, A^m e_i \rangle > 0,$$

where $\{e_1, \ldots, e_n\}$ denotes the canonical basis of $\mathbb{R}^n$.
(iv) *The directed graph $G(A)$ of A is strongly connected.*

Proof Proof of $(i) \Leftrightarrow (ii)$. Let $m > 0$ be a given integer and $\varepsilon > 0$. By using the binomial formula we have

$$(\varepsilon I + A)^m = \sum_{k=0,\ldots,m} C_n^k \varepsilon^{n-k} A^k$$

with $A^0 = I$. Next we can find two numbers $0 < c_- < c_+$ such that

$$c_-(I + A + A^2 + \cdots + A^m) \leq (\varepsilon I + A)^m \leq c_+(I + A + A^2 + \cdots + A^m).$$

The proofs of $(i) \Leftrightarrow (iii)$ and $(i) \Leftrightarrow (iv)$ are left as an exercise. $\square$

The following theorem can be found in the book of Horn and Johnson [161, Theorem 8.5.3, p. 517].

Theorem 4.37 *A non-negative matrix A is primitive if and only if G(A) is strongly connected and the greatest common divisor of the lengths of all paths from P_i to itself is one.*

Remark 4.38 Horn and Johnson [161, Corollary 8.5.9, p. 520] proved by using graph theory applied to $G(A)$ that the matrix A is primitive if and only if

$$A^{n^2} \gg 0.$$

Remark 4.39 Observe that if A is primitive then A is irreducible. The converse is false. Indeed, consider the Leslie matrix $A = \begin{bmatrix} 0 & 1 \\ 1 & 0 \end{bmatrix}$. Then one has

$$I + A \gg 0.$$

So A is irreducible. But A is not primitive since $A^{2n} = I, \quad \forall n \in \mathbb{N}$.

In Figure 4.3 the first primitive graphs correspond, for example, to the matrices

$$\begin{pmatrix} 1/2 & 0 & 1 \\ 1/2 & 0 & 0 \\ 0 & 1 & 0 \end{pmatrix} \text{ and } \begin{pmatrix} 0 & 1 & 1 \\ 1 & 0 & 0 \\ 0 & 1 & 0 \end{pmatrix}$$

while the irreducible and non-irreducible graphs correspond to the matrices

$$\begin{pmatrix} 0 & 0 & 1 \\ 1 & 0 & 0 \\ 0 & 1 & 0 \end{pmatrix} \text{ and } \begin{pmatrix} 0 & 1 & 0 \\ 1 & 0 & 0 \\ 0 & 1 & 0 \end{pmatrix}.$$

Our next theorem is concerned with primitive matrices.

Theorem 4.40 *Let $A \in M_n(\mathbb{R})$ be a non-negative and primitive matrix. Then the conclusions of Theorem 4.25 and Corollary 4.29 hold.*

Exercise 4.41 Prove Theorem 4.40. Reconsider the arguments given in the proof of Theorem 4.25 for a matrix A which now is only primitive.

Hint: By using the Jordan reduction again we can prove that for each integer $n > 0$

$$\sigma(A^n) = \{\lambda^n : \lambda \in \sigma(A)\},$$

and of course one has $|\lambda^n| = |\lambda|^n$, for all $\lambda \in \mathbb{C}$.

As already mentioned, the matrix

$$A = \begin{bmatrix} 0 & 1 \\ 1 & 0 \end{bmatrix}$$

is irreducible but not primitive. The characteristic equation is

$$\det(\lambda I - A) = \lambda^2 - 1, \forall \lambda \in \mathbb{C}.$$

Graphs of primitive matrices

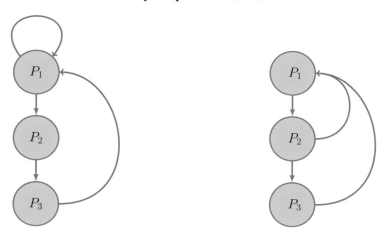

Graph of a (non-primitive) irreducible matrix   **Graph of a non-irreducible matrix**

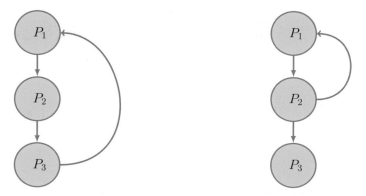

Fig. 4.3: *In this figure we show some examples of graphs $G(A)$ of primitive, irreducible and non-irreducible matrices.*

Therefore the spectrum of A reads as

$$\sigma(A) = \{-1, 1\}.$$

So the peripheral spectrum of A is not reduced to its spectral radius $r(A) = 1$.
  More generally the same result holds for the following $n \times n$ Leslie matrix

$$L_n = \begin{bmatrix} 0 & 0 & \cdots & 0 & \beta \\ \pi & 0 & \cdots & \cdots & 0 \\ 0 & \pi & 0 & & \vdots \\ \vdots & \ddots & \ddots & \ddots & 0 \\ 0 & \cdots & 0 & \pi & 0 \end{bmatrix} \in M_n(\mathbb{R}),$$

for some parameters $\beta > 0$ and $\pi > 0$. Note that one has

$$L_n^n = \beta \pi^{n-1} I.$$

So for all eigenvalues $\lambda \in \sigma(L)$, we have

$$\lambda^n = \beta \pi^{n-1}.$$

Therefore the spectrum and the peripheral spectrum of L coincide.

Our next result is concerned with irreducible matrices.

Theorem 4.42 *Let $A \in M_n(\mathbb{R})$ be a non-negative and irreducible matrix. Then the following properties hold:*

(i) $r(A) > 0$.
(ii) $r(A)$ *is an eigenvalue of A.*
(iii) *There exists $v_r \gg 0$ (a right eigenvector of A) and $v_l \gg 0$ (a left eigenvector of A) such that*
$$Av_r = r(A)v_r \text{ and } v_l^T A = r(A)v_l^T.$$

(iv) $r(A)$ *is a simple eigenvalue of A.*

Moreover, if A is not primitive, then the peripheral spectrum of A contains some eigenvalues distinct from $r(A)$.

Exercise 4.43 Prove Theorem 4.42.

Hint 1: Let $\varepsilon > 0$ be given so that the matrix $A + \varepsilon I$ is primitive and

$$\lambda \in \sigma(A) \Leftrightarrow \lambda + \varepsilon \in \sigma(A + \varepsilon I).$$

Hint 2: For the last part of the theorem, assume by contradiction that the peripheral spectrum of A contains no other eigenvalue than $r(A)$. Then as above conclude that

$$\lim_{k \to +\infty} \frac{1}{r(A)^k} A^k = \Pi \gg 0$$

(where $\Pi = v_r v_l^T$), which implies that A is primitive.

Example 4.44 In Figure 4.4 we plot the spectrum of

$$L_4 = \begin{bmatrix} 0 & 0 & 0 & \beta \\ \pi & 0 & 0 & 0 \\ 0 & \pi & 0 & 0 \\ 0 & 0 & \pi & 0 \end{bmatrix}.$$

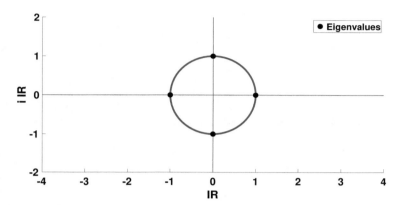

Fig. 4.4: *In this figure we plot the spectrum of the above Leslie matrix L_4 with $\pi = 1$ and $\beta = 1$.*

In Figure 4.5 we plot the spectrum of

$$\widehat{L}_4 = \begin{bmatrix} 0 & 0 & \beta & \beta \\ \pi & 0 & 0 & 0 \\ 0 & \pi & 0 & 0 \\ 0 & 0 & \pi & 0 \end{bmatrix}.$$

The major difference between L_4 and $\widehat{L}_4$ is that $\widehat{L}_4$ is primitive while L_4 is only irreducible.

4.5 Applications of the Perron–Frobenius Theorem

4.5.1 Application to Leslie's model

In this section, we reconsider the Leslie matrix introduced in Chapter 1. Consider the Leslie model

$$U^{t+1} = LU^t, \text{ for all } t \geq 0, \text{ with } U^0 = U_0 \in \mathbb{R}_+^{m+1},$$

where the Leslie matrix L is given by

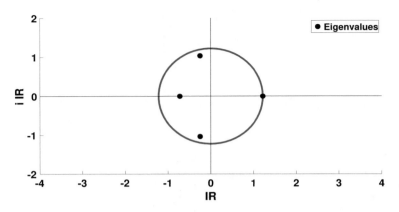

Fig. 4.5: *In this figure we plot the spectrum of the above Leslie matrix* $\widehat{L}_4$ *with* $\pi = 1$ *and* $\beta = 1$.

$$
L = \begin{bmatrix}
\beta_0 & \beta_1 & \cdots & \cdots & \beta_m \\
\pi_0 & 0 & \cdots & \cdots & 0 \\
0 & \pi_1 & 0 & & \vdots \\
\vdots & \ddots & \ddots & \ddots & 0 \\
0 & \cdots & 0 & \pi_{m-1} & 0
\end{bmatrix}.
$$

Here we assume that

$$\beta_j \geq 0, \quad \forall j = 0, \ldots, m$$

and

$$\pi_j > 0, \quad \forall j = 0, \ldots, m - 1.$$

By computing the powers of the Leslie matrix

$$
\widehat{L} = \begin{bmatrix}
0 & 0 & \cdots & 0 & 1 \\
1 & 0 & \cdots & \cdots & 0 \\
0 & 1 & 0 & & \vdots \\
\vdots & \ddots & \ddots & \ddots & 0 \\
0 & \cdots & 0 & 1 & 0
\end{bmatrix} \in M_{m+1}(\mathbb{R}),
$$

one obtains the following lemma.

Lemma 4.45 *The matrix L is irreducible if* $\beta_m > 0$.

The following proposition is also a consequence of Theorem 4.37. This result is due to Demetrius [75].

Proposition 4.46 *Assume that* $\beta_m > 0$ *and that there exists an integer* $j_0 \in \{0, 1, \ldots, m - 1\}$ *such that*

$$\beta_{j_0} > 0 \ and \ \beta_{j_0+1} > 0.$$

Then L is a primitive matrix.

Proof It is also instructive to prove the above proposition by considering the renewal equation for $t > m - 1$

$$U_0(t + 1) = \beta_0 U_0(t) + \beta_1 \pi_0 U_0(t - 1) + \cdots + \beta_m \pi_0 \times \pi_{m-1} U_0(t - (m - 1)).$$

The proof is left to the reader. □

From the above results and the Perron–Frobenius theorem, the following lemma follows.

Theorem 4.47 *Assume that $\beta_m > 0$. Then the spectral radius $r(L) > 0$ is the unique positive solution of the λ-equation*

$$1 = \frac{1}{\lambda} \left[\beta_0 + \beta_1 \frac{\pi_0}{\lambda} + \beta_2 \frac{\pi_0}{\lambda} \frac{\pi_1}{\lambda} + \cdots + \beta_m \frac{\pi_0}{\lambda} \frac{\pi_1}{\lambda} \times \cdots \times \frac{\pi_{m-1}}{\lambda} \right].$$

Moreover, the right eigenvector of L associated with $r(L)$ is given by

$$U_r := \begin{pmatrix} 1 \\ \frac{\pi_0}{r(L)} \\ \frac{\pi_0}{r(L)} \frac{\pi_1}{r(L)} \\ \vdots \\ \frac{\pi_0}{r(L)} \frac{\pi_1}{r(L)} \times \cdots \times \frac{\pi_{m-1}}{r(L)} \end{pmatrix}.$$

Furthermore, setting

$$R_0 := \beta_0 + \beta_1 \pi_0 + \beta_2 \pi_0 \pi_1 + \cdots + \beta_m \pi_0 \pi_1 \times \cdots \times \pi_{m-1},$$

we have following alternatives:

(i) *If $R_0 > 1$ then $r(L) > 1$.*
(ii) *If $R_0 = 1$ then $r(L) = 1$.*
(iii) *If $R_0 < 1$ then $r(L) < 1$.*

If we assume in addition that L is primitive, then for each initial distribution $U_0 > 0$ the solution of the difference equation

$$U(t + 1) = LU(t), \forall t \geq 0, \ and \ U(0) = U_0 > 0,$$

satisfies the following asymptotic behavior

$$\lim_{t \to +\infty} \frac{1}{U(t)_0 + U(t)_1 + \ldots + U(t)_m} U(t) = \frac{1}{U_{r0} + U_{r1} + \ldots + U_{rm}} U_r.$$

Figure 4.6, taken from Chapter 1, illustrates this last convergence result to the right eigenvector.

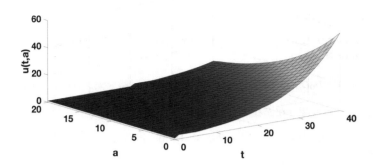

Fig. 4.6: *In this figure we plot a solution* $t \to u(t, a)$ *of the Leslie model* $a \in [0, 20]$. *The reproduction function* $\beta(a) = 0.8 * \Delta a$ *if* $a > 5$ *and* $\beta(a) = 0$ *otherwise. The survival rate is* $\pi(a) = \exp(-0.1 * \Delta a)$. *The initial distribution is constant equal to* 1. *We observe that it takes* 40 *years for the distribution of population to grow exponentially.*

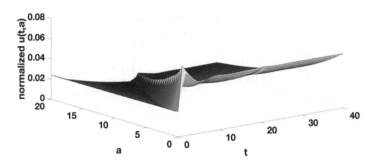

Fig. 4.7: *In this figure we plot a normalized solution* $t \to u(t, a)/\Sigma_{i=0,\ldots,20} u(t, i)$ *of the Leslie model* $a \in [0, 20]$. *The reproduction function is defined by* $\beta(a) = 0.8 * \Delta a$ *if* $a > 5$ *and* $\beta(a) = 0$ *otherwise. The survival rate is* $\pi(a) = \exp(-0.1 * \Delta a)$. *The initial distribution is constant equal to* 1. *We observe the convergence of the normalized distribution when the time becomes large enough.*

Note that since $\beta_m > 0$, the matrix L is irreducible (see Lemma 4.45). Hence, due to the Perron–Frobenius theorem (see Theorem 4.37, Theorem 4.42 and its corollary), to prove the above theorem, it is sufficient to check the first assertion on the spectral radius $r(L) > 0$. To see this, note that the equation

$$U \in \mathbb{R}^{m+1} \setminus \{0\} \text{ and } r(L)U = LU,$$

which can be rewritten as $\lambda = r(L) > 0$, satisfies the equation

$$1 = \frac{1}{\lambda} \left[\beta_0 + \beta_1 \frac{\pi_0}{\lambda} + \beta_2 \frac{\pi_0}{\lambda} \frac{\pi_1}{\lambda} + \ldots + \beta_m \frac{\pi_0}{\lambda} \frac{\pi_1}{\lambda} \times \ldots \times \frac{\pi_{m-1}}{\lambda} \right] =: f(\lambda).$$

Next, since $\beta_m > 0$, we have

$$\lim_{\lambda \to 0} f(\lambda) = +\infty \quad \text{and} \quad \lim_{\lambda \to +\infty} f(\lambda) = 0,$$

and since f is decreasing on $(0, \infty)$, the above equation has a unique solution $\lambda_0 > 0$, that is, $\lambda_0 = r(L)$.

Remark 4.48 Leslie's model was used by Song to understand how to control the growth of the population in China. The number $N_i(t)$ is the number of females in age class i. Assume that β_i is the average number of newborns per female in age class i, which has been estimate over one year. Assume that π_i is the fraction of females surviving from age class i to age class $i+1$. Then (by using the characteristic equation) one can derive the growth rate $r(L)$. Song's work on population control led to the one-child policy in China [331, 332]. More information can be found in Greenhalgh [120, 121].

More recently, since the growth rate $r(L)$ has been reduced by the one-child policy, the expected distribution of the population v_r has changed. When we normalize v_r (i.e. divide by $v_{r0} + v_{r1} + \cdots + v_{rm}$) we obtain the expected distribution of population of China. That is, one can compute the expected fraction of young people, middle-aged people, and old people in the population. Since the expected number of old people is now too large compared to the expected number of middle-aged people (or working people), the authorities decided to change the one-child policy, and a second child is now allowed in China. Of course, some further analysis is needed to understand the consequences of such a change.

4.5.2 Application to the space-time discrete diffusion process

In this section we consider the space-time discrete heat equation with Neumann homogeneous boundary conditions. As discussed in Chapter 1, if $\Delta t > 0$ and $\Delta x > 0$ denote respectively the time and space step, the discrete heat equation reads for $t \geq 0$ as

$$u(t + \Delta t) = u(t) + \frac{\varepsilon \Delta t}{\Delta x^2} D \, u(t) \quad \text{with } u(0) = u_0 \in \mathbb{R}_+^N.$$

Herein the matrix D is given by

$$D = \begin{pmatrix} -1 & 1 & 0 & \dots & \dots & 0 \\ 1 & -2 & 1 & \ddots & & \vdots \\ 0 & 1 & -2 & \ddots & \ddots & \vdots \\ \vdots & \ddots & \ddots & & \ddots & 0 \\ \vdots & & \ddots & 1 & -2 & 1 \\ 0 & \dots & & 0 & 1 & -1 \end{pmatrix}.$$

To understand the dynamical behavior of the difference equation, we first investigate some basic properties of the matrix D.

Lemma 4.49 *Assume that* $p := 2\frac{\varepsilon \Delta t}{\Delta x^2} < 1$. *Then the matrix* $I + \frac{\varepsilon \Delta t}{\Delta x^2} D$ *is non-negative and primitive.*

Remark 4.50 The condition $2\frac{\varepsilon \Delta t}{\Delta x^2} < 1$ is called the *CFL (Courant–Friedrichs–Lax)* condition.

It is readily checked that

$$D\mathbb{1} = 0 \text{ and } \mathbb{1}^T D = 0^T.$$

Hence we get

$$\left(I + \frac{\varepsilon \Delta t}{\Delta x^2} D \right) \mathbb{1} = \mathbb{1} \text{ and } \mathbb{1}^T \left(I + \frac{\varepsilon \Delta t}{\Delta x^2} D \right) = \mathbb{1}^T,$$

and applying the Perron–Frobenius theorem we deduce that the following lemma holds.

Lemma 4.51 *Assume that* $p = 2\frac{\varepsilon \Delta t}{\Delta x^2} < 1$. *Then the spectral radius of the matrix* $I + \frac{\varepsilon \Delta t}{\Delta x^2} D$ *is given by*

$$r\left(I + \frac{\varepsilon \Delta t}{\Delta x^2} D \right) = 1.$$

Moreover, for each $u_0 \geq 0$ *one has*

$$\sum_{i=1}^N u(t)_i = \sum_{i=1}^N u_{0i}, \quad \forall t \geq 0,$$

which means that the total number of individuals is constant, and

$$\lim_{n \to +\infty} u(t) = \left(\sum_{i=1}^N u_{0i} \right) \begin{pmatrix} 1/N \\ 1/N \\ \vdots \\ 1/N \end{pmatrix},$$

which means that the individuals are equally redistributed between the cities.

Proof Since by assumption $p < 1$ we deduce by applying Theorem 4.37 that the matrix $M = (I + \frac{\varepsilon \Delta t}{\Delta x^2} D)$ is primitive. Therefore, by using the Perron–Frobenius theorem, we know that there exists a $v_l \gg 0$ such that

$$v_l^T M = r(M) v_l^T.$$

But

$$v_l^T \mathbb{1} = v_l^T M \mathbb{1} = r(M) v_l^T \mathbb{1}.$$

Therefore $r(M) = 1$. The result follows by using the fact that the dimension of the right and left eigenspace of M associated with 1 is one. Therefore the right eigenspace of M associated to 1 is $\mathbb{R}\mathbb{1}$ and the left eigenspace of M associated to 1 is $\mathbb{R}\mathbb{1}^T$.   □

Figure 4.8 illustrates this convergence result.

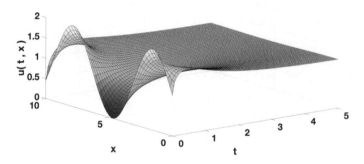

Fig. 4.8: *In this figure we plot a heat equation with $x \in [0, 10]$. The diffusion coefficient is equal to $\varepsilon = 2$. The initial distribution is constant equal to $u_0(x) = 1 + \sin(x)$. We observe the quite rapid convergence to the constant distribution.*

Exercise 4.52 Assume that $2\frac{\varepsilon \Delta t}{\Delta x^2} < 1$. Consider the implicit numerical scheme given by

$$u(t + \Delta t) = u(t) + \frac{\varepsilon \Delta t}{\Delta x^2} D\, u(t + \Delta t),$$

yielding the following linear difference equation

$$\left(I - \frac{\varepsilon \Delta t}{\Delta x^2} D \right) u(t + \Delta t) = u(t), \quad \forall t \geq 0 \text{ and } u(0) = u_0.$$

Prove that if $2\frac{\varepsilon \Delta t}{\Delta x^2} < 1$, then the matrix $(I - \frac{\varepsilon \Delta t}{\Delta x^2} D)$ is invertible and the matrix $(I - \frac{\varepsilon \Delta t}{\Delta x^2} D)^{-1}$ is strictly positive.

4.5.3 The Perron–Frobenius theorem for linear ordinary differential equations

In this part, we come back to the positivity property of the solutions of linear differential equations and we describe some further properties as a consequence of the Perron–Frobenius theorem. Our result reads as follows.

Theorem 4.53 *Let $A \in M_n(\mathbb{R})$ be a given matrix such that for all $\delta > 0$ large enough $\delta I + A$ is a non-negative and primitive matrix. Then the following properties hold:*

(i) *For each $t > 0$ one has*

$$e^{At} \gg 0.$$

(ii) *The spectral bound of A, $s(A) := \max\{\mathrm{Re}(\lambda) : \lambda \in \sigma(A)\}$, is a simple eigenvalue of the matrix A.*

(iii) *For each $\lambda \in \sigma(A) \backslash \{s(A)\}$ one has*

$$\mathrm{Re}(\lambda) < s(A).$$

(iv) *There exist two vectors $v_r \gg 0$ and $v_l \gg 0$ such that*

$$v_l^T A = s(A) v_l^T \text{ and } A v_r = s(A) v_r.$$

(v) *If Π is the projector given by $\Pi(x) := \frac{\langle v_l, x \rangle}{\langle v_l, v_r \rangle} v_r$ for $x \in \mathbb{R}^n$, then we have*

$$\Pi e^{At} = e^{At} \Pi = e^{s(A)t} \Pi, \quad \forall t \geq 0,$$

and there exist two constants $\chi > 0$ and $M \geq 1$ such that

$$\|e^{-s(A)t} e^{At} (I - \Pi)\| \leq M e^{-\chi t} \|(I - \Pi)\|, \quad \forall t \geq 0.$$

Remark 4.54 In the above theorem, the diagonal elements of A can have any sign, while all the off-diagonal elements of A are non-negative.

Proof *Proof of (i).* Let $\delta > 0$ be such that $\delta I + A$ is non-negative and primitive. Then we have

$$e^{At} = e^{-\delta t} e^{(A+\delta I)t} = e^{-\delta t} \sum_{k=0}^{+\infty} \frac{((A + \delta I)t)^k}{k!} \gg 0, \quad \forall t > 0.$$

Sketch of the proof for (ii)–(iv). To prove (ii) implies (iv), it is sufficient to apply the Perron–Frobenius theorem to the primitive matrix $(A + \delta I)$ and to observe that one has

$$\lambda \in \sigma(A) \Leftrightarrow \lambda + \delta \in \sigma(A + \delta I).$$

Now assertion (v) is a direct consequence of (ii)–(iv). □

Example 4.55 We reconsider the heat equation, but now we assume the time is continuous while the space is discrete. In other words, we assume that the individuals are located at some discrete positions. Then we can consider the ordinary differential equation

$$u'(t) = \frac{\gamma}{2} Du(t), \forall t \geq 0, \text{ and } u(0) = u_0 \geq 0,$$

where D has been defined in the previous section and $u(t)_i$ is the number of individuals in position i. Then for $i = 2, \ldots, N - 1$

$$u_i(t)' = \frac{\gamma}{2} (u_{i+1} + u_{i-1}) - \gamma u_i$$

with

$$u_1(t)' = \frac{\gamma}{2} (u_2 - u_1)$$

and

$$u_N(t)' = \frac{\gamma}{2} (u_{N-1} - u_N).$$

Here the parameter $\gamma > 0$ is the leaving rate of individuals at position i. In other words, the time spent in position i follows the exponential law with average

$$T = \frac{1}{\gamma}.$$

By applying Theorem 4.53 we obtain the following lemma.

Lemma 4.56 *For each $u_0 \geq 0$ we have*

$$\lim_{t \to +\infty} u(t) = (u_{01} + u_{02} + \cdots + u_{0N}) \begin{pmatrix} 1/N \\ 1/N \\ \vdots \\ 1/N \end{pmatrix}.$$

4.5.4 Stability criteria for linear ordinary differential equations

The stability criteria stated in this part are commonly used in population dynamics. In the context of epidemic models, such criteria have been extensively used in the literature. We refer to Diekmann, Heesterbeek and Metz [88] and to Van den Driessche and Watmough [93]. One can also find some infinite-dimensional versions of this result, for which we refer to Thieme [340].

Example 4.57 In order to illustrate this stability result, let us consider the following continuous-time Leslie model

$$\frac{\mathrm{d}}{\mathrm{d}t} \begin{pmatrix} U_0(t) \\ U_1(t) \end{pmatrix} = L \begin{pmatrix} U_0(t) \\ U_1(t) \end{pmatrix} \tag{4.4}$$

wherein the matrix L takes the form

$$L := \begin{pmatrix} \beta_0 - \mu_0 & \beta_1 \\ \eta_0 & -\mu_1 \end{pmatrix}$$

for some given parameters $\beta_0 \geq 0, \beta_1 > 0, \eta_0 > 0, \mu_0 > 0, \mu_1 > 0$.
Set

$$A = \begin{pmatrix} -\mu_0 & 0 \\ 0 & -\mu_1 \end{pmatrix} \text{ and } B = \begin{pmatrix} \beta_0 & \beta_1 \\ \eta_0 & 0 \end{pmatrix}.$$

Then we have

$$\begin{aligned} B(-A)^{-1} &= \begin{pmatrix} \beta_0 & \beta_1 \\ \eta_0 & 0 \end{pmatrix} \times \begin{pmatrix} \mu_0^{-1} & 0 \\ 0 & \mu_1^{-1} \end{pmatrix} \\ &= \begin{pmatrix} \beta_0 \mu_0^{-1} & \beta_1 \mu_1^{-1} \\ \eta_0 \mu_0^{-1} & 0 \end{pmatrix}. \end{aligned}$$

The matrix $B(-A)^{-1}$ is irreducible, and by using Lemma 4.47 we deduce that $r(B(-A)^{-1}) < 1$ if

$$R_0 := \beta_0 \mu_0^{-1} + \beta_1 \mu_1^{-1} \eta_0 \mu_0^{-1} < 1.$$

It follows from Theorem 4.58 that (4.4) is stable (i.e. $s(L) < 0$) if $R_0 < 1$.

Theorem 4.58 (Stability) *Let $A, B \in M_n(\mathbb{R})$ be two given matrices with $\delta I + A \geq 0$ for some $\delta \geq 0$ and $B \geq 0$. Assume that $\mathrm{s}(A) < 0$ or equivalently the equilibrium 0 is exponentially asymptotically stable for the system*

$$X'(t) = AX(t).$$

Assume in addition that the matrix $B(-A)^{-1}$ is non-negative and irreducible and satisfies

$$r\left(B(-A)^{-1}\right) < 1.$$

Then one has $\mathrm{s}(A + B) < 0$ or equivalently the equilibrium 0 is exponentially asymptotically stable for the system

$$X'(t) = (A + B)X(t).$$

Proof Let us prove that $\mathrm{s}(A + B) < 0$. With that aim, let $\lambda \in \mathbb{C}$ be given with $\mathrm{Re}(\lambda) \geq 0$. Observe first that since for all $(x, y) \in \mathbb{R}^n \times \mathbb{R}^n$ one has

$$(\lambda I - (A + B))x = y \Leftrightarrow [I - B(\lambda I - A)^{-1}](\lambda I - A)x = y,$$

it follows that the matrix $(\lambda I - (A + B))$ is invertible if and only if the matrix $[I - B(\lambda I - A)^{-1}]$ is invertible. Let us now prove that we can find a new norm $\|\cdot\|_1$ on $\mathbb{R}^n$ such that

$$\sup_{\|x\|_1 \leq 1} \|B(\lambda I - A)^{-1}x\|_1 < 1, \quad \forall \lambda \in \{\nu \in \mathbb{C} : \mathrm{Re}(\nu) \geq 0\}.$$

Since $B \geq 0$ and $\mathrm{e}^{At} \geq 0$ for all $t \geq 0$, it follows from the resolvent formula and the definition of the modulus that for all $x \in \mathbb{R}^n$ one has

$$\left|B(\lambda I - A)^{-1}x\right| = \left|B \int_0^{+\infty} e^{-\lambda t} e^{At} x \, dt\right| \le B \int_0^{+\infty} e^{-\mathrm{Re}(\lambda)t} e^{At} |x| \, dt.$$

Now since $\mathrm{Re}(\lambda) \ge 0$ we obtain

$$|B(\lambda I - A)x| \le B \int_0^{+\infty} e^{At} |x| \, dt = B(-A)^{-1}|x|, \quad \forall x \in \mathbb{R}^n.$$

Since the matrix $B(-A)^{-1}$ is irreducible, the Perron–Frobenius theorem applies and ensures that we can find $v_g \gg 0$ such that

$$v_g^T B(-A)^{-1} = r\left(B(-A)^{-1}\right) v_g^T.$$

Define

$$\|x\|_1 := \langle v_g, |x|\rangle = v_g^T |x|, \quad \forall x \in \mathbb{R}^n.$$

Then $\|\cdot\|_1$ is a norm on $\mathbb{R}^n$ and one has

$$\|B(\lambda I - A)x\|_1 = v_g^T |B(\lambda I - A)x| \le v_g^T B(-A)^{-1}|x| = r\left(B(-A)^{-1}\right) \|x\|_1, \ \forall x \in \mathbb{R}^n.$$

Finally, since by assumption one has $r\left(B(-A)^{-1}\right) < 1$, the result follows. $\qquad\square$

Example 4.59 In order to illustrate this stability result, let us consider the following continuous-time Leslie model

$$\frac{\mathrm{d}}{\mathrm{d}t} \begin{pmatrix} U_0(t) \\ U_1(t) \\ \vdots \\ U_m(t) \end{pmatrix} = L \begin{pmatrix} U_0(t) \\ U_1(t) \\ \vdots \\ U_m(t) \end{pmatrix} \tag{4.5}$$

wherein the matrix L takes the form

$$L = \begin{pmatrix} \beta_0 - \mu_0 & \beta_1 & \cdots & \cdots & \beta_m \\ \eta_0 & -\mu_1 & 0 & \cdots & 0 \\ 0 & \eta_1 & -\mu_2 & \ddots & \vdots \\ \vdots & \ddots & \ddots & \ddots & 0 \\ 0 & \cdots & 0 & \eta_{m-1} & -\mu_m \end{pmatrix}.$$

for some given parameters $\beta_i \ge 0$, $i = 0, \ldots, m$, $\beta_m > 0$, $\eta_i > 0$, $\mu_i > 0$, $i = 0, \ldots, m$.

Set

$$A = \begin{pmatrix} -\mu_0 & 0 & \cdots & 0 \\ 0 & -\mu_1 & \ddots & \vdots \\ \vdots & \ddots & \ddots & 0 \\ 0 & \cdots & 0 & -\mu_m \end{pmatrix} \quad \text{and} \quad B = \begin{pmatrix} \beta_0 & \beta_1 & \cdots & \cdots & \beta_m \\ \eta_0 & 0 & 0 & \cdots & 0 \\ 0 & \eta_1 & 0 & \ddots & \vdots \\ \vdots & \ddots & \ddots & \ddots & 0 \\ 0 & \cdots & 0 & \eta_{m-1} & 0 \end{pmatrix}.$$

Then we have

$$
B(-A)^{-1} = \begin{pmatrix} \beta_0 & \beta_1 & \cdots & & \cdots & \beta_m \\ \eta_0 & 0 & 0 & \cdots & & 0 \\ 0 & \eta_1 & 0 & \ddots & & \vdots \\ \vdots & \ddots & \ddots & & \ddots & 0 \\ 0 & \cdots & 0 & \eta_{m-1} & & 0 \end{pmatrix} \times \begin{pmatrix} \mu_0^{-1} & 0 & \cdots & 0 \\ 0 & \mu_1^{-1} & \ddots & \vdots \\ \vdots & \ddots & \ddots & 0 \\ 0 & \cdots & 0 & \mu_m^{-1} \end{pmatrix}
$$

$$
= \begin{pmatrix} \beta_0\mu_0^{-1} & \beta_1\mu_1^{-1} & \cdots & & \cdots & \beta_m\mu_m^{-1} \\ \eta_0\mu_0^{-1} & 0 & 0 & \cdots & & 0 \\ 0 & \eta_1\mu_1^{-1} & 0 & \ddots & & \vdots \\ \vdots & & \ddots & \ddots & & 0 \\ 0 & & \cdots & 0 & \eta_{m-1}\mu_{m-1}^{-1} & 0 \end{pmatrix}.
$$

Since $\beta_m > 0$, the matrix $B(-A)^{-1}$ is irreducible, and by using the Lemma 4.47 we deduce $r(B(-A)^{-1}) < 1$ if

$$
R_0 := \widehat{\beta}_0 + \widehat{\beta}_1\pi_0 + \widehat{\beta}_2\pi_0\pi_1 + \cdots + \widehat{\beta}_m\pi_0\pi_1 \times \cdots \times \pi_{m-1} < 1,
$$

where

$$
\widehat{\beta}_j = \beta_j\mu_j^{-1}
$$

and

$$
\pi_j = \eta_j\mu_j^{-1}.
$$

It follows from Theorem 4.58 that (4.5) is stable (i.e. $s(L) < 0$) if $R_0 < 1$.

4.6 Remarks and Notes

Positivity of linear EDO systems in Banach spaces

Definition 4.60 A closed and convex subset X_+ of a Banach space X is called a *positive cone* of X if the following properties are satisfied:

(i) $\lambda X_+ \subset X_+, \forall \lambda \geq 0$;
(ii) $X_+ \cap (-X_+) = \{0\}$.

Similarly as for $\mathbb{R}^n$, by using the positive cone X_+ one can define a partial order on X as follows

$$
x \geq y \iff x - y \in X_+,
$$
$$
x > y \iff x - y \in X_+ \setminus \{0\},
$$
$$
x \gg y \iff x - y \in \mathring{X}_+,
$$

wherein $\mathring{X}_+$ is the interior of X_+.

Remark 4.61 In a Banach space the interior of the positive cone is not necessarily non-empty. Indeed,

(i) The interior of the positive cone $C_+([0,1],\mathbb{R})$ is not empty in $C([0,1],\mathbb{R})$) (Hint: The function $u(x) = 1, \forall x \in [0,1]$ belongs to the interior of the cone);

(ii) The interior of the positive cone $L_+^1((0,1),\mathbb{R})$ is empty in $L^1((0,1),\mathbb{R})$ (Hint: The function $u(x) = 1$, for almost every $x \in [0,1]$, does not belong to the interior of the cone).

Definition 4.62 A Banach space X endowed with such a partial order $\geq$ is said to be *partially ordered*. We will say that a bounded linear operator $A \in \mathcal{L}(X)$ is *positive* (or for short $A \geq 0$) if

$$Ax \geq 0, \quad \forall x \geq 0, \text{ that is, } AX_+ \subset X_+.$$

Theorem 4.63 *Let $A \in \mathcal{L}(X)$ be a bounded linear operator on a partially ordered Banach space X. Then*

$$e^{At} \geq 0, \quad \forall t \geq 0,$$

if and only if there exists a $\lambda_0 > 0$ large enough such that $[\lambda_0, \infty) \subset \rho(A)$ and

$$(\lambda I - A)^{-1} \geq 0, \quad \forall \lambda \geq \lambda_0.$$

Proof The proof of this theorem is similar to that of Theorem 4.11. This proof uses the fact that the positive cone is closed and we leave it as an exercise. $\square$

Further reading about the Perron–Frobenius theorem

The Perron–Frobenius theorem presented in this chapter was proved by Perron [275] and Frobenius [111, 112]. This is one of the most classical results about the spectrum of matrices. We refer to the books of Gantmacher [114], Seneta [311], Minc [256], and Horn and Johnson [161] for more results on non-negative matrices.

The Krein–Rutman theorem

The Perron–Frobenius theorem has several infinite-dimensional extensions. Below we present the Krein–Rutman theorem, which is an infinite-dimensional version of this theorem in some ordered Banach spaces endowed with a solid positive cone, that is, a positive cone with non-empty interior.

To present this result, let us first recall the definition of a compact operator.

Definition 4.64 Let $(X, \|\cdot\|_X)$ be a Banach space. Let $A \in \mathcal{L}(X)$ be a bounded linear operator on the Banach space X. Then A is said to be a *compact operator* if the closure of $A(B)$ is a compact subset of X for every bounded subset B of X.

As mentioned above, there are several extensions of the Perron–Frobenius theorem in Banach spaces. The main assumption of the Krein–Rutman theorem is that the interior of the positive cone X_+ is non-empty. We refer to [2, 74, 191, 307, 330, 333] for various proofs and more results on this subject.

Theorem 4.65 (Krein–Rutman) *Let* $(X, \|\cdot\|_X)$ *be a Banach space partially ordered with a positive cone* X_+ *with non-empty interior. Let* $A \in \mathcal{L}(X)$ *be a compact bounded linear operator on X such that*

$$Ax \gg 0, \ \forall x > 0 \text{ or equivalently } A(X_+ \setminus \{0\}) \subset \mathring{X}_+.$$

Then the following properties are satisfied

(i) *The spectral radius of A, which is defined by*

$$r(A) = \lim_{n \to \infty} \|A^n\|_{\mathcal{L}(X)}^{1/n},$$

is strictly positive and is a simple eigenvalue of A (i.e. $\dim(N(r(A)I - A))) = 1$ *and* $N((r(A)I - A)) = N\left((r(A)I - A)^2\right)$*).*
(ii) *There exists a* $u \in \text{Int}(X_+)$ *such that* $Au = r(A)u$.
(iii) *If* $\lambda \in \mathbb{C}$ *is an eigenvalue of A with* $|\lambda| = r(A)$, *then* $\lambda = r(A)$.
(iv) *If* $\lambda \in \mathbb{C}$ *is an eigenvalue of A such that there exists a* $u \in X_+ \setminus \{0\}$ *with* $Au = \lambda u$, *then* $\lambda = r(A)$.

Note that the compactness of the linear operator A can be weakened by working with the essential spectral radius and the measure of non-compactness. More general versions of the above result can also be stated for Banach spaces partially ordered by a cone with an empty interior. We refer the interested readers to the monographs of Schaefer [307], and to those of Meyer-Nieberg [255]. See also [245, 268].

Random linear systems

To quote a few results involving random linear difference equations, we refer to the paper of Cohen and Newman [64] for a nice discussion of examples and counterexamples related to the growth of solutions of a non-autonomous difference equation of the form

$$N(n + 1) = A(n)N(n), \forall n \in \mathbb{N}, \text{ and } N(0) = x \in \mathbb{R}^n,$$

where $A(n)$ is an n by n random matrix (i.e. all elements are random variables).
The authors investigate the growth of the solution, that is, the function of x:

$$\lambda(x) = \lim_{n \to +\infty} \frac{\ln(\|N(n)\|)}{n}.$$

For the most advanced readers, we also refer to the work of Lian and Lu [204] on Lyapunov exponents and invariant manifolds for random dynamical systems in a Banach space.

4.7 MATLAB Codes

Figure 4.2

```
1  M=[1/10  2/10  3/10  4/10;4/10  1/10  2/10  3/10;  3/10
       4/10  1/10  2/10;
2  2/10  3/10  4/10  1/10     ]
3
4  clf;
5  hold on;
6  eig(M)
7  p1=plot(eig(M),'or','DisplayName',  'Eigenvalues',  '
       MarkerFaceColor','r',  'MarkerSize',  15)
8
9  x=-4:0.1:4;
10  y=0*x;
11  p2=plot(x,y,'k','LineWidth',1);
12  p3=plot(y,x,'k','LineWidth',1);
13
14  legend([p1],{'Eigenvalues'});
15  xlabel('IR');
16  ylabel('i IR');
17  set(gca,'YLim',[-1  1])
18  set(gca,'XLim',[-1  3])
19
20
21  set(gca,'fontweight','bold','FontSize',30);
22  ax=gca;
23  ax.YAxis.Exponent=0;
```

Figure 4.4

```
1  p=1;
2  b=1;
3  M=[0  0  0  b;p  0  0  0;  0  p  0  0;  0  0  p  0     ];
4  clf;
5
6  hold on;
```

```
7   t =0:0.1:2.1*pi;
8   plot(max(abs(eig(M)))*exp(i*t),'r','LineWidth',5)
9
10  p1=plot(eig(M),'ok','DisplayName', 'Eigenvalues',  '
        MarkerFaceColor','k', 'MarkerSize', 15);
11
12  x=-3:0.1:3;
13  y=0*x;
14  plot(x,y,'k','LineWidth',1);
15  plot(y,x,'k','LineWidth',1);
16  xlabel('R');
17  ylabel('iR');
18
19  set(gca,'YLim',[-2  2])
20  set(gca,'XLim',[-3  3])
21  legend([p1],{'Eigenvalues'});
22  set(gca,'fontweight','bold','FontSize',30);
23  ax=gca;
24  ax.YAxis.Exponent=0;
```

Part II
Nonlinear Differential Equations

Chapter 5
Nonlinear Differential Equations

5.1 Introduction

In this chapter we will be interested in nonlinear (autonomous) differential equations. We will consider

$$\frac{du}{dt} = F(u(t)), \quad \forall t \geq 0 \text{ and } u(0) = u_0 \in \mathbb{R}^n, \tag{5.1}$$

where $F : \mathbb{R}^n \to \mathbb{R}^n$ is Lipschitz continuous on bounded sets.

Definition 5.1 We will say that a function $u \in C([0, \tau], \mathbb{R}^n)$ is a *solution* of the differential equation (5.1) if u satisfies the integral equation

$$u(t) = u_0 + \int_0^t F(u(\sigma)) \, d\sigma, \text{ for all } t \in [0, \tau].$$

Definition 5.2 Let $F : \mathbb{R}^n \to \mathbb{R}^n$ be a map. We will say that F is *Lipschitz continuous on bounded sets* of $\mathbb{R}^n$ if for each constant $M > 0$ there exists a constant $k = k(M) > 0$ such that

$$\|F(x) - F(y)\| \leq k\|x - y\|,$$

whenever $x, y \in \mathbb{R}^n$ with $\|x\| \leq M$ and $\|y\| \leq M$.

Recall the fundamental formula of differential calculus.

Lemma 5.3 *Let $F : \mathbb{R}^n \to \mathbb{R}^n$ be a continuously differentiable map (or C^1-map). Then we have for each $x, y \in \mathbb{R}^n$*

$$F(x) - F(y) = \int_0^1 DF(\sigma x + (1 - \sigma)y)(x - y) \, d\sigma.$$

Proof Let $\psi : [0, 1] \to \mathbb{R}^n$ be the map defined by

$$\psi(s) = F(\sigma x + (1 - \sigma)y) \text{ for all } \sigma \in [0, 1].$$

We have

$$\psi'(\sigma) = DF(\sigma x + (1-\sigma)y)(x-y)$$

and the result comes from

$$\psi(1) - \psi(0) = \int_0^1 \psi'(\sigma)d\sigma.$$

The proof is complete.   □

Corollary 5.4 *Let $F : \mathbb{R}^n \to \mathbb{R}^n$ be a C^1-map. Then F is Lipschitz on bounded sets.*

Remark 5.5 The result is only true for C^1-maps $F : X \to X$ on a finite-dimensional Banach space X, since we need the closed unit ball to be compact. Nevertheless, in many infinite-dimensional examples, the map considered is Lipschitz on bounded sets.

Proof Let $x, y \in \mathbb{R}^n$ with $\|x\| \le M$ and $\|y\| \le M$. We have

$$F(x) - F(y) = \int_0^1 DF(\sigma x + (1-\sigma)y)(x-y)d\sigma,$$

hence

$$\|F(x) - F(y)\| \le \sup_{\sigma \in [0,1]} \|DF(\sigma x + (1-\sigma)y)\|_{\mathcal{L}(\mathbb{R}^n)} \|x-y\|$$

and

$$\|F(x) - F(y)\| \le \sup_{\|z\| \le M} \|DF(z)\|_{\mathcal{L}(\mathbb{R}^n)} \|x-y\|.$$

By assumption the map $x \to DF(x)$ is continuous from $\mathbb{R}^n$ in $\mathcal{L}(\mathbb{R}^n)$, so we deduce that

$$k(M) = \sup_{\|z\| \le M} \|DF(z)\|_{\mathcal{L}(\mathbb{R}^n)} < +\infty.$$

The proof is complete.   □

Recall that $F : \mathbb{R}^n \to \mathbb{R}^n$ is said to be *locally Lipschitz continuous* if for each $x \in \mathbb{R}^n$ we can find two constants $\varepsilon > 0$ and $k > 0$ such that

$$\|F(y) - F(z)\| \le k\|y-z\|$$

whenever $\|z - x\| \le \varepsilon$ and $\|y - x\| \le \varepsilon$.

Exercise 5.6 Prove that a map $F : \mathbb{R}^n \to \mathbb{R}^n$ is locally Lipschitz continuous if and only if F is Lipschitz on bounded sets. (Hint: Start by considering the segment $sY + (1-s)X$ with $s \in [0,1]$.)

5.2 The Logistic Equation

The so-called *logistic equation* was introduced in population dynamics by Bernoulli (1760) [28] and Verhulst (1838) [347] to model the limitation of growth in a natural population. Let $N(t)$ be the total number of individuals. The equation reads as follows

$$\frac{dN}{dt} = \underbrace{bN(t)}_{\text{flux of newborn}} - \underbrace{(m + \chi N(t)) N(t)}_{\text{flux of exit or death}}, \quad \forall t \geq 0 \text{ and } N(0) = N_0 \geq 0, \quad (5.2)$$

where $b \geq 0$ is the birth rate, $m \geq 0$ is the mortality rate and $\chi \geq 0$ is an additional mortality term. In the logistic model the death rate $m + \chi N(t)$ increases proportionally to the size of the population.

The growth of the population when the population is small is $\lambda = b - m$. In the logistic equation, we use a nonlinear growth rate $\Lambda(N(t)) := \lambda - \chi N(t)$ which depends on the total number of individuals in the population. By using the nonlinear growth rate the logistic equation can be rewritten as

$$N'(t) = \Lambda(N(t)) N(t), \quad \forall t \geq 0 \text{ and } N(0) = N_0 \geq 0.$$

Assume that $\lambda > 0$ and $\chi > 0$, and set

$$\kappa := \frac{\lambda}{\chi}.$$

Remark 5.7 The solution is given by

$$N(t) = N_0 \exp\left(\int_0^t \Lambda(N(\sigma)) d\sigma\right), \forall t \geq 0.$$

Therefore $t \to \Lambda(N(t))$ can be regarded as a time-dependent growth rate.

The quantity κ is called the *carrying capacity* of the population and

$$N'(t) = \lambda N(t)\left(1 - \frac{N(t)}{\kappa}\right), \quad \forall t \geq 0 \text{ and } N(0) = N_0 \geq 0.$$

In this example we have

$$f(x) := \lambda x \left(1 - \frac{x}{\kappa}\right)$$

and the map f is C^1 (hence continuous on bounded subsets of $\mathbb{R}$), but f is not Lipschitz continuous on $\mathbb{R}$.

The map f is not Lipschitz continuous: Indeed, we have

$$f'(x) = \lambda\left(1 - \frac{2x}{\kappa}\right)$$

therefore

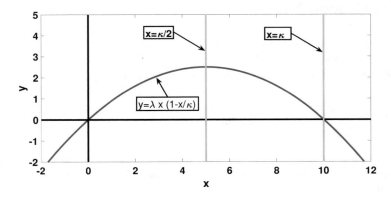

Fig. 5.1: *In this figure we plot the logistic map for $\lambda = 1$ and $\kappa = 10$.*

$$f(x) - f(y) = \int_y^x f'(z)\mathrm{d}z$$

and for $x \geq y \geq \frac{\kappa}{2}$

$$|f(x) - f(y)| = \int_y^x |f'(z)|\,\mathrm{d}z \geq |f'(y)||x - y|$$

since $f'(x) \leq 0$ for each $x \in \left[\frac{\kappa}{2}, +\infty\right)$ and since the map $x \to |f'(x)| = \lambda\left(\frac{2x}{\kappa} - 1\right)$ is increasing. But

$$|f'(y)| \to +\infty, \quad \text{when } y \to +\infty,$$

so f is not Lipschitz continuous on $\mathbb{R}$.

Explicit solutions: For each $N_0 \geq 0$ the solution of the logistic equation (5.2) is explicitly given by

$$N(t) := \frac{\mathrm{e}^{\lambda t} N_0}{1 + \frac{\lambda}{\kappa} \int_0^t \mathrm{e}^{\lambda\sigma} N_0\, \mathrm{d}\sigma}, \quad \forall t \geq 0.$$

Indeed, we have for each $t \geq 0$,

$$N'(t) = \lambda N(t) - \mathrm{e}^{\lambda t} N_0 \times \frac{\lambda}{\kappa} \times \frac{\mathrm{e}^{\lambda t} N_0}{(1 + \frac{\lambda}{\kappa} \int_0^t \mathrm{e}^{\lambda\sigma} N_0\mathrm{d}\sigma)^2}$$

$$N'(t) = \lambda N(t) - \frac{\lambda}{\kappa} \frac{(\mathrm{e}^{\lambda t} N_0)^2}{(1 + \frac{\lambda}{\kappa} \int_0^t \mathrm{e}^{\lambda\sigma} N_0\, \mathrm{d}l)^2}$$

thus

$$N'(t) = \lambda N(t) - \frac{\lambda}{\kappa} N^2(t).$$

Semiflow generated by (5.2): We can also verify that the family of nonlinear maps $\{U(t)\}_{t \geq 0}$ defined on $[0, +\infty)$ by

$$U(t)x = \frac{e^{\lambda t} x}{1 + \frac{\lambda}{\kappa} \int_0^t e^{\lambda \sigma} x \, d\sigma}$$

is a nonlinear semiflow on $[0, +\infty)$.

Maximal semiflow: We define the maximal time of existence of solution as follows

$$\tau(x) = \sup \left\{ t \geq 0 : \sup_{s \in [0,t]} |U(s)x| < +\infty \right\}.$$

Assume that $\lambda > 0$ and $\kappa > 0$ and consider the formula for $U(t)x$ ($x \in \mathbb{R}$). Then we have the following

Case 1: If $x \geq 0$, we have

$$1 + \frac{1}{\kappa} \int_0^t e^{\lambda \sigma} x \, d\sigma \geq 1, \quad \forall t \geq 0,$$

so

$$\tau(x) = +\infty, \quad \forall x \geq 0,$$

and $t \to U(t)x$ is defined on $[0, +\infty)$. The solution starting from x is a global solution.

Case 2: If $x < 0$, since $\lambda > 0$, we can find $\tau(x) > 0$ such that

$$1 + \frac{\lambda}{\kappa} \int_0^{\tau(x)} e^{\lambda \sigma} x \, d\sigma = 0$$
$$\Leftrightarrow 1 + \frac{x}{\kappa}(e^{\lambda \tau(x)} - 1) = 0$$
$$\Leftrightarrow e^{\lambda \tau(x)} = 1 - \frac{\kappa}{x}$$

so here we have

$$\tau(x) := \frac{1}{\lambda} \ln \left(1 - \frac{\kappa}{x} \right),$$

and

$$U(t)x = \frac{e^{\lambda t} x}{1 + \frac{\lambda}{\kappa} \int_0^t e^{\lambda \sigma} x \, d\sigma} \to -\infty, \quad \text{as } t \nearrow \tau(x).$$

Figure 5.2 summarizes the behavior of the solutions of the logistic equation.

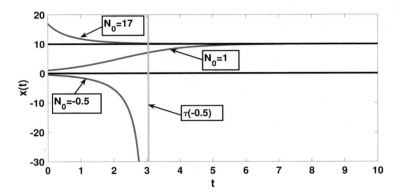

Fig. 5.2: *In this figure we plot three solutions starting from $N_0 = -0.5, 1, 17$ of the logistic equation for $\lambda = 1$ and $\kappa = 10$.*

5.3 The n-Dimensional Logistic Equation

The n-dimensional logistic equation reads as follows

$$\begin{cases} \dfrac{\mathrm{d}U(t)}{\mathrm{d}t} = AU(t) - \rho(U(t))U(t), & \text{for } t \geq 0, \\ U(0) = x \in \mathbb{R}^n, \end{cases}$$

where $A \in M_n(\mathbb{R})$ is an n by n real matrix and $\rho : \mathbb{R}^n \to \mathbb{R}$ is a continuous map which is positively homogeneous. That is,

$$\rho(\lambda x) = \lambda \rho(x), \forall \lambda \geq 0, \forall x \in \mathbb{R}^n.$$

Define

$$\tau(x) := \sup \left\{ t > 0 : \left(1 + \int_0^s \rho\left(e^{A\sigma}x\right) \mathrm{d}\sigma \right) > 0, \forall s \in [0, t] \right\} \in (0, +\infty].$$

Then the solution of the n-dimensional logistic equation is given explicitly by

$$U(t)x = \frac{e^{At}x}{1 + \int_0^t \rho\left(e^{A\sigma}x\right) \mathrm{d}\sigma}, \quad \forall t \in [0, \tau(x)).$$

One may observe that if $\tau(x) < +\infty$ and $x \neq 0$ then

$$\lim_{t \nearrow \tau(x)} \frac{\|e^{At}x\|}{1 + \int_0^t \rho\left(e^{A\sigma}x\right) \mathrm{d}\sigma} = +\infty,$$

that is, the solution blows up when t approaches $\tau(x)$. In other words, $\tau(x)$ is the blow-up time of the solution starting from x.

Assume for example that $\rho(x) = \sum_{i=1}^{n} v_i x_i = \langle v, x \rangle$, where $v \geq 0$. Assume that the matrix $A \in M_n(\mathbb{R})$ satisfies

$$A + \delta I \geq 0$$

for some $\delta > 0$. Then by using the results in Chapter 4 we know that

$$e^{At} \geq 0, \quad \forall t \geq 0.$$

This implies that

$$\tau(x) = +\infty, \quad \forall x \geq 0.$$

Therefore the solution of the n-dimensional logistic equation is given by

$$U(t)x = \frac{e^{At}x}{1 + \int_0^t \langle v, e^{A\sigma} x \rangle \, d\sigma}$$

and is well defined for each $t > 0$ as long as $x \geq 0$. In other words, no blow-up occurs whenever $x \geq 0$. Of course, a blow-up may of course occur when x is no longer positive.

5.4 The Bernoulli–Verhulst Equation

The Bernoulli–Verhulst equation is the following

$$N'(t) = N(t) \left(\lambda - \frac{|N(t)|^\theta}{\kappa} \right), \forall t \geq 0, \text{ and } N(0) = N_0 > 0,$$

where $\lambda \in \mathbb{R}$, $\kappa > 0$ and $\theta > 0$.

Assume that $N(t) > 0$, $\forall t \geq 0$. Set

$$V(t) := N(t)^{-\theta}.$$

We have

$$V'(t) = -\theta N(t)^{-\theta-1} N'(t) = -\theta N(t)^{-\theta} \left(\lambda - \frac{N(t)^\theta}{\kappa} \right),$$

and

$$V'(t) = -\theta \lambda N(t)^{-\theta} + \frac{\theta}{\kappa},$$

hence

$$V'(t) = -\theta \lambda V(t) + \frac{\theta}{\kappa}, \forall t \geq 0 \text{ and } V(0) = V_0.$$

Therefore by using the variation of constant formula, we obtain

$$V(t) = e^{-\theta \lambda t} V_0 + \int_0^t e^{-\theta \lambda (t-s)} \frac{\theta}{\kappa} \, ds, \quad \forall t \geq 0.$$

Hence

$$V(t) = e^{-\theta\lambda t}V_0 + \int_0^t e^{-\theta\lambda l}\frac{\theta}{\kappa}dl$$

and

$$V(t) = e^{-\theta\lambda t}V_0 - \frac{1}{\theta\lambda}\frac{\theta}{\kappa}\left[e^{-\theta\lambda t} - 1\right] = e^{-\theta\lambda t}v_0 + \frac{1}{\lambda\kappa}\left[1 - e^{-\theta\lambda t}\right].$$

Finally, since

$$V(t) = N(t)^{-\theta} \Leftrightarrow N(t) = V(t)^{-\frac{1}{\theta}},$$

we obtain

$$N(t) = \left(e^{-\theta\lambda t}N_0^{-\theta} + \int_0^t e^{-\theta\lambda l}\frac{\theta}{\kappa}dl\right)^{-\frac{1}{\theta}} = e^{\lambda t}N_0\left(1 + \frac{\theta}{\kappa}\int_0^t e^{\theta\lambda(t-l)}N_0^\theta dl\right)^{-\frac{1}{\theta}}.$$

So starting from a positive initial value we obtain for all $t \geq 0$,

$$N(t) = \frac{e^{\lambda t}N_0}{\left(1 + \frac{\theta}{\kappa}\int_0^t e^{\theta\lambda(t-l)}N_0^\theta dl\right)^{\frac{1}{\theta}}}.$$

Now rewriting the Bernoulli–Verhulst equation as

$$N'(t) = N(t)\left(\lambda - \frac{1}{\kappa}(N^2(t))^{\frac{\theta}{2}}\right), \quad t \geq 0, \text{ and } N(0) = N_0 \in \mathbb{R}$$

with a real-valued initial condition, we can define the solution as

$$N(t) = \frac{e^{\lambda t}N_0}{\left(1 + \frac{\theta}{\kappa}\int_0^t e^{\theta\lambda\sigma}|N_0|^\theta d\sigma\right)^{\frac{1}{\theta}}} = \frac{e^{\lambda t}N_0}{\left(1 + \frac{\theta}{\kappa}\int_0^t e^{\theta\lambda\sigma}(N_0^2)^{\frac{\theta}{2}}d\sigma\right)^{\frac{1}{\theta}}}.$$

Remark 5.8 Assume that $\lambda \neq 0$. We can rewrite the Bernoulli–Verhulst equation as

$$N'(t) = \lambda N(t)\left(1 - \left(\frac{N(t)}{N_\infty}\right)^\theta\right), \forall t \geq 0, \text{ and } N(0) = N_0 \in (0, N_\infty],$$

where $N_\infty > 0$ and $\theta > 0$.

Set

$$W(t) := \frac{1}{N(t)^\theta} - \frac{1}{N_\infty^\theta} \Leftrightarrow N(t) = \left(\frac{1}{W(t) + \frac{1}{N_\infty^\theta}}\right)^{1/\theta}$$

and

$$W'(t) = -\theta N(t)^{-\theta-1}N'(t) = -\theta\lambda W(t).$$

Therefore

$$W(t) = \exp\left(-\theta\lambda t\right)\left[\frac{1}{N_0^\theta} - \frac{1}{N_\infty^\theta}\right],$$

thus

$$N(t)^\theta = \cfrac{1}{\exp(-\theta \lambda t)\left[\cfrac{1}{N_0^\theta} - \cfrac{1}{N_\infty^\theta}\right] + \cfrac{1}{N_\infty^\theta}} = \cfrac{\exp(\theta \lambda t)\, N_0^\theta}{1 + (\exp(\theta \lambda t) - 1)\,\cfrac{N_0^\theta}{N_\infty^\theta}}$$

hence we obtain

$$N(t) = \cfrac{\exp(\lambda t)\, N_0}{\left[1 + (\exp(\theta \lambda t) - 1)\,\cfrac{N_0^\theta}{N_\infty^\theta}\right]^{1/\theta}} = \cfrac{\exp(\lambda t)\, N_0}{\left[1 + \cfrac{\theta \lambda}{N_\infty^\theta} \int_0^t \exp(\theta \lambda s)\, N_0^\theta \, ds\right]^{1/\theta}}.$$

We can observe that $N(t)$ is a nonlinear transformation of an exponentially growing solution $W(t)$.

5.5 The *n*-Dimensional Bernoulli–Verhulst Equation

The *n*-dimensional Bernoulli–Verhulst equation is the following

$$u'(t) = Au(t) - \rho\,(u(t))^\theta\, u(t), \quad \forall t \geq 0 \text{ with } u(0) = x \in \mathbb{R}^n,$$

where $A \in M_n(\mathbb{R})$ is an n by n real matrix, and $\rho : \mathbb{R}^n \to [0, +\infty)$ is a continuous map which is positively homogeneous. That is,

$$\rho(\lambda x) = \lambda \rho(x), \forall \lambda \geq 0, \forall x \in \mathbb{R}^n.$$

Theorem 5.9 *The solution to the n-dimensional Bernoulli–Verhulst equation is given by the explicit formula*

$$u(t) = \frac{e^{At} x}{\left(1 + \theta \int_0^t \rho\left(e^{Al}x\right)^\theta dl\right)^{\frac{1}{\theta}}}, \forall t \geq 0.$$

Proof Set $X(t) = U(t)x$. We have

$$u'(t) = \frac{A e^{At} x}{\left(1 + \theta \int_0^t \rho\left(e^{Al}x\right)^\theta dl\right)^{\frac{1}{\theta}}} - \frac{1}{\theta} e^{At} x \left(1 + \theta \int_0^t \rho\left(e^{Al}x\right)^\theta dl\right)^{-\frac{1}{\theta}-1} \theta \rho\left(e^{At}x\right)^\theta,$$

and by using the fact that ρ is positively homogeneous we obtain

$$u'(t) = Au(t) - \frac{e^{At} x}{\left(1 + \theta \int_0^t \rho\left(e^{Al}x\right)^\theta dl\right)^{\frac{1}{\theta}}} \rho \left(\frac{e^{At} x}{\left(1 + \theta \int_0^t \rho\left(e^{Al}x\right)^\theta dl\right)^{\frac{1}{\theta}}}\right)^\theta.$$

The proof is complete.   □

5.6 Non-Uniqueness of Solutions

Consider the equation

$$x'(t) = |x(t)|^{\frac{1}{2}}, \quad \forall t \geq 0 \text{ and } x(0) = x_0.$$

We will prove that this equation admits several solutions passing through the same point at time $t = 0$.

Case 1: If $x_0 > 0$

$$\frac{x'(t)}{\sqrt{x(t)}} = 1 \Leftrightarrow x(t) = \left(\sqrt{x_0} + \frac{t}{2}\right)^2, \quad \forall t \geq -2\sqrt{x_0}.$$

Case 2: If $x_0 < 0$

$$x(t) = -\left(\sqrt{|x_0|} - \frac{t}{2}\right)^2, \quad \forall t < 2\sqrt{|x_0|}.$$

Let us choose $t_1 < t_0$ with $t_0 := -2\sqrt{x_0}$ and define

$$u(t) = \begin{cases} \left(\sqrt{x_0} + \dfrac{t}{2}\right)^2 & \text{if } t > t_0, \\ 0 & \text{if } t \in [t_1, t_0], \\ -\left(\dfrac{t_1 - t}{2}\right)^2 & \text{if } t < t_1. \end{cases}$$

One can prove that $u(t)$ is a solution. The non-uniqueness of solution follows since we can choose t_1 arbitrarily smaller than t_0.

5.7 Maximal Semiflow

Definition 5.10 Consider a map $\tau : \mathbb{R}^n \to (0, +\infty]$ (maximal time of existence) and a map $U : D_\tau \to \mathbb{R}^n$ with

$$D_\tau := \{(t, x) \in [0, +\infty] \times \mathbb{R}^n : 0 \leq t < \tau(x)\}.$$

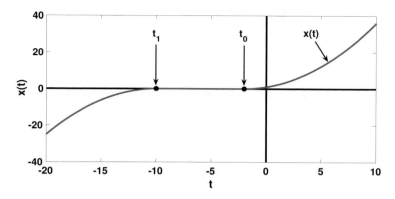

Fig. 5.3: *Example of a solution of the equation* $x'(t) = |x(t)|^{\frac{1}{2}}$.

Set

$$U(t)x := U(t, x) \quad \forall (t, x) \in D_\tau.$$

We will say that U is a *maximal semiflow* on $\mathbb{R}^n$ if the following properties are satisfied.

(i) $\tau(U(t)x) + t = \tau(x), \forall x \in \mathbb{R}^n, \forall t \in [0, \tau(x))$.

(ii) $U(0)x = x, \quad \forall x \in \mathbb{R}^n$.

(iii) $U(t)U(s)x = U(t + s)x, \quad \forall t, s \in [0, \tau(x))$ with $t + s < \tau(x)$.

(iv) If $\tau(x) < +\infty$ then

$$\lim_{t \nearrow \tau(x)} \|U(t)x\| = +\infty.$$

We will say that U is *continuous* if D_τ is relatively open in $[0, +\infty) \times \mathbb{R}^n$ and the map $(t, x) \to U(t)x$ is continuous from D_τ into $\mathbb{R}^n$.

Example 5.11 Consider

$$\begin{cases} \dfrac{du(t)}{dt} = u(t)^2 & \forall t \geq 0 \\ u(0) = u_0 > 0. \end{cases}$$

We have

$$u(t) = \frac{x}{1 - \int_0^t x ds} = \frac{x}{1 - tx}.$$

Which gives

$$\tau(x) = \begin{cases} \dfrac{1}{x} & \text{if } x > 0, \\ +\infty & \text{if } x = 0, \\ +\infty & \text{if } x < 0. \end{cases}$$

Definition 5.12 We will say that the map $\tau : \mathbb{R}^n \to (0, +\infty]$ is *lower semi-continuous* (or *lsc*) if for each $x_0 \in \mathbb{R}^n$ and each $\tau^* \in (0, \tau(x_0))$ there exists an $\eta = \eta(x_0, \tau^*) > 0$ such that for each $y \in \mathbb{R}^n$

$$\|x_0 - y\| \le \eta \Rightarrow \tau^* \le \tau(y).$$

In other words, τ is lower semi-continuous if and only if for each $x_0 \in \mathbb{R}^n$ we have

$$\liminf_{y \to x_0} \tau(y) \ge \tau(x_0).$$

We will see that the maximal time of existence of solutions is a lower semi-continuous map. This property is illustrated in Figure 5.4.

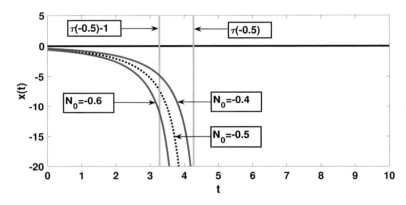

Fig. 5.4: *In this figure we consider the initial condition $u_0 = -0.5$ for the logistic equation. The solution starting from $u_0 = -0.5$ exists until the blow-up time $\tau(-0.5)$. If we choose, for example, the time $\tau^* = \tau(-0.5) - 1$ then the solutions starting from $u_0 = -0.4$ and $u_0 = -0.6$ exist until a time that is larger than τ^*. This is the lower semi-continuity of the maximal time of existence of solutions.*

5.8 Existence and Uniqueness of a Maximal Continuous Semiflow

Consider

$$\begin{cases} \dfrac{dU(t)x}{dt} = F(U(t)x), & \forall t \ge 0 \\ U(0)x = x \in \mathbb{R}^n. \end{cases} \tag{5.3}$$

The following theorem is the main result of this chapter.

Theorem 5.13 *Assume that $F : \mathbb{R}^n \to \mathbb{R}^n$ is Lipschitz continuous on bounded sets. Then there exists a unique map $\tau : \mathbb{R}^n \to (0, +\infty]$ which is lower semi-continuous and a unique maximal semiflow $U : D_\tau \to \mathbb{R}^n$ such that for any $x \in \mathbb{R}^n$ the function $t \to U(t)x \in C([0, \tau(x)), \mathbb{R}^n)$ is the unique solution of (5.3). That is, $u(t) = U(t)x$ is the unique continuous function satisfying*

$$u(t) = x + \int_0^t F(u(s))\mathrm{d}s, \quad \forall t \in [0, \tau(x)).$$

Moreover, D_τ is relatively open in $[0, +\infty) \times \mathbb{R}^n$. That is, for each $(t_0, x_0) \in D_\tau$ there exists an $\varepsilon > 0$ such that for each $(t, x) \in [0, \infty) \times \mathbb{R}^n$

$$|t - t_0| + \|x - x_0\| \le \varepsilon \Rightarrow (t, x) \in D_\tau.$$

Finally, the map $(t, x) \to U(t)x$ is continuous from D_τ into $\mathbb{R}^n$.

Lemma 5.14 (Uniqueness) *For each $x \in \mathbb{R}^n$, equation (5.3) admits at most one solution $u \in C([0, \tau], \mathbb{R}^n)$ (with $\tau > 0$).*

Proof Assume that there are two solutions $u, v \in C([0, \tau], \mathbb{R}^n)$ of (5.3) with $u(0) = v(0) = x$. Define

$$t_0 := \sup \{t \ge 0; u(l) = v(l), \quad \forall l \in [0, t]\}.$$

Assume that $t_0 < \tau$. Then for all $t \ge t_0$ we have

$$u(t) - v(t) = \int_0^t F(u(l))\mathrm{d}l - \int_0^t F(v(l))\mathrm{d}l = \int_{t_0}^t [F(u(l)) - F(v(l))]\,\mathrm{d}l.$$

Let

$$M := \sup_{t \in [0, \tau]} \|u(t)\| + \|v(t)\| < +\infty.$$

For all $t \in [t_0, \tau]$ we have

$$
\begin{aligned}
\|u(t) - v(t)\| &\le \int_{t_0}^t \|F(u(l)) - F(v(l))\|\mathrm{d}l \\
&\le k(M) \int_{t_0}^t \|u(l) - v(l)\|\mathrm{d}l \\
&\le k(M)(t - t_0) \sup_{l \in [t_0, t]} \|u(l) - v(l)\|.
\end{aligned}
$$

Next we fix $\varepsilon > 0$ such that $k(M)\varepsilon < 1$. We obtain

$$\sup_{t \in [t_0, t_0 + \varepsilon]} \|u(t) - v(t)\| \le k(M)\varepsilon \sup_{t \in [t_0, t_0 + \varepsilon]} \|u(t) - v(t)\|$$

so

$$\sup_{t \in [t_0, t_0 + \varepsilon]} \|u(t) - v(t)\| = 0.$$

This is in contradiction with the definition of t_0. □

Lemma 5.15 (Local existence) *For each $M > 0$ and each $\beta > 0$ there exists a $\tau = \tau(M, \beta) > 0$ such that, for each $x \in \mathbb{R}^n$ with $\|x\| \leq M$, system (5.3) has a unique solution $u \in C([0, \tau], \mathbb{R}^n)$ which satisfies*

$$\|u(t)\| \leq M(1 + \beta), \quad \forall t \in [0, \tau].$$

Proof Let $M > 0$ and $\beta > 0$ be fixed. Let $x \in \mathbb{R}^n$ with $\|x\| \leq M$. Define

$$\Psi(u)(t) := x + \int_0^t F(u(l)) \mathrm{d}l, \quad \forall t > 0.$$

Consider

$$E = \{u \in C([0, \tau], \mathbb{R}^n) : \|u(t)\| \leq (1 + \beta)M, \forall t \in [0, \tau]\}.$$

The set E is a complete metric space endowed with the usual distance

$$d(u, v) := \|u - v\|_\infty = \sup_{t \in [0, \tau]} \|u(t) - v(t)\|.$$

Let $u \in E$, we have for all $t \in [0, \tau]$

$$\begin{aligned}
\|\Psi(u)(t)\| &\leq \|x\| + \int_0^t \|F(u(l))\| \mathrm{d}l \\
&\leq M + \int_0^t \left[\|F(u(l)) - F(0)\| + \|F(0)\| \right] \mathrm{d}l \\
&\leq M + \tau \|F(0)\| + \tau k(M(1 + \beta))M(1 + \beta).
\end{aligned}$$

We want

$$\Psi(E) \subset E,$$

that is,

$$M + \tau \left[\|F(0)\| + k(M(1 + \beta))M(1 + \beta) \right] \leq (1 + \beta)M,$$

which equivalent to

$$\tau \left[\|F(0)\| + k(M(1 + \beta))M(1 + \beta) \right] \leq \beta M. \tag{5.4}$$

Therefore, we can choose $\tau > 0$ small enough to satisfy (5.4). Moreover, if $u, v \in E$ we have

$$\begin{aligned}
\|\Psi(u)(t) - \Psi(v)(t)\| &\leq \int_0^t \|F(u(l)) - F(v(l))\| \mathrm{d}l \\
&\leq \tau k(M(1 + \beta))\|u - v\|_\infty.
\end{aligned}$$

By choosing $\tau > 0$ small enough inequality (5.4) is satisfied and we have

$$\tau k(M(1 + \beta))(1 + \beta)M \leq \beta M \implies \tau k(M(1 + \beta)) \leq \frac{\beta}{1 + \beta} < 1.$$

So if we fix

$$0 < \tau < \frac{\beta M}{1 + \|F(0)\| + k(M(1 + \beta))(1 + \beta)M}$$

the map Ψ maps E into itself and $\Psi : E \to E$ is a contraction. $\qquad \square$

Define for each $x \in \mathbb{R}^n$

$\tau(x) :=$

$\sup \{t > 0 :$ there exists a solution $u \in C([0, t], \mathbb{R}^n)$ to (5.3) with $u(0) = x\}$.

The above local existence result implies that

$$\tau(x) > 0, \quad \forall x \in \mathbb{R}^n.$$

Lemma 5.16 *Equation (5.4) generates a unique maximal semiflow $U : D_\tau \to \mathbb{R}^n$ on $\mathbb{R}^n$ such that the map $t \to U(t, x)$ is the unique solution of*

$$U(t, x) := x + \int_0^t F(U(s, x)) \mathrm{d}s, \quad \forall t \in [0, \tau(x)), \forall x \in \mathbb{R}^n.$$

Proof Let $x \in \mathbb{R}^n$. We have for all $t \in [0, \tau(x))$ and $r \in [0, t]$,

$$\begin{aligned} U(t)x &= x + \int_0^t F(U(s)x) \mathrm{d}s \\ &= x + \int_0^r F(U(s)x) \mathrm{d}s + \int_r^t F(U(s)x) \mathrm{d}s \\ &= U(r)x + \int_r^t F(U(s)x) \mathrm{d}s. \end{aligned}$$

So for each $t \geq r$ we have

$$U(t)x = U(r)x + \int_0^{t-r} F(U(r + l)x) \mathrm{d}l.$$

Setting

$$V(t) := U(t + r), \quad \forall t \in [0, \tau(x) - r),$$

we obtain

$$V(t) = U(r)x + \int_0^t F(V(l)) \mathrm{d}l, \quad \forall t \in [0, \tau(x) - r),$$

and by uniqueness of solutions we have

$$V(t) = U(t)U(r)x, \quad \forall t, r \in [0, \tau(x)) \text{ with } t \leq \tau(x) - r.$$

So we deduce that

$$U(t)x = U(t - r)U(r)x, \quad \forall t, r \in [0, \tau(x))$$

and

$$\tau(x) - r \leq \tau(U(r)x),$$

since the map $V(t) = U(t)U(r)x$ is defined on $[r, \tau(x) - r]$ and is a solution starting from $U(r)x$ at time $t = 0$.

Let $r < \tau(x)$ be given. Define

$$v(t) = \begin{cases} U(t-r)U(r)x, \ \forall t \in [r, r + \tau(U(r)x)) \\ U(t)x, \ \forall t \in [0, r]. \end{cases}$$

We obtain

$$v(t) = x + \int_0^t F(v(l))\mathrm{d}l, \quad \forall t \in [0, r + \tau(U(r)x)) \,.$$

So v is a solution and by definition of the maximal time of existence $\tau(x)$ we have

$$\tau(x) \geq r + \tau(U(r)x).$$

We conclude that

$$\tau(x) = r + \tau(U(r)x), \quad \forall r \in [0, \tau(x)),$$

and

$$U(t)x = U(t-r)U(r)x, \quad \forall t, r \in [0, \tau(x)).$$

It remains to prove that if $\tau(x) < +\infty$ then

$$\lim_{t \nearrow \tau(x)} \|U(t)x\| = +\infty.$$

Assume that $\tau(x) < +\infty$ and

$$\lim_{t \nearrow \tau(x)} \|U(t)x\| < +\infty.$$

Then we can find $M > 0$ and a sequence $\{t_m\}_{m \geq 0} \subset [0, \tau(x))$ such that

$$\lim_{m \to \infty} t_m = \tau(x),$$

and

$$\|U(t_m)x\| \leq M, \quad \forall m \geq 0.$$

By using the local existence result with (for example) $\beta = 2$ we can find a constant $\tau^* = \tau^*(M, \beta) > 0$ such that for each integer $m \geq 0$

$$\tau(x) = t_m + \tau(U(t_m)x) \geq t_m + \tau^*.$$

Now when m goes to infinity, we obtain $\tau(x) \geq \tau(x) + \tau^*$, which is impossible (since $\tau^* > 0$). $\qquad\square$

Lemma 5.17 *We have the following properties*

(i) *The map $x \to \tau(x)$ is lower semi-continuous on $\mathbb{R}^n$.*
(ii) *For each $x \in \mathbb{R}^n$, each $\hat{\tau} \in (0, \tau(x))$ and each sequence $\{x_m\}_{m \geq 0} \subset \mathbb{R}^n \to x$ we have*

$$\lim_{m \to \infty} \sup_{t \in [0, \hat{\tau}]} \|U(t)x_m - U(t)x\| = 0.$$

(iii) *The subset*
$$D_\tau = \{(t,x) \in [0,+\infty) \times \mathbb{R}^n : 0 \le t < \tau(x)\}$$

is open in $[0,+\infty) \times \mathbb{R}^n$ *(for the induced topology).*
(iv) *The map* $(t,x) \to U(t)x$ *is continuous from* D_τ *into* $\mathbb{R}^n$.

Proof Let $x \in \mathbb{R}^n$. Consider a sequence $\{x_m\}_{m \ge 0} \subset \mathbb{R}^n \to x$. Let $\hat\tau \in (0, \tau(x))$ be fixed. Set
$$\xi := 2 \sup_{t \in [0,\hat\tau]} \|U(t)x\| + 1$$

and define

$$\hat\tau_m := \sup \{t \in (0, \tau(x_m)) : \|U(l)x_m\| \le 2\xi, \quad \forall l \in [0,t]\}.$$

Let $\varepsilon > 0$ be such that
$$\xi_1 := \varepsilon K(2\xi) < 1.$$

We have for each $t, r \in [0, \min(\hat\tau_m, \hat\tau))$ with $t \ge r$

$$\|U(t)x_m - U(t)x\| = \|U(r)x_m - U(r)x - \int_r^t F(U(l)x_m) - F(U(l)x)\mathrm{d}l\|$$
$$\le \|U(r)x_m - U(r)x\| + (t-r)K(2\xi) \sup_{l \in [r,t]} \|U(l)x_m - U(l)x\|$$

and if we assume in addition that

$$r \le t \le \varepsilon + r$$

then we obtain

$$\sup_{t \in [r,r+\varepsilon]} \|U(t)x_m - U(t)x\| \le \|U(r)x_m - U(r)x\| + \xi_1 \sup_{l \in [r,r+\varepsilon]} \|U(l)x_m - U(l)x\|.$$

So for each $r \in [0, \min(\hat\tau_m, \hat\tau) - \varepsilon]$ we have

$$\sup_{t \in [r,r+\varepsilon]} \|U(t)x_m - U(t)x\| \le \left(\frac{1}{1-\xi_1}\right) \|U(r)x_m - U(r)x\|$$

and we deduce that

$$\lim_{m \to +\infty} \sup_{t \in [0,\min(\hat\tau_m,\hat\tau)]} \|U(t)x_m - U(t)x\| = 0.$$

We also have

$$\sup_{t \in [0,\min(\hat\tau_m,\hat\tau)]} \|U(t)x_m\| \le \sup_{t \in [0,\min(\hat\tau_m,\hat\tau)]} \|U(t)x_m - U(t)x\| + \sup_{t \in [0,\min(\hat\tau_m,\hat\tau)]} \|U(t)x\|$$
$$\le \sup_{t \in [0,\min(\hat\tau_m,\hat\tau)]} \|U(t)x_m - U(t)x\| + \xi,$$

therefore when m goes to $+\infty$ we obtain

$$\limsup_{m\to\infty} \sup_{t\in[0,\min(\hat{\tau}_m,\hat{\tau})]} \|U(t)x_m\| \le \xi.$$

Assume that there exists a sub-sequence $\left\{\hat{\tau}_{m_p}\right\}_{p\ge0}$ such that

$$\hat{\tau}_{m_p} \le \hat{\tau}, \quad \forall p \ge 0.$$

We have for all p large enough

$$\sup_{t\in[0,\hat{\tau}_{m_p}]} \|U(t)x_{m_p}\| < 2\xi,$$

which contradicts the definition of $\hat{\tau}_{m_p}$. So we deduce that

$$\liminf_{m\to+\infty} \hat{\tau}_m > \hat{\tau}$$

and

$$\lim_{m\to\infty} \sup_{t\in[0,\hat{\tau}]} \|U(t)x_m - U(t)x\| = 0.$$

The proof is complete.   □

5.9 Notes and Remarks

More about the logistic equation

The logistic equation was first proposed by Bernoulli [28] in 1760 as a phenomeno-logical model to describe the cumulative number of cases produced by an epidemic. Bernoulli's original paper was written in French, but his results were reconsidered in English by Dietz and Heesterbeek [90]. The logistic equation was later applied to population growth by Verhulst [347] in 1838, where the growth rate decreases with the size of population and the amount of available resources. The equation was rediscovered in 1911 by McKendrick [253] in his study of the growth of bacteria in broth and experimentally tested using a technique for nonlinear parameter estimation. Another scientist, Lotka [217], derived the equation again in 1925, calling it the law of population growth.

In 1959 Richards [289] generalized the logistic equation, and proposed a model for the growth of plants. This model takes the following form

$$u'(t) = \lambda u(t)^\alpha \left(1 - \left(\frac{u(t)}{N_\infty}\right)^\beta\right), \forall t \ge 0 \text{ and } u(s) = x \in [0, \infty),$$

where $\lambda > 0$, $N_\infty > 0$, $\alpha > 0$ and $\beta > 0$ are given parameters.

This model no longer has an explicit formula for its solution. The interested reader can find more information about the long history of the generalized logistic equation in the survey paper by Tsoularis and Wallace [342].

Model with birth limitations

In the context of cell population dynamics, the process of *contact inhibition* means that cells stop dividing whenever their local environment is too crowded (see Ducrot et al. [95]). This corresponds to a birth limitation, which is described by the following equation

$$N'(t) = \underbrace{\frac{bN(t)}{1 + \chi N(t)}}_{\text{flux of newborn}} - \underbrace{mN(t)}_{\text{flux of exit or death}}, \quad \forall t \geq 0 \text{ and } N(0) = N_0 \geq 0, \quad (5.5)$$

where $b > 0$, $m > 0$ and $\chi > 0$.

This equation is equivalent to the logistic equation via a nonlinear change of variable in time. Indeed, consider the solution $t \to L(t)$ of the equation

$$L'(t) = (1 + \chi N(L(t))), \forall t \geq 0 \text{ and } L(0) = 0$$

and define

$$V(t) := N(L(t)).$$

Then by computing the derivative of $V(t)$, we obtain

$$V'(t) = N'(L(t))L'(t) = \left[\frac{bN(L(t))}{1 + \chi N(L(t))} - mN(L(t))\right](1 + \chi N(L(t)))$$

and we deduce that V satisfies the logistic equation

$$V'(t) = bV(t) - mV(t)(1 + \chi V(t)), \forall t \geq 0 \text{ and } V(0) = N_0 \geq 0. \quad (5.6)$$

Conversely, set

$$L'(t) = (1 + \chi V(t))), \forall t \geq 0 \text{ and } L(0) = 0 \Leftrightarrow L(t) = \int_0^t (1 + \chi V(s))\mathrm{d}s, \forall t \geq 0,$$

and define

$$N(t) = V(L^{-1}(t)).$$

Then

$$N'(t) = V'(L^{-1}(t)) \, L^{-1\,\prime}(t)$$

$$= \frac{V'(L^{-1}(t))}{L'(L^{-1}(t))}$$

$$= \frac{bV(L^{-1}(t)) - mV(L^{-1}(t))(1 + \chi V(L^{-1}(t)))}{1 + \chi V(L^{-1}(t))}.$$

We deduce that $t \to N(t)$ is a solution of (5.5). Moreover, the birth limitations in (5.5) can be regarded as a version of the logistic equation after a nonlinear change of variable in time.

Remark 5.18 We do not have an explicit formula for the solution of (5.5). We have an explicit formula for $V(t)$ and for $L(t)$, but we don't have an explicit formula for $L^{-1}(t)$.

The time-dependent logistic equation

We can also look at the following non-autonomous version of the logistic equation

$$u'(t) = \lambda(t)u(t) - \gamma(t)u(t)^2, \forall t \geq s \text{ and } u(s) = x \in [0, \infty). \tag{5.7}$$

The solution is given by

$$u(t) = \frac{e^{\int_s^t \lambda(\sigma)d\sigma} x}{1 + \int_s^t \gamma(\sigma)e^{\int_s^\sigma \lambda(\hat{\sigma})d\hat{\sigma}} d\sigma}, \qquad \forall t \geq s. \tag{5.8}$$

The solution of the logistic equation is well defined by this formula as long as the denominator does not cross 0.

Parameterized systems

Consider a system of ordinary differential equation parameterized by $\lambda \in \mathbb{R}^p$

$$\frac{du_\lambda}{dt} = F(\lambda, u_\lambda(t)), \quad \forall t \geq 0 \text{ and } u_\lambda(0) = x \in \mathbb{R}^n, \tag{5.9}$$

where $F : \mathbb{R}^p \times \mathbb{R}^n \to \mathbb{R}^n$ is Lipschitz on bounded sets.

Since F is regular enough with respect to λ, we can incorporate the parameter into the state variable. Namely, we can consider the following equation

$$\begin{cases} \gamma'(t) = 0, \\ u'_\lambda(t) = F(\gamma(t), u_\lambda(t)) \end{cases} \tag{5.10}$$

with initial values

$$u_\lambda(0) = x \text{ and } \gamma(0) = \lambda.$$

Then by applying Theorem 5.13 to the system 5.10 and by using the notation

$$\tau_\lambda(x) := \tau(\lambda, x),$$

we obtain the following result.

Theorem 5.19 *Assume that* $F : \mathbb{R}^p \times \mathbb{R}^n \to \mathbb{R}^n$ *is Lipschitz on bounded sets. Then there exists a lower semi-continuous map* $\tau : \mathbb{R}^p \times \mathbb{R}^n \to (0, +\infty]$ *and a unique maximal continuous semiflow* $U_\lambda : D_{\tau_\lambda} \to \mathbb{R}^n$, *with*

$$D_\lambda = \{(t, x) \in [0, \infty) \times \mathbb{R}^n : 0 \le t < \tau_\lambda(x)\}.$$

Moreover, for each $x \in \mathbb{R}^n$, $t \to U_\lambda(t)x \in C([0, \tau_\lambda(x)), \mathbb{R}^n)$ *is the unique continuous function satisfying*

$$U_\lambda(t)x = x \int_0^t F(\lambda, U_\lambda(\sigma)) d\sigma, \quad \forall t \in [0, \tau_\lambda(x))$$

and the subset

$$D = \{(t, \lambda, x) \in [0, \infty) \times \mathbb{R}^p \times \mathbb{R}^n : 0 \le t \le \tau(\lambda, x)\}$$

is relatively open in $[0, \infty) \times \mathbb{R}^p \times \mathbb{R}^n$. *That is, for each* $(t, \lambda, x) \in D$ *there exists an* $\varepsilon > 0$ *such that*

$$|t - s| + \|\lambda - \gamma\| + \|x - y\| \le \varepsilon \text{ and } (s, \gamma, y) \in [0, \infty) \times \mathbb{R}^p \times \mathbb{R}^n \Rightarrow (s, \gamma, y) \in D.$$

Furthermore, the map $(t, \lambda, x) \to U_\lambda(t)x$ *is continuous from* D *to* $\mathbb{R}^n$.

Exercise 5.20 Assume that $F : \mathbb{R}^p \times \mathbb{R}^n \to \mathbb{R}^n$ is (only) continuous and for each λ the map $x \to F(\lambda, x)$ is Lipschitz on bounded sets. By using

$$F(\lambda, x) = F(\lambda_0, x) - [F(\lambda, x) - F(\lambda_0, x)]$$

and by extending the proof of Theorem 5.13, prove that $(\lambda, x) \to \tau(\lambda, x)$ is lower semi-continuous and the map $(\lambda, x) \to U_\lambda(t)x$ is continuous.

Non-autonomous systems

A system of ordinary differential equations is called *non-autonomous* when the right-hand side is time-dependent. That is,

$$\frac{du}{dt} = F(t, u(t)), \quad \forall t \ge s \text{ and } u(s) = x \in \mathbb{R}^n, \tag{5.11}$$

where $s \in \mathbb{R}$ is the initial time and $F : \mathbb{R} \times \mathbb{R}^n \to \mathbb{R}^n$ is Lipschitz continuous on bounded sets.

Definition 5.21 Let $s \in \mathbb{R}$ and $\tau > 0$. We say that a function $u \in C([s, s + \tau], \mathbb{R}^n)$ is a *solution* of the differential equation (5.11) if u satisfies the integral equation

$$u(t) = x + \int_s^t F(\sigma, u(\sigma)) \, d\sigma, \quad \forall t \in [s, s + \tau].$$

Definition 5.22 Consider two maps $\tau : \mathbb{R} \times \mathbb{R}^n \to (0, +\infty]$ and $U : D_\tau \to \mathbb{R}^n$, where

$$D_\tau = \left\{ (t, s, x) \in \mathbb{R}^2 \times \mathbb{R}^n : s \leq t < s + \tau(s, x) \right\}.$$

We say that U is a *maximal non-autonomous semiflow* on $\mathbb{R}^n$ if U satisfies the following properties

(i) $\tau(r, U(r, s)x) + r = \tau(s, x) + s, \ \forall s \in \mathbb{R}, \quad \forall x \in \mathbb{R}^n, \ \forall r \in [s, s + \tau(s, x))$.

(ii) $U(s, s)x = x, \ \forall s \in \mathbb{R}, \ \forall x \in \mathbb{R}$.

(iii) $U(t, r)U(r, s)x = U(t, s)x, \ \forall s \in \mathbb{R}, \quad \forall x \in X_0, \ \forall t, r \in [s, s + \tau(s, x))$ with $t \geq r$.

(iv) If $\tau(s, x) < +\infty$, then

$$\lim_{t \to (s + \tau(s, x))^-} \|U(t, s)x\| = +\infty.$$

In order to present a theorem on the existence and uniqueness of solutions to equation (5.11), we make the following assumption.

Assumption 5.23 Assume that $F : \mathbb{R} \times \mathbb{R}^n \to \mathbb{R}^n$ is a continuous map, and for each $s \in \mathbb{R}$, each $\sigma > 0$ and each $\xi > 0$ there exists a $K(s, \sigma, \xi) > 0$ such that

$$\|F(t + s, x) - F(t + s, y)\| \leq K(s, \sigma, \xi) \|x - y\|$$

whenever $t \in [0, \sigma]$, $y, x \in X_0$ with $\|x\| \leq \xi$ and $\|y\| \leq \xi$.

Set

$$D = \left\{ (t, s, x) \in \mathbb{R}^2 \times X_0 : t \geq s \right\}.$$

One can find a proof of the following theorem in Magal and Ruan [237, Theorem 5.2].

Theorem 5.24 *Let Assumption 5.23 be satisfied. Then there exist a map* $\tau : \mathbb{R} \times \mathbb{R}^n \to (0, +\infty]$ *and a maximal non-autonomous semiflow* $U : D_\tau \to \mathbb{R}^n$ *such that for each* $x \in \mathbb{R}^n$ *and each* $s \geq \mathbb{R}$, $U(\cdot, s)x \in C([s, s + \tau(s, x)), \mathbb{R}^n)$ *is a unique maximal solution of* (5.11). *Moreover,* D_τ *is open in* D *and the map* $(t, s, x) \to U(t, s)x$ *is continuous from* D_τ *into* $\mathbb{R}^n$.

Exercise 5.25 Prove Theorem 5.24 by extending the arguments of Theorem 5.13.

Autonomous reformulation of non-autonomous systems

Assume that F is more regular, namely that $(t, x) \rightarrow F(t, x)$ is Lipschitz continuous on bounded sets. Then we can transform the system (5.11) into the following autonomous system for all $t \geq 0$

$$\begin{cases} u'(t) = F(v(t), u(t)), \\ v'(t) = 1, \end{cases} \tag{5.12}$$

where the initial value is

$$u(0) = x \in \mathbb{R}^n \text{ and } v(0) = s \in \mathbb{R}.$$

We can apply Theorem 5.13 to the system (5.12). We deduce that the system (5.12) generates a semiflow

$$\Pi(t) \begin{pmatrix} s \\ x \end{pmatrix} = \begin{pmatrix} u(t) \\ v(t) \end{pmatrix} = \begin{pmatrix} U(t + s, s, x) \\ V(t + s, s, x) \end{pmatrix}, \quad \forall t \in [0, \tau(x, s))$$

where $\tau(x, s) \in (0, \infty]$ is the time of blow-up for the solution starting from the initial value (x, s).

By solving the first equation (5.12) we obtain

$$v(t) = t + s.$$

Therefore, by using the semi-flow property for $\Pi(t)\Pi(t') = \Pi(t + t')$, we deduce that

$$U(t + t' + s, s, x) = U(t + t' + s, t' + s, U(t' + s, s, x)).$$

Maximal flows

Consider again the ordinary differential equation

$$\begin{cases} u'(t) = F(u(t)), \quad \forall t \geq 0, \\ u(0) = x \in \mathbb{R}^n, \end{cases}$$

then we can try to extend the solution backwards in time (i.e. for negative time) by setting

$$u(t) = v(-t), \quad \forall t \leq 0,$$

where $t \rightarrow v(t)$ is the unique solution of

$$\begin{cases} v'(t) = -F(v(t)), \quad \forall t \geq 0, \\ v(0) = x \in \mathbb{R}^n. \end{cases}$$

Then

$$u'(t) = -v'(-t) = F(v(-t)) = F(u(t)), \quad \forall t \le 0.$$

We conclude that the problem is unchanged for negative time, and it is sufficient to replace F with $-F$ and apply the result for the problem forward in time.

Definition 5.26 We consider two maps $\tau^+ : \mathbb{R}^n \to (0, +\infty]$ (the *blow-up time forward in time*) and $\tau^- : \mathbb{R}^n \to (0, +\infty]$ (the *blow-up time backwards in time*) and $U : D_{\tau^\pm} \to \mathbb{R}^n$, where

$$D_{\tau^\pm} := \{(t, x) \in \mathbb{R} \times \mathbb{R}^n : -\tau^-(x) < t < \tau^+(x)\}.$$

We will say that U is a *maximal flow* on $\mathbb{R}^n$ if the following properties are satisfied:

(i) $\pm\tau^\pm(U(t)x) + t = \pm\tau^\pm(x)$, $\forall x \in \mathbb{R}^n$, $\forall t \in (-\tau^-(x), \tau^+(x))$;
(ii) $U(0)x = x$, $\forall x \in \mathbb{R}^n$;
(iii) $U(t)U(s)x = U(t + s)x$, whenever $x \in \mathbb{R}^n$, $t, s \in (-\tau^-(x), \tau^+(x))$ and $t + s \in (-\tau^-(x), \tau^+(x))$;
(iv) If $\tau^+(x) < +\infty$ (respectively $\tau^-(x) < +\infty$) then

$$\lim_{t \to \tau^+(x)^-} \|U(t)x\| = +\infty \text{ (respectively } \lim_{t \to -\tau^-(x)^+} \|U(t)x\| = +\infty).$$

We will say that U is *continuous* if $D_{\tau^\pm}$ is open in $\mathbb{R} \times \mathbb{R}^n$ and the map $(t, x) \to U(t)x$ is continuous from $D_{\tau^\pm}$ into $\mathbb{R}^n$.

As a direct consequence of Theorem 5.13 we obtain the following result.

Theorem 5.27 *Let $F : \mathbb{R}^n \to \mathbb{R}^n$ be a map which is Lipschitz continuous on bounded subsets of $\mathbb{R}^n$. Then there exist two unique lower semi-continuous maps $\tau^\pm : \mathbb{R}^n \to (0, +\infty]$ a unique maximal continuous flow $U : D_{\tau^\pm} \to \mathbb{R}^n$ such that for each $x \in \mathbb{R}^n$, $u(\cdot) := U(\cdot)x \in C((-\tau^-(x), \tau^+(x)), \mathbb{R}^n)$ is the unique solution of the fixed-point problem*

$$u(t) = x + \int_0^t F(u(s)x)\mathrm{d}s, \quad \forall t \in (-\tau^-(x), \tau^+(x)).$$

Remark 5.28 For the logistic equation (5.2) we have

$$\tau^+(x) := \begin{cases} \infty, & \text{if } x \ge 0, \\ \frac{1}{\lambda} \ln\left(1 - \frac{\kappa}{x}\right), & \text{if } x < 0, \end{cases}$$

and

$$\tau^-(x) := \begin{cases} \infty, & \text{if } x \le \kappa, \\ -\frac{1}{\lambda} \ln\left(1 - \frac{\kappa}{x}\right), & \text{if } x > \kappa. \end{cases}$$

Semiflow and blow-up time in Banach spaces

The results presented in this chapter can be extended to the abstract Cauchy problem

$$u'(t) = Au(t) + F(u(t)), \forall t \geq 0, \text{ and } u(0) = x \in X, \tag{5.13}$$

where $A : D(A) \subset X \to X$ is a linear operator on a Banach space X and $F : \overline{D(A)} \to X$.

The first problem with such an equation is that

$$u(t) \notin D(A).$$

Therefore we need to introduce a weaker notion of solution than the classical one.

Definition 5.29 A *mild solution* of (5.13) is a continuous map $u \in C([0, \tau], X)$ satisfying

$$\int_0^t u(s)\mathrm{d}s \in D(A), \quad \forall t \in [0, \tau] \tag{5.14}$$

and

$$u(t) = x + A \int_0^t u(s)\mathrm{d}s + \int_0^t F(u(s))\mathrm{d}s, \quad \forall t \in [0, \tau]. \tag{5.15}$$

We will say that $u \in C([0, \tau], X)$ is a *classical solution* (or *strong solution*) if

$$u(t) \in D(A), \quad \forall t \in [0, \tau],$$
$$u \in C^1([0, \tau], X), \text{ and}$$
$$u'(t) = Au(t) + F(u(t)), \quad \forall t \in [0, \tau].$$

Whenever the domain of A is dense in X, that is, if

$$\overline{D(A)} = X,$$

then we can use the semigroup theory if A is a Hille–Yosida operator (see Theorem 2.45 in the remarks and notes of Chapter 2). In this case, A is the infinitesimal generator of a C_0- semigroup $\{T_A(t)\}_{t \geq 0} \subset \mathcal{L}(X)$ and the mild solution of (5.13) is given by

$$u(t) = T_A(t)x + \int_0^t T_A(t - s)F(u(s))\mathrm{d}s, \quad \forall t \geq 0.$$

We refer to the books of Pazy [274] and Cazenave and Haraux [51] for densely defined Cauchy problems. We refer to Henry [149] for a presentation of the case of a sectorial operator A (i.e. corresponding to a parabolic equation whenever the linear operator A corresponds to a diffusion). We refer to Magal [237, Section 5] and [236] for more results in the case when A is not densely defined and $F(x)$ is replaced by a non-autonomous $F(t, x)$.

An abstract logistic equation

The explicit solution of the logistic equation also extends to the Banach case

$$u'(t) = Au(t) + x^*(u(t))u(t), \forall t \geq 0, \text{ and } u(0) = x \in X$$

where $x^* : X \to \mathbb{R}$ is a continuous linear form on a Banach space X and $A : D(A) \subset X \to X$ is a linear operator on X. Then we have the mild solution

$$u(t) = T_A(t)x + \int_0^t T_A(t-s)x^*(u(\sigma))u(\sigma)\mathrm{d}\sigma,$$

which is given by

$$u(t) = \frac{T_A(t)x}{1 + \int_0^t x^*(T_A(\sigma)x)\mathrm{d}\sigma}.$$

More results can be found in Magal [228].

Nonlinear Volterra integral equations

The existence and uniqueness results of this chapter can be extended to nonlinear Volterra integral equations of the form

$$u(t) = F(t) + \int_0^t G(t-a)h(u(a))\,\mathrm{d}a,$$

where $t \in [0, \infty) \to F(t) \in \mathbb{R}^n$, $a \in (0, \infty) \to G(a) \in M_n(\mathbb{R})$, are continuous maps and we assume that

$$\int_0^\tau \|G(a)\|\mathrm{d}a < \infty, \quad \forall \tau > 0.$$

Moreover, the map $h : \mathbb{R}^n \to \mathbb{R}^n$ is Lipschitz continuous on bounded sets.

Remark 5.30 If we assume that $a \to G(a)$ blows up at $a = 0$ we can cover the fractional differential equations.

We refer to the book of Burton [41] for more results in this direction.

5.10 MATLAB Codes

Figure 5.1

```
1
2  lambda=1;
3  k=10;
4  x=-10:0.01:100;
5  x=x';
6  y=f(0,x,lambda,k);
7
8  clf;
9  plot(x,y,'r','LineWidth',5)
10 hold on;
11 plot(x,0*x,'k',0*x,x,'k','LineWidth',5)
12
13 aux=ones(size(x))
14
15 plot(lambda*k*aux,x,'g',lambda*k*aux/2,x,'g','
       LineWidth',5)
16
17 xlabel('x');
18 ylabel('y');
19
20
21 set(gca,'XLim',[-2  12])
22 set(gca,'YLim',[-2  5])
23
24 set(gca,'fontweight','bold','FontSize',30);
25 ax=gca;
26
27 function dy=f(t,x,lambda,k)
28 n=size(x);
29 dy=zeros(n);
30 dy=x.*(lambda-x/k);
31 end
```

Figure 5.2

```
1
2  lambda=1;
3  k=10;
4
5  deltaT=0.05;
```

```
 6   T=10;
 7
 8   X0=[1];
 9   t0 =0: deltaT :T;
10   [ t1 , x1 ]= ode45 (@f, t0 ,X0,[] , lambda , k ) ;
11
12   clf ;
13   plot ( t1 , x1 , ' r ' , ' LineWidth ' ,5)
14   hold  on ;
15
16   plot ( t0 ,0* t0 , 'k ' , ' LineWidth ' ,5)
17
18   X0=[ 17 ];
19
20   [ t2 , x2 ]= ode45 (@f, t0 ,X0,[] , lambda , k ) ;
21   plot ( t2 , x2 , ' r ' , ' LineWidth ' ,5)
22
23   aux1=ones ( size ( t0 ) ) ;
24
25   plot ( t0 , lambda* k* aux1 , 'k ' , ' LineWidth ' ,5)
26   X0=[ −0.5 ];
27
28   [ t2 , x2 ]= ode45 (@f, t0 ,X0,[] , lambda , k ) ;
29   plot ( t2 , x2 , ' r ' , ' LineWidth ' ,5)
30
31
32   tau =(1/ lambda )* log (1 − lambda* k /X0) ;
33
34   x = −30:0.1:20;
35   aux=ones ( size ( x ) ) ;
36
37   plot ( tau* aux , x , ' g ' , ' LineWidth ' ,5) ;
38   xlabel ( ' t ' ) ;
39   ylabel ( ' x ( t ) ' ) ;
40
41
42   set ( gca , 'YLim ' ,[ −30  20])
43
44
45
46   set ( gca , ' fontweight ' , ' bold ' , ' FontSize ' ,30) ;
47   ax=gca ;
48
49   function  dy=f( t , x , lambda , k )
50   n= size ( x ) ;
51   dy= zeros ( n ) ;
```

```
52  dy=x.*(lambda-x/k);
53  end
```

Figure 5.3

```
1
2   x=1;
3
4   t1=-2*x^0.5-8;
5
6   t=-50:0.1:40;
7   n=size(t)
8   y=zeros(n);
9
10
11  for  i=1:n(2)
12      y(i)=f(t(i),x,t1);
13  end
14  clf;
15  plot(t,0*t,'k','LineWidth',5);
16  hold on;
17
18  plot(0*t,t,'k','LineWidth',5);
19
20
21  plot(t,y,'r','LineWidth',5);
22
23  plot(t1,0,'ok', 'MarkerFaceColor','k', 'MarkerSize',
        15)
24
25  plot(-2*x^0.5,0,'ok', 'MarkerFaceColor','k', '
        MarkerSize', 15)
26
27  xlabel('t');
28  ylabel('x(t)');
29
30
31  set(gca,'XLim',[-20  10])
32  set(gca,'YLim',[-40  40])
33  set(gca,'fontweight','bold','FontSize',30);
34  ax=gca;
35
36
37
38  function y=f(t,x,t1)
```

```
39
40  if  ( t >=-2*x^0.5)
41       y =( x^0.5+ t /2 )^2;
42  else
43       if  ( t > t1 )
44            y =0;
45       else
46            y =-(( t1 - t )/2 )^2;
47       end
48  end
49  end
```

Figure 5.4

```
1   lambda =0.6;
2   k =10;
3
4   deltaT =0.05;
5   T =10;
6   t0 =0: deltaT : T;
7
8   clf ;
9
10
11
12
13
14
15  X0 =[ -0.5];
16  [ t2 , x2 ]= ode45 (@f, t0 , X0,[ ] , lambda , k ) ;
17  plot ( t2 , x2 , ': k ' , 'LineWidth' ,5)
18  hold  on ;
19
20  plot ( t0 ,0* t0 , 'k' , 'LineWidth' ,5)
21
22  tau =(1/ lambda )* log (1 - lambda * k / X0) ;
23  x = -30:0.1:20;
24  aux = ones ( size ( x ) ) ;
25  plot ( tau * aux , x , 'g' , 'LineWidth' ,5) ;
26
27
28  plot (( tau -1)* aux , x , 'g' , 'LineWidth' ,5) ;
29
30  X0 =[ -0.6];
31  [ t2 , x2 ]= ode45 (@f, t0 , X0,[ ] , lambda , k ) ;
```

```
32  plot(t2,x2,'r','LineWidth',5)
33
34
35  X0=[-0.4];
36  [t2,x2]=ode45(@f,t0,X0,[],lambda,k);
37  plot(t2,x2,'r','LineWidth',5)
38
39
40
41
42  xlabel('t');
43  ylabel('x(t)');
44
45  set(gca,'YLim',[-20  5])
46  set(gca,'fontweight','bold','FontSize',30);
47  ax=gca;
48
49  function dy=f(t,x,lambda,k)
50  n=size(x);
51  dy=zeros(n);
52  dy=x.*(lambda-x/k);
53  end
```

Chapter 6
The Linearized Stability Principle and the Hartman–Grobman Theorem

First, we reconsider the logistic equation around the trivial equilibrium 0. Recall from Chapter 5 that the logistic equation takes the following form

$$N'(t) = \lambda N(t)\left(1 - \frac{N(t)}{\kappa}\right), \quad \forall t \geq 0 \text{ and } N(0) = N_0 \geq 0, \tag{6.1}$$

where $\lambda > 0$ and $\kappa > 0$ are given parameters. Figure 6.1 summarizes the behavior of the solutions of the above logistic equation, depending on the sign of the initial data N_0.

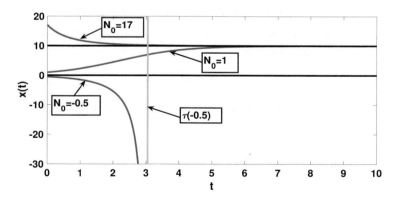

Fig. 6.1: *In this figure we plot three solutions starting from $N_0 = -0.5, 1, 17$ of the logistic equation for $\lambda = 1$ and $\kappa = 10$.*

The main difficulty in defining the linearized equation around 0 for the logistic equation is that finite time blow-up occurs for all negative initial data. Now set $U = U(t, x)$, the maximal semiflow associated to (6.1) (here $x \in \mathbb{R}$ denotes the initial data). This map $x \mapsto U(t, x)$ is not defined for all $t \geq 0$ whenever $x < 0$. Indeed, we can explicitly compute the solution as follows

A. Ducrot et al., *Differential Equations and Population Dynamics I*, Lecture Notes on Mathematical Modelling in the Life Sciences, https://doi.org/10.1007/978-3-030-98136-5_6

$$U(t, x) = \frac{e^{\lambda t} x}{1 + \frac{\lambda}{\kappa} \int_0^t e^{\lambda \sigma} x \, d\sigma}, \qquad \forall t \in [0, \tau(x)), \tag{6.2}$$

wherein $\tau(x)$ is the maximal existence time given by

$$\tau(x) := \frac{1}{\lambda} \ln \left(1 - \frac{\kappa}{x} \right).$$

We observe that due to the lower semi-continuity of the map $x \to \tau(x)$ (time of blow-up if finite), and since $\tau(0) = \infty$, for each $\widehat{\tau} > 0$, we can find $\varepsilon > 0$ such that

$$x \in (-\varepsilon, \varepsilon) \Rightarrow \tau(x) > \widehat{\tau}.$$

Now the map $x \mapsto U(t, x)$ is well defined on $(t, x) \in [0, \widehat{\tau}] \times (-\varepsilon, \varepsilon)$ and we can try to differentiate this map with respect to x. By using the explicit formula (6.2) we obtain that

$$\partial_x U(t, x) = \frac{e^{\lambda t} \left[1 + \frac{\lambda}{\kappa} \int_0^t e^{\lambda \sigma} x \, d\sigma \right] - e^{\lambda t} x \left[\frac{\lambda}{\kappa} \int_0^t e^{\lambda \sigma} \, d\sigma \right]}{\left[1 + \frac{\lambda}{\kappa} \int_0^t e^{\lambda \sigma} x \, d\sigma \right]^2},$$

so that with $x = 0$

$$\partial_x U(t, 0) = e^{\lambda t}, \qquad \forall t \in [0, \widehat{\tau}].$$

The derivative of the function $t \mapsto V(t)y := \partial_x U(t, 0)y = e^{\lambda t} y$ becomes the solution of

$$V'(t)y = \lambda V(t)y, \forall t \geq 0, \text{ and } V(0)y = y. \tag{6.3}$$

Observe that by computing the derivative at $N = 0$ of the right-hand side of (6.1) (i.e. $f(N) = \lambda N(1 - \frac{N}{\kappa})$) we obtain

$$f'(0) = \lambda.$$

Therefore, (6.3) is called the linearized equation of (6.1) at $N = 0$.

6.1 The Linearized Equation Around a Solution

In this section we are concerned with general n-dimensional ordinary differential equations of the form

$$\frac{du(t)}{dt} = F(u(t)), \; t \geq 0 \text{ and } u(0) = x \in \mathbb{R}^n. \tag{6.4}$$

Here and below $n \geq 1$ denotes some given and fixed integer while $F : \mathbb{R}^n \to \mathbb{R}^n$ is some smooth map.

The first result describes the derivative of the maximal semiflow generated by (6.4), denoted below by $U = U(t, x)$, while $x \mapsto \tau(x)$ is the maximal time of existence.

Theorem 6.1 *Assume that $F : \mathbb{R}^n \to \mathbb{R}^n$ is of class C^1 on $\mathbb{R}^n$. Then for each $x_0 \in \mathbb{R}^n$ and each $\tau \in [0, \tau(x_0))$ there exists an $\varepsilon = \varepsilon(\tau, x_0) > 0$ such that the map $x \mapsto U(t, x)$ is defined for each $t \in [0, \tau]$ on the open ball $B_{\mathbb{R}^n}(x_0, \varepsilon) = \{x \in \mathbb{R}^n : \|x - x_0\| < \varepsilon\}$. Moreover, for each $t \in [0, \tau]$, the map $x \mapsto U(t, x)$ is continuously differentiable and if we set*

$$V(t)y = \partial_x U(t, x_0)y, \forall t \in [0, \tau],$$

then $t \mapsto V(t)y$ becomes the solution of the following non-autonomous ordinary differential equation

$$\begin{cases} \dfrac{dV(t)y}{dt} = DF\left(U(t, x_0)\right)(V(t)y), & \forall t \in [0, \tau], \\ V(0)y = y. \end{cases}$$

Moreover, for each $t \in [0, \tau]$, the map $x \mapsto \partial_x U(t, x)$ is continuous.

Proof For each $t \in [0, \tau]$, we have

$$U(t, x_0 + h) - U(t, x_0)$$

$$= \left[x_0 + h + \int_0^t F\left(U(l, x_0 + h)\right) dl\right] - \left[x_0 + \int_0^t F\left(U(l, x_0)\right) dl\right]$$

$$= h + \int_0^t \left[F\left(U(l, x_0 + h)\right) - F\left(U(l, x_0)\right)\right] dl$$

and

$$V(t)h = h + \int_0^t DF(U(l, x_0))(V(s)h)ds.$$

We deduce that

$$U(t, x_0 + h) - U(t, x_0) - V(t)h =$$

$$\int_0^t \left[F(U(s, x_0 + h)) - F(U(s, x_0)) - DF(U(s, x_0))(V(s)h)\right]ds =$$

$$\int_0^t \left\{F(U(s, x_0 + h)) - F(U(s, x_0)) - DF(U(s, x_0))\left[U(s, x_0 + h) - U(s, x_0)\right]\right\} ds$$

$$+ \int_0^t DF(U(s, x_0))\left[U(s, x_0 + h) - U(s, x_0) - V(s)h\right]ds.$$

Define

$$W(t)(h) = U(t, x_0 + h) - U(t, x_0) - V(t)h,$$

and observe that it satisfies

$$W(t)(h) =$$

$$\int_0^t F(U(s, x_0 + h)) - F(U(s, x_0)) - DF(U(s, x_0))[U(s, x_0 + h) - U(s, x_0)]ds$$

$$+ \int_0^t DF(U(s, x_0))(W(s)h)ds.$$

Next set

$$\kappa := \sup_{t \in [0, \tau]} \|DF(U(s, x_0))\|_{\mathcal{L}(\mathbb{R}^n)} < +\infty,$$

which is finite because $x \mapsto DF(x)$ and $t \to U(t, x_0)$ are both continuous.

By using the fundamental formula of differential calculus (see Lemma 5.3), we have

$$F(U(s, x_0 + h)) - F(U(s, x_0)) =$$

$$\int_0^1 DF\big(sU(t, x_0 + h) + (1 - s)U(t, x_0)\big)\big(U(t, x_0 + h) - U(t, x_0)\big)\, ds,$$

and we obtain

$$\|W(t)h\| \le \int_0^t \|H(s)\|ds + \kappa \int_0^t \|W(s)h\|ds, \qquad (6.5)$$

with

$$H(t) := \int_0^1 \big[DF(sU(t, x_0 + h) + (1 - s)U(t, x_0)) - DF(U(t, x_0))\big]\big[U(t, x_0 + h) - U(t, x_0)\big]ds.$$

Thanks to the semiflow property (i.e. $U(t)U(s) = U(t + s)$) and by continuity of the map $(t, x) \to U(t, x)$, it is sufficient to prove the result for $\tau > 0$ small enough.

Let $\tau \in (0, \frac{1}{1+\kappa})$ be given. From (6.5) we have

$$\sup_{t \in [0, \tau]} \|W(t)h\| \le \tau \sup_{t \in [0, \tau]} \|H(t)\| + \kappa\tau \sup_{t \in [0, \tau]} \|W(t)h\|$$

hence

$$\sup_{t \in [0, \tau]} \|W(t)h\| \le \frac{\tau}{1 - \kappa\tau} \sup_{t \in [0, \tau]} \|H(t)\|. \qquad (6.6)$$

Finally, we have

$$U(t, x_0 + h) - U(t, x_0) = h + \int_0^t [F(U(s, x_0 + h)) - F(U(s, x_0))]\, ds$$
$$= h + \int_0^t \int_0^1 DF[lU(s, x_0 + h) + (1 - l)U(s, x_0)](U(s, x_0 + h) - U(s, x_0))dlds$$

so that for each $t \in [0, \tau]$ we get

$$\|U(t, x_0 + h) - U(t, x_0)\| \le \|h\| + \int_0^t \widehat{\kappa}\|U(s, x_0 + h) - U(s, x_0)\|ds. \qquad (6.7)$$

Here we have set

$$\widehat{\kappa} := \sup_{t \in [0,\tau] \text{ and } l \in [0,1]} \|DF(lU(t, x_0 + h) + (1 - l)U(t, x_0)))\|_{\mathcal{L}(\mathbb{R}^n)}.$$

Now by using the continuity of the map $(t, x) \rightarrow U(t, x)$ and taking $\varepsilon > 0$ small enough, we have $\widehat{\kappa} \leq \kappa + 1$. Hence, taking the supremum of both sides of (6.7) yields

$$\sup_{t \in [0,\tau]} \|U(t, x_0 + h) - U(t, x_0)\| \leq \frac{\|h\|}{1 - \widehat{\kappa}\tau},$$

so that

$$\sup_{t \in [0,\tau]} \|H(t)\| \leq \frac{\|h\|\varepsilon(h)}{1 - \widehat{\kappa}\tau}, \tag{6.8}$$

with

$$\varepsilon(h) := \sup_{t \in [0,\tau] \text{ and } s \in [0,1]} \|DF(sU(t, x_0+h)+(1-s)U(t, x_0))) - DF(U(t, x_0))\|_{\mathcal{L}(\mathbb{R}^n)}.$$

Since

$$\varepsilon(h) \underset{h \to 0}{\rightarrow} 0,$$

the result follows by combining (6.6) and (6.8).   □

6.2 Exponential Stability of an Equilibrium

Assume that $\overline{x}$ is an equilibrium. Then it satisfies

$$U(t, \overline{x}) = \overline{x}, \ \forall t \geq 0.$$

In this case the function of time

$$V(t)y = \partial_x U(t, \overline{x})y$$

is the unique solution of the linearized equation

$$\begin{cases} \dfrac{dV(t)y}{dt} = DF(\overline{x})(V(t)y), & \forall t \in [0, \tau], \\ V(0)y = y. \end{cases}$$

Theorem 6.2 (Exponential stability) *Let F be a C^1-map on $\mathbb{R}^n$. Assume that there exists an $\overline{x} \in \mathbb{R}^n$ such that*

$$F(\overline{x}) = 0$$

and

$$s(DF(\overline{x})) < 0.$$

Then for each $\eta \in (0, -s(DF(\overline{x})))$, there exist two constants $\varepsilon = \varepsilon(\eta) > 0$ and $M := M(\eta) \geq 0$ such that

$$\tau(x) = +\infty, \forall x \in B_{\mathbb{R}^n}(\overline{x}, \varepsilon),$$

and

$$\|U(t, x) - \overline{x}\| \le e^{-\eta t} M \|x - \overline{x}\|, \quad \forall t \ge 0, \forall x \in B_{\mathbb{R}^n}(\overline{x}, \varepsilon).$$

Remark 6.3 Recall that by definition

$$s(DF(\overline{x})) = \max\{\text{Re}(\lambda) : \lambda \in \sigma(DF(\overline{x}))\}.$$

Therefore $s(DF(\overline{x}))$, the spectral bound of $DF(\overline{x})$, is negative if and only if all the eigenvalues of $DF(\overline{x})$ have a strictly negative real part.

Proof By using the change of variable $\widetilde{x} = x - \overline{x}$ we can replace $\overline{x}$ by 0. Set

$$A := DF(0) \text{ and } G(x) = F(x) - Ax.$$

Let $\eta \in (0, -s(A))$ be fixed. Let $\widehat{\eta} \in (\eta, -s(A))$ be given. We can rewrite the ordinary differential equation

$$X'(t) = F(X(t))$$

as

$$X'(t) = AX(t) + G(X(t)).$$

Consider now the equivalent norm

$$|x| = \sup_{t \ge 0} e^{\widehat{\eta} t} \left\| e^{At} x \right\|.$$

Since $\widehat{\eta} < -s(A)$, we deduce that this norm is well defined, since

$$s(A + \widehat{\eta}I) = s(A) + \widehat{\eta} < 0.$$

So by the exponential stability Theorem 3.17, we have

$$\lim_{t \to +\infty} e^{\widehat{\eta} t} e^{At} = \lim_{t \to +\infty} e^{[A + \widehat{\eta}I]t} = 0.$$

It is readily checked that

$$\|x\| \le |x| \le M \|x\|, \quad \forall x \in \mathbb{R}^n, \tag{6.9}$$

and

$$\left| e^{At} x \right| \le \sup_{s \ge 0} e^{\widehat{\eta} s} \left\| e^{A(s+t)} x \right\| = e^{-\widehat{\eta} t} \sup_{s \ge 0} e^{\widehat{\eta}(s+t)} \left\| e^{A(s+t)} x \right\| \le e^{-\widehat{\eta} t} |x|,$$

hence

$$\left| e^{At} x \right| \le e^{-\widehat{\eta} t} |x|, \quad \forall t \ge 0, \quad \forall x \in \mathbb{R}^n. \tag{6.10}$$

Let $\varepsilon_0 > 0$ be given. By using the local existence result provided in Lemma 5.15, there exists a $\tau_0 = \tau_0(\varepsilon_0) > 0$ such that for each $x \in B_{\mathbb{R}^n}(0, \varepsilon_0)$ one has

$$\|U(t,x)\| \leq 2\varepsilon_0, \quad \forall t \in [0, \tau_0].$$

Observe that for each $x \in B(0, \varepsilon_0)$ and each $t \in [0, \tau_0]$ we have

$$U(t,x) = U(t,x) - 0 = U(t,x) - U(t,0) = \int_0^1 \partial_x U(t, sx)x\,ds,$$

and by computing the derivative of the semiflow with respect to the initial value (see Theorem 6.1) we have

$$\partial_x U(t,x)y = e^{At}y + \int_0^t e^{A(t-\sigma)} DG(U(\sigma,x)) \left[\partial_x U(\sigma,x)y\right] d\sigma,$$

for each $t \in [0, \tau_0]$, $x \in B(0, \varepsilon_0)$ and each $y \in \mathbb{R}^n$.

Therefore, we obtain

$$|\partial_x U(t,x)|_{\mathcal{L}(\mathbb{R}^n)} \leq \left|e^{At}\right|_{\mathcal{L}(\mathbb{R}^n)}$$
$$+ \int_0^t \left|e^{A(t-s)}\right|_{\mathcal{L}(\mathbb{R}^n)} |DG(U(s,x))|_{\mathcal{L}(\mathbb{R}^n)} |\partial_x U(s,x)|_{\mathcal{L}(\mathbb{R}^n)}\,ds,$$

which implies

$$|\partial_x U(t,x)|_{\mathcal{L}(\mathbb{R}^n)} \leq e^{-\widehat{\eta}t} + \int_0^t e^{-\widehat{\eta}(t-s)} |DG(U(s,x))|_{\mathcal{L}(\mathbb{R}^n)} |\partial_x U(s,x)|_{\mathcal{L}(\mathbb{R}^n)}\,ds.$$
(6.11)

Let $\delta \in (0, \widehat{\eta} - \eta)$ be given and fixed. Since by assumption G is a C^1-map, we have

$$\lim_{x \to 0} |DG(x)|_{\mathcal{L}(\mathbb{R}^n)} = 0,$$

and reducing $\varepsilon_0 > 0$ if necessary one may assume

$$|DG(x)|_{\mathcal{L}(\mathbb{R}^n)} \leq \delta, \quad \forall x \in B(0, 2\varepsilon_0),$$

and (6.11) becomes

$$|\partial_x U(t,x)|_{\mathcal{L}(\mathbb{R}^n)} \leq e^{-\widehat{\eta}t} + \int_0^t \delta e^{-\widehat{\eta}(t-s)} |\partial_x U(s,x)|_{\mathcal{L}(\mathbb{R}^n)}\,ds.$$

Setting

$$X(t) := e^{\widehat{\eta}t} |\partial_x U(t,x)|_{\mathcal{L}(\mathbb{R}^n)}, \quad \forall t \in [0, \tau_0],$$

we obtain

$$X(t) \leq 1 + \int_0^t \delta X(s)ds,$$

and by using the integral form of Gronwall's lemma (see Lemma 8.8), we deduce that

$$X(t) \leq e^{\delta t}, \quad \forall t \in [0, \tau_0],$$

that is, since $-\widehat{\eta} + \delta \leq -\eta$,

$$|\partial_x U(t,x)|_{\mathcal{L}(\mathbb{R}^n)} = e^{-\widehat{\eta}t} X(t) \leq e^{[-\widehat{\eta}+\delta]t} \leq e^{-\eta t}.$$

We deduce that for each $t \in [0, \tau_0]$ and each $x \in B(0, \varepsilon_0)$ we have

$$|U(t,x)| = \left| \int_0^1 \partial_x U(t, sx) x \, ds \right| \leq \int_0^1 |DU(t)(sx) x| \, dt \leq e^{-\eta t} |x|.$$

As a consequence, when $\mathbb{R}^n$ is endowed with the norm $|\cdot|$ we have

$$|U(t,x)| \leq e^{-\eta t} |x|, \quad \forall x \in B(0, \varepsilon_0), \quad \forall t \in [0, \tau_0].$$

We may always assume that $B(0, \varepsilon_0)$ is the ball for the new norm $|\cdot|$ and the result follows by induction and by using again the semiflow property (i.e. $U(t + s) = U(t)U(s), \forall t, s \geq 0$ with $t + s \leq \tau(\cdot)$). $\qquad \square$

6.3 The Hartman–Grobman Theorem for a Hyperbolic Equilibrium

The following fixed-point theorem can be proved by using index theory (see for example Deimling [74]).

Theorem 6.4 (Brouwer's fixed-point theorem) *Let $F : C \to C$ be a continuous map on a compact and convex subset C of $\mathbb{R}^n$. Then there exists an $\overline{x} \in C$ such that $F(\overline{x}) = \overline{x}$.*

Remark 6.5 Brouwer's fixed-point theorem has an infinite dimensional version called the Schauder's fixed-point theorem.

Theorem 6.6 (Hartman–Grobman) *Consider an ordinary differential of the form*

$$U'(t)x = AU(t)x + G(U(t)x), \forall t \geq 0, \text{ and } U(0)x = x,$$

where $A \in M_n(\mathbb{R})$, and $G : \mathbb{R}^n \to \mathbb{R}^n$ is a continuously differentiable map satisfying

$$G(0) = 0, \text{ and } DG(0) = 0_{M_n(\mathbb{R})}.$$

Assume that 0 is hyperbolic (i.e. the spectrum of A does not contain any purely imaginary eigenvalue), that is,

$$\sigma(A) \cap i\mathbb{R} = \emptyset.$$

Then there exists a number $\varepsilon > 0$ such that for any map $G : \mathbb{R}^n \to \mathbb{R}^n$ such that

$$\|G\|_{\mathrm{Lip}} \leq \varepsilon \text{ and } \|G\|_\infty := \sup_{x \in \mathbb{R}^n} \|G(x)\| < +\infty,$$

there exists a map $\Lambda : \mathbb{R}^n \to \mathbb{R}^n$ (a nonlinear change of variables) which is continuous and invertible with

$$\Lambda(0) = 0,$$

and which satisfies

$$\Lambda^{-1}U(t)\Lambda = e^{At}, \quad \forall t \in \mathbb{R}.$$

Remark 6.7 By using a truncation procedure, we can obtain the same result locally in a neighborhood of 0.

Proof We first assume there exists such an invertible and continuous function $\Lambda : \mathbb{R}^n \to \mathbb{R}^n$ of the form

$$\Lambda = I + \Psi$$

and $\Psi \in BC(\mathbb{R}^n)$ (i.e. bounded and continuous functions on $\mathbb{R}^n$ into itself)

$$\|\Psi\|_\infty < +\infty.$$

We should have for any $t \geq 0$ and $x \in \mathbb{R}^n$:

$$U(t)(x + \Psi(x)) = e^{At}x + \Psi(e^{At}x). \tag{6.12}$$

Then using the variation of constant formula

$$U(t)x = e^{A(t-s)}U(s)x + \int_s^t e^{A(t-l)}G(U(s)x)\,ds \text{ for } t \geq s,$$

we derive

$$U(t)(x + \Psi(x)) = \begin{cases} e^{At}(x + \Psi(x)) + \int_0^t e^{A(t-l)}G(U(l)(x + \Psi(x)))\,dl \text{ for } t \geq 0, \\ e^{At}(x + \Psi(x)) - \int_t^0 e^{A(t-l)}G(U(l)(x + \Psi(x)))\,ds \text{ for } t \leq 0, \end{cases}$$

therefore, we should have

$$e^{At}x + \Psi(e^{At}x) = \begin{cases} e^{At}(x + \Psi(x)) + \int_0^t e^{A(t-l)}G(U(l)(x + \Psi(x)))\,dl \text{ for } t \geq 0, \\ e^{At}(x + \Psi(x)) - \int_t^0 e^{A(t-l)}G(U(l)(x + \Psi(x)))\,ds \text{ for } t \leq 0. \end{cases}$$

Now by projecting the above formula on X_u for $t > 0$ it follows that

$$e^{-A_u t}\Pi_u\Psi(e^{At}x) = \Pi_u\Psi(x) + \int_0^t e^{-A_u l}\Pi_u G\left(e^{Al}x + \Psi(e^{Al}x)\right)\,dl$$

and since Ψ is bounded, letting $t \to +\infty$ leads us to

$$\Pi_u\Psi(x) = -\int_0^{+\infty} e^{-A_u l}\Pi_u G\left(e^{Al}x + \Psi(e^{Al}x)\right)\,dl.$$

Similarly, projecting on X_s for $t < 0$, yields

$$e^{-A_s t}\Pi_s\Psi(e^{At}x) = \Pi_s\Psi(x) - \int_t^0 e^{-A_s l}\Pi_s G\left(e^{Al}x + \Psi(e^{Al}x)\right)\,ds$$

and by using again the fact Ψ is bounded we obtain, letting $t \to -\infty$, that

$$\Pi_s \Psi(x) = \int_{-\infty}^{0} e^{-A_s l} \Pi_s G \left(e^{Al} x + \Psi(e^{Al} x) \right) ds.$$

By combining both formulations, we obtain a fixed-point problem for the function Ψ

$$\Psi = \Phi(\Psi) \tag{6.13}$$

where

$$\Phi(\Psi)(x) := \int_{-\infty}^{0} e^{-A_s l} \Pi_s G \left(e^{Al} x + \Psi(e^{Al} x) \right) ds$$
$$- \int_{0}^{+\infty} e^{-A_u l} \Pi_u G \left(e^{Al} x + \Psi(e^{Al} x) \right) dl.$$

The map Φ maps $BC(\mathbb{R}^n)$ into itself and by using the fact that $G(0) = 0$ we obtain

$$\left\| \Phi(\Psi) - \Phi(\widehat{\Psi}) \right\|_{\infty} \leq (M_s + M_u) \int_{0}^{+\infty} e^{-\eta l} dl \, \|G\|_{\text{Lip}} \left\| \Psi - \widehat{\Psi} \right\|_{\infty}.$$

The existence and the uniqueness of $\Psi \in BC(\mathbb{R}^n)$ follows by applying the Banach contraction fixed-point theorem (whenever $\|G\|_{\text{Lip}}$ is small enough). We leave as an exercise the converse implication, namely that a fixed point Ψ of (6.13) satisfies (6.12).

It is remains to prove that a continuous $\Lambda = I + \Psi$ satisfying (6.12) is invertible and that Λ^{-1} is also continuous.

Claim 1: The map $\Lambda = I + \Psi$ is onto. Indeed, let $z \in \mathbb{R}^n$ be given. Then the equation

$$z = x + \Psi(x)$$

is equivalent to

$$x = z - \Psi(x) =: \Theta(x)$$

and since Θ is bounded, Brouwer's fixed-point theorem implies that Θ has a fixed-point, namely there exists an $x \in \mathbb{R}^n$ with $z = x + \Psi(x)$.

Claim 2: The map $\Lambda = I + \Psi$ is one to one. Let $x, y \in \mathbb{R}^n$ be given and assume that $\Lambda(x) = \Lambda(y) =: z$. This implies

$$U(t)z = \Lambda(e^{At} x) = \Lambda(e^{At} y).$$

This rewrites as

$$e^{At} x + \Psi \left(e^{At} x \right) = e^{At} y + \Psi \left(e^{At} y \right)$$
$$\Leftrightarrow e^{At} (x - y) = \Psi \left(e^{At} y \right) - \Psi \left(e^{At} x \right)$$
$$\Leftrightarrow (x - y) = e^{-At} \left[\Psi \left(e^{At} y \right) - \Psi \left(e^{At} x \right) \right]$$

and since Ψ is bounded projecting on the unstable and stable spaces X_u and X_s, we deduce that

$$\|\Pi_u (x - y)\| = \lim_{t \to +\infty} \left\| e^{-A_u t} \Pi_u \left[\Psi \left(e^{At} y \right) - \Psi \left(e^{At} x \right) \right] \right\| = 0$$

while

$$\|\Pi_s (x - y)\| = \lim_{t \to -\infty} \left\| e^{-A_s t} \Pi_u \left[\Psi \left(e^{At} y \right) - \Psi \left(e^{At} x \right) \right] \right\| = 0.$$

Since $\mathbb{R}^n = \Pi_u(\mathbb{R}^n) \oplus \Pi_s(\mathbb{R}^n)$, this means that $x = y$.

Claim 3: The function Λ^{-1} is continuous.

To see this let $\{z_m\}_{m \in \mathbb{N}} \subset \mathbb{R}^n$ be a sequence which converges to some point $z \in \mathbb{R}^n$. Set

$$x_m = \Lambda^{-1}(z_m).$$

Then we have

$$z_m = x_m + \Psi(x_m)$$

and it follows that $\{x_m\}_{m \in \mathbb{N}}$ is bounded. Therefore, we can find a sub-sequence $x_{m_p} \to x$, and by taking the limit in the above inequality we obtain

$$z = x + \Psi(x).$$

Therefore $x = \Lambda^{-1}(z)$. Now since all sub-sequences of $\{x_m\}_{m \in \mathbb{N}}$ converge to $\Lambda^{-1}(z)$, it follows that $\{x_m\}_{m \in \mathbb{N}} \to \Lambda^{-1}(z)$. The proof is completed. $\qquad\square$

6.4 Notes and Remarks

Linearized stability

The stability of equilibrium points has been studied by Desch and Schappacher [81] in the general framework of nonlinear and Fréchet-differentiable semiflows. Applications to densely and non-densely defined abstract Cauchy problems have been studied by Thieme [337] and by Magal and Ruan [238].

The Hartman–Grobman theorem

The theorem presented in this chapter was first proved by Grobman [129] in 1959 and rediscovered by Hartman [145] in 1960. The problem was reconsidered for discrete- and continuous-time dynamical systems for both finite and infinite-dimensional settings by several authors. We refer for instance to Quandt [286], Bates and Lu [26], and Rodrigues and Solà-Morales [292].

The study of the smooth local conjugacy problem for a finite-dimensional dynamical system goes back to Poincaré's 1890 article [279] on the three-body problem. Poincaré and Dulac in 1903 [103] proved the following.

Theorem 6.8 (Poincaré-Dulac) *Let $F : \mathbb{R}^n \rightarrow \mathbb{R}^n$ be an analytic diffeomorphism (i.e. bijective and F and F^{-1} are both analytic) such that $F(0) = 0$ and*

$$F(x) = Ax + G(x),$$

where

$$A \in M_n(\mathbb{R}) \text{ and } G(x) = O(\|x\|^2) \text{ as } \|x\| \rightarrow 0.$$

We assume in addition that

(i) *(**Arithmetic condition**) Assume that the eigenvalues $\lambda_1, \lambda_2, \ldots, \lambda_n$ of A satisfy the non-resonant condition*

$$\lambda_i \neq \lambda_1^{k_1} \times \lambda_2^{k_2} \times \ldots \times \lambda_n^{k_n}, \text{ for all } k = k_1 + k_2 + \cdots + k_n \geq 2,$$

where

$$(k_1, \ldots, k_n) \subset \mathbb{N}^n.$$

(ii) *(**Geometric condition**) There exists a half-plane determined by a line passing by the origin so that all eigenvalues belong to this half-plan. In other words, the eigenvalues belong to the Poincaré domain, that is*

$$0 \notin \overline{\mathrm{co}}(\sigma(A)).$$

Then there exists an analytic local diffeomorphism Λ such that

$$\Lambda F \Lambda^{-1} = A.$$

This problem was reconsidered recently by Zhang, Lu and Zhang [387] for maps in Banach spaces.

Chapter 7
Positivity and Invariant Sub-Regions

The goal of this chapter is to give a necessary and sufficient condition for the positivity of all the solutions of an ordinary differential equation, starting from positive initial values. This turns out to be a very natural question, in particular (but not only) for applications in population dynamics. In that case, most of the models are concerned with population densities, which are non-negative quantities.

7.1 Main Result

We have already considered this problem for linear ordinary differential equations in Chapter 4. Recall that for linear systems, the positive cone $\mathbb{R}_+^n$ is invariant as soon as the following condition holds on the matrix A of the linear system

$$A + \lambda I \geq 0$$

for some $\lambda \geq 0$ large enough.

The theorem presented below, namely Theorem 7.1, extends this condition to nonlinear equations. This theorem says that the semiflow generated by a function F, which is Lipschitz continuous on bounded sets, is positive if and only if for each $M > 0$ there exists some $\lambda \in \mathbb{R}$ large enough such that the map $F + \lambda I$ is positive on the positive element ball of center 0 and radius M, that is, on the ball intersected with the positive cone $\mathbb{R}_+^n$.

Hereafter when $F : \mathbb{R}^n \to \mathbb{R}^n$ is a function which is Lipschitz continuous on bounded sets, we will denote by $U(t)$ the semiflow generated by F. In other words $t \to U(t)x$ is the solution to the equation

$$\begin{cases} \dfrac{\mathrm{d}U(t)x}{\mathrm{d}t} = F\big(U(t)x\big), & t \geq 0, \\ U(0)x = x \in \mathbb{R}^n. \end{cases}$$

Recall that it follows from Theorem 5.13 that $U(t)x$ is well defined on the time interval $[0, \tau(x))$, where $\tau : \mathbb{R}^n \to (0, +\infty]$ is a lower semi-continuous function.

A. Ducrot et al., *Differential Equations and Population Dynamics I*, Lecture Notes on Mathematical Modelling in the Life Sciences, https://doi.org/10.1007/978-3-030-98136-5_7

Theorem 7.1 (Positivity) *Assume that $F : \mathbb{R}^n \to \mathbb{R}^n$ is Lipschitz continuous on bounded sets. Then the following properties are equivalent*

(i) *For each $M > 0$, there exists a $\lambda = \lambda(M) > 0$ such that*

$$F(x) + \lambda x \geq 0, \ \forall x \in B_{\mathbb{R}^n}(0, M) \cap \mathbb{R}^n_+.$$

(ii) *For each $x \geq 0$ and each $i = 1, \dots, n$,*

$$x_i = 0 \ \Rightarrow \ F_i(x) \geq 0.$$

(iii) *For each $x \geq 0$ one has*

$$U(t)x \geq 0, \ \forall t \in [0, \tau(x)).$$

Remark 7.2 The condition (ii) is usually called the *tangential condition*.

Proof The proof of this theorem involves 3 steps. We first show that (i) implies (iii), then that (iii) yields (ii) and finally that (ii) implies (i).

Proof of (i) $\Rightarrow$ (iii). Let $x \in \mathbb{R}^n_+$ be given. We first observe that a continuous function $t \to U(t)x$ is a solution of

$$U(t)x = x + \int_0^t F(U(s)x)\mathrm{d}s, \ \text{for all } t \in [0, \tau(x))$$

if and only if it satisfies

$$U(t) = \mathrm{e}^{-\lambda t}x + \int_0^t \mathrm{e}^{-\lambda(t-s)}(\lambda I + F)(U(s)x)\mathrm{d}s, \ \text{for all } t \in [0, \tau(x)).$$

Let $\tau > 0$ and $M > \|x\|$ be given and set

$$E_\tau := \{u \in C([0, \tau], \mathbb{R}^n) : u(t) \geq 0 \text{ and } \|u(t)\| \leq M, \text{ for all } t \in [0, \tau]\}.$$

Since $\mathbb{R}^n_+$ is closed, E_τ is a complete metric space endowed with the distance

$$d(u, v) = \sup_{t \in [0, \tau]} \|u(t) - v(t)\|.$$

Let $\lambda = \lambda(M) > 0$ be such that

$$(\lambda I + F)(x) \geq 0,$$

whenever $x \geq 0$ with $\|x\| \leq M$.

Define the map $\Gamma : C([0, \tau], \mathbb{R}^n) \to C([0, \tau], \mathbb{R}^n)$ by

$$\Gamma(u)(t) := \mathrm{e}^{-\lambda t}x + \int_0^t \mathrm{e}^{-\lambda(t-s)}(\lambda I + F)(u(s))\mathrm{d}s \geq 0, \ \text{for all } t \in [0, \tau],$$

for each $u \in C([0, \tau], \mathbb{R}^n)$.

First observe that we have for all $u \in E_\tau$ and $t \in [0, \tau]$

$$\|\Gamma(u)(t)\| \leq e^{-\lambda t}\|x\| + \int_0^t e^{-\lambda(t-s)}\|(\lambda I + F)(u(s)) - (\lambda I + F)(0)\|ds$$

$$+ \int_0^t e^{-\lambda(t-s)}\|F(0)\|ds$$

$$\leq e^{-\lambda t}\|x\| + \int_0^t e^{-\lambda(t-s)}(k(M) + \lambda)M + \|F(0)\|ds$$

$$\leq \|x\| + \tau\big[(k(M) + \lambda)M + \|F(0)\|\big],$$

where $k(M)$ denotes the Lipschitz constant of F on the ball $B_{\mathbb{R}^n}(0, M)$. Therefore when $\tau > 0$ is small enough such that

$$\|x\| + \tau\big[(k(M) + \lambda)M + \|F(0)\|\big] < M,$$

we obtain

$$\Gamma(E_\tau) \subset E_\tau.$$

Moreover, the map Γ is $\widehat{k}$-Lipschitz continuous with

$$\widehat{k} = \tau(k(M) + \lambda).$$

By reducing $\tau > 0$ sufficiently, if necessary, we can assume that $\widehat{k} < 1$ and it follows that Γ has a unique fixed point in E_τ whenever $\tau > 0$ is small enough.

We deduce that for each $x \in \mathbb{R}_+^n$ there exists a $\tau_+ > 0$ such that

$$U(t)x \in \mathbb{R}_+^n, \text{ for all } t \in [0, \tau_+] \cap [0, \tau(x)).$$

Set

$$\tau_+(x) := \sup\{t \in [0, \tau(x)) : U(s)x \in \mathbb{R}_+^n, \text{ for all } s \in [0, t]\}.$$

We know that

$$\tau_+(x) > 0, \text{ for all } x \in \mathbb{R}_+^n.$$

Assume that

$$\tau_+(x) < \tau(x).$$

Since $\mathbb{R}_+^n$ is closed we have

$$\lim_{t \to \tau_+(x)^-} U(t)x = U(\tau_+(x))x \geq 0.$$

By using the semiflow property, for each $t \in [\tau_+(x), \tau(x))$ we have

$$U(t)x = U(t - \tau_+(x))x_1$$

with

$$x_1 := U(\tau_+(x)) \geq 0.$$

But from the first part of the proof there exists a time $\tau_+(x_1) > 0$ such that

$$U(t)(x_1) \geq 0, \text{ for all } t \in [0, \tau_+(x_1)],$$

and therefore
$$U(t)x \in \mathbb{R}_+^n, \text{ for all } t \in [0, \tau_1(x_1) + \tau_+(x)).$$

This contradicts the definition of $\tau_+(x)$ and the equality $\tau_+(x) = \tau(x)$ follows.

Proof of (iii) $\Rightarrow$ (ii). Consider the duality product

$$\langle x^*, x \rangle = \sum_{i=1}^n x_i^* x_i, \text{ for all } x, x^* \in \mathbb{R}^n.$$

Let $x, x^* \in \mathbb{R}_+^n$ be given. Note that for each $t \in (0, \tau(x))$ we have

$$U(t)x = x + \int_0^t F(U(l)x)dl,$$

therefore by using the fact that $x \to \langle x^*, x \rangle$ is continuous, by taking the duality product of the above equality we obtain

$$\langle x^*, U(t)x \rangle = \langle x^*, x \rangle + \int_0^t \langle x^*, F(U(l)x) \rangle dl$$

and if we assume in addition $\langle x^*, x \rangle = 0$ we obtain

$$0 \le \frac{1}{t} \langle x^*, U(t)x \rangle = \frac{1}{t} \int_0^t \langle x^*, F(U(l)x) \rangle dl.$$

Therefore by taking the limit when t goes to 0 we obtain

$$\langle x^*, F(x) \rangle \ge 0.$$

We conclude that for each $x \ge 0$ and each $x^* \ge 0$

$$\langle x^*, x \rangle = 0 \implies \langle x^*, F(x) \rangle \ge 0.$$

By replacing x^* by each element of the canonical basis $\{e_1, \cdots, e_n\}$ we obtain (ii).

Proof of (ii) $\Rightarrow$ (i). For each $x \in \mathbb{R}_+^n$ we can define

$$\underline{\lambda}(x) := \inf\{\lambda > 0 : \lambda x + F(x) \ge 0\}.$$

Indeed (ii) implies that $F(0) \ge 0$, so that $\underline{\lambda}(0) = 0$. Moreover for each $x > 0$

$$\underline{\lambda}(x) = \max_{i=1,..,n : x_i \neq 0} -\frac{F_i(x)}{x_i}.$$

Let $M \ge \|x\|$ be given. Assume for example that $x_i > 0$ for some i. Then we have

$$\frac{F_i(x)}{x_i} = \frac{F_i(x) - F_i(z)}{x_i} + \frac{F_i(z)}{x_i}$$

with

$$z = (x_1, x_2, \cdots, x_{i-1}, 0, x_{i+1}, \cdots, x_n).$$

So, since $z_i = 0$, (ii) applies and ensures that we have

$$F_i(z) \geq 0.$$

It follows that

$$\frac{F_i(x)}{x_i} \geq -k(M) \frac{\|x - z\|}{|x_i|} = -k(M) \|e_i\|,$$

where $k(M)$ is the Lipschitz constant of F on $B(0, M)$ and $e_i = (0, ..., 0, 1, 0, ..., 0)$.
We deduce that

$$\underline{\lambda}(x) \leq k(M) \max_{i=1,..,n} \|e_i\|,$$

and the result follows.   □

In the following result, we observe that the positivity of the semiflow implies that the interior region of the positive cone also stays invariant by the semiflow.

Proposition 7.3 *Assume that $F : \mathbb{R}^n \to \mathbb{R}^n$ is Lipschitz continuous on bounded sets and assume that*

$$U(t)x \geq 0, \quad \forall t \in [0, \tau(x)), \text{ for all } x \geq 0.$$

Then

$$U(t)x \gg 0, \quad \forall t \in [0, \tau(x)), \text{ for all } x \gg 0.$$

Proof Let $x \gg 0$ and $\tau \in (0, \tau(x))$ be given. Set $M := \sup_{t \in [0,\tau]} \|U(t)x\|$ and let $\lambda = \lambda(M) > 0$ denote the constant arising in condition (i) of Theorem 7.1. Then one has

$$U(t)x = e^{-\lambda t}x + \underbrace{\int_0^t e^{-\lambda(t-s)}(\lambda I + F)(U(s)x)\mathrm{d}s}_{\geq 0}, \quad \forall t \in [0, \tau],$$

hence

$$U(t)x \geq e^{-\lambda t}x \gg 0, \text{ for all } t \in [0, \tau].$$

7.2 Examples

Example 7.4 In the scalar case

$$u'(t) = f(u(t)), \forall t \geq 0 \text{ and } u(0) = x \in \mathbb{R}$$

for some function $f \in C^1(\mathbb{R})$. Then the condition becomes

$$x \geq 0 \Rightarrow u(t) \geq 0, \quad \forall t \geq 0$$

if and only if

$$f(0) \geq 0.$$

In many examples, the following proposition is sufficient to prove the positivity of the solutions.

Proposition 7.5 *Let $F = (F_1, \cdots, F_n) : \mathbb{R}^n \to \mathbb{R}^n$ be a function such that there exist two maps $G : \mathbb{R}^n \to \mathbb{R}^n$ and $H : \mathbb{R}^n \to \mathbb{R}^n$ that are Lipschitz continuous on bounded sets and such that*

$$F_i(x) = G_i(x) + x_i H_i(x), \text{ for all } i = 1, \ldots, n, \text{ and } x \in \mathbb{R}^n$$

with

$$G(x) \geq 0 \text{ whenever } x \geq 0.$$

Then the maximal semiflow $U = U(t)$ generated by the following system on $\mathbb{R}^n$

$$\frac{\mathrm{d}u(t)}{\mathrm{d}t} = F(u(t)),$$

satisfies

$$U(t)x \geq 0, \text{ for all } t \in [0, \tau(x)), \quad \forall x \in \mathbb{R}^n_+.$$

Proof To prove this proposition, we check condition (i) of Theorem 7.1. With that aim, it is sufficient to prove that for each real number $M > 0$ we can find a $\lambda = \lambda(M) > 0$ such that

$$\lambda x_i + x_i H_i(x) \geq 0$$

whenever $i = 1, \ldots, n$, $x \geq 0$ and $\|x\| \leq M$. Therefore, it is sufficient to choose

$$\lambda(M) = \max_{i=1,\ldots,n} \sup_{0 \leq x \text{ and } \|x\| \leq M} H_i(x) < +\infty.$$

Example 7.6 Consider, for example, the classical SIR epidemic model

$$\begin{cases} \dfrac{\mathrm{d}S}{\mathrm{d}t} = \lambda - \mu S - \beta SI \\[2mm] \dfrac{\mathrm{d}I}{\mathrm{d}t} = \beta SI - (\mu + \eta)I \\[2mm] \dfrac{\mathrm{d}R}{\mathrm{d}t} = \eta I - \mu R \end{cases}$$

where $\lambda, \mu, \beta, \eta \geq 0$ are given non-negative parameters.
Then to prove the positivity of the solutions by applying the above proposition, it is sufficient to observe that one can choose

$$G\begin{pmatrix} S \\ I \\ R \end{pmatrix} = \begin{pmatrix} \lambda \\ \beta SI \\ \eta I \end{pmatrix}$$

and

$$H\begin{pmatrix} S \\ I \\ R \end{pmatrix} = \begin{pmatrix} -\mu - \beta I \\ -(\mu + \eta) \\ -\mu \end{pmatrix}.$$

7.3 Invariance of a Sub-Region by Using an Outward Normal Vector Condition

Assumption 7.7 Let $\Omega \subset \mathbb{R}^n$ be a bounded open set with C^2 boundary $\partial\Omega$.

Define

$$d(x, \partial\Omega) := \inf_{y \in \partial\Omega} \|x - y\|.$$

The following Lemma is a consequence of Foote [110, Theorem 1].

Lemma 7.8 *Let Assumption 7.7 be satisfied. There exists a neighborhood U of $\partial\Omega$ in $\overline{\Omega}$ such that $\delta(x) := d(x, \partial\Omega)$ is of class C^2 in $U\backslash\partial\Omega$. Moreover, for every $x \in U$ there exists a unique point $P_{\partial\Omega}(x) \in \partial\Omega$ such that*

$$\delta(x) = \|x - P_{\partial\Omega}(x)\|.$$

The map $P_{\partial\Omega} : U \to \partial\Omega$ is called the projection on $\partial\Omega$.

By combining the above Lemma and a result of Ambrosio [6, Theorem 1, p. 11] we obtain the following lemma.

Lemma 7.9 *Let Assumption 7.7 be satisfied and let U be the neighborhood introduced in Lemma 7.8. For each $x \in U$ we have*

$$\nabla\delta(x) = \frac{x - P_{\partial\Omega}(x)}{\|x - P_{\partial\Omega}(x)\|} = -\nu(P_{\partial\Omega}(x)),$$

where $\nu(y)$ is the outer normal vector of Ω at $y \in \partial\Omega$.

We consider the following non-autonomous differential equation on $\Omega \subset \mathbb{R}^n$

$$\begin{cases} u'(t) = f(t, u(t)), & \text{for all } t \geq 0, \\ u(0) = u_0 \in \Omega. \end{cases} \tag{7.1}$$

Assumption 7.10 We assume that the vector field $f : [0, +\infty) \times \mathbb{R}^n \to \mathbb{R}^n$ is directed inwards on the boundary of Ω, that is,

$$\nu(x) \cdot f(t, x) \leq 0 \text{ for all } t \geq 0 \text{ and } x \in \partial\Omega,$$

where $\nu(x)$ is the outer normal vector of Ω at $x \in \partial\Omega$. We assume moreover that for all $T > 0$ there exists a constant $K = K(T)$ such that the vector field f satisfies

$$|f(t, x) - f(t, y)| \leq K|x - y| \text{ for all } x, y \in \overline{\Omega} \text{ and } t \in [0, T].$$

Definition 7.11 Let $\{U(t)\}_{t \in [0,\infty)}$ be a family of maps from Ω into itself. We say that $\{U(t)\}_{t \in I}$ is a *semiflow* if

$$U(0) = \text{Id and } U(t + s) = U(t) \circ U(s), \quad \forall t, s \in [0, \infty).$$

We will say that U is *continuous* if the map $(t, x) \to U(t)x$ is a continuous map from $[0, \infty) \times \Omega$ into Ω.

The following theorem is a generalization of a result found in [31, Theorem 2.1].

Theorem 7.12 (Positive invariance of Ω) *Let Assumptions 7.7 and 7.10 be satisfied. Then the solution of (7.1) $t \to u(t)$ stays in Ω and never touches the boundary of Ω for all $t \geq 0$ (i.e. moving forward in time). There exists a unique continuous semiflow $\{U(t)\}_{t \geq 0}$ on Ω such that $u(t) = U(t)x$ is the solution of (7.1) on $[0, +\infty)$.*

Remark 7.13 The above invariant theorem has been successfully used to study the hyperbolic Keller–Segel equation in [113]. In the aforementioned work, the problem was handled by using integration along the characteristic lines, which turn out to be the solutions of some ordinary differential equations. The invariance theorem presented above has been used to prove that the characteristic lines do not escape the domain Ω on which the PDE is posed.

Proof We prove this theorem by contradiction. Let $t^* \in (0, +\infty)$ be the first time when $u(t)$ reaches the boundary $\partial\Omega$, i.e.,

$$t^* = \inf\{t \geq 0 : \delta(u(t)) = 0\}.$$

We can find $\theta > 0$ such that $u(t) \in U \cap \overline{\Omega}$ for any $t \in [t^* - \theta, t^*]$, where U is the neighborhood introduced in Lemma 7.8. Since $t \to u(t)$ is C^1, the mapping $t \mapsto \delta(u(t))$ is C^1 on $[t^* - \theta, t^*]$. By Lemma 7.9, we have

$$\frac{d}{dt}\delta(u(t)) = x'(t) \cdot \nabla\delta(u(t)) = -f(t, u(t)) \cdot v(y(t)), \qquad (7.2)$$

where v is the outward normal vector and $y(t) := P_{\partial\Omega}(u(t))$ is the projection of $u(t)$ onto $\partial\Omega$. By Assumption 7.10, we have

$$-f(t, u(t)) \cdot v(y(t)) = \big(f(t, y(t)) - f(t, u(t))\big) \cdot v(y(t)) - f(t, y(t)) \cdot v(y(t))$$
$$\geq \big(f(t, y(t)) - f(t, u(t))\big) \cdot v(y(t)).$$

Hence (7.2) becomes

$$\frac{d}{dt}\delta(u(t)) = -f(t, u(t)) \cdot v(y(t))$$
$$\geq \big(f(t, y(t)) - f(t, u(t))\big) \cdot v(y(t))$$
$$\geq -|f(t, y(t)) - f(t, u(t))|\,|v(y(t))|$$
$$\geq -K|y(t) - u(t)| = -K\delta(u(t)), \quad t \in [t^* - \theta, t^*],$$

which yields

$$\delta(u(t)) \geq \delta(x(t^* - \theta))e^{-K(t - t^* + \theta)}, \quad \forall t \in [t^* - \theta, t^*].$$

Since by construction $\delta(x(t^* - \theta)) > 0$, this implies $\delta(x(t^*)) > 0$ and we obtain a contradiction. $\qquad\square$

7.4 Notes and Remarks

Further references

The invariance of a sub-region for differential equations has a long history. We refer to the seminal work of Nagumo [265] in 1942. This topic became very active in the late '60s and the early '70s, both for finite and infinite-dimensional problems. We refer to the works of Yorke [377], Brezis [37] and Hartman [146] on ordinary differential equations and to those of Walter [356], Martin [248] and Redheffer and Walter [287] for extensions to ordinary differential equations in ordered Banach spaces. We also refer to the book of Aubin [16] for a nice survey on this topic.

Various extensions to partial differential equations have been obtained. We refer for instance to Redheffer and Walter [288], to Chueh, Conley and Smoller [58] and to Martin [249], for parabolic equations in particular. We also refer to the monograph of Smoller [330] for further results on positively invariant of regions for parabolic systems, roughly based on comparison arguments, and to the book of Protter and Weinberger [283] for results on the maximum principle for various types of PDEs (elliptic, parabolic and hyperbolic).

We refer the reader to Martin and Smith [250] for further results on differential inequalities and invariant sets for abstract functional differential equations and reaction-diffusion systems with time delays, and their comparison.

The book of Pavel and Motreanu [273] is also concerned with this topic, and includes an extensive study of densely defined semi-linear Cauchy problems. Let us also quote the works of Thieme [337] and Magal, Seydi and Wang [240], who derived conditions for a closed convex subset for semi-linear non-densely defined Cauchy problems with Hille–Yosida and non-Hille–Yosida linear operators.

Existence and uniqueness of solutions on the positive cone only

The results and the methodologies presented in this chapter can be adapted to handle the ODE problem posed on a positive cone only. To explain this we consider the following example of an ordinary differential equation posed on the two-dimensional positive quadrant $[0, +\infty)^2$

$$\frac{dU(t)}{dt} = F(U(t)),$$

where the function $F : [0, +\infty)^2 \to \mathbb{R}^2$ is defined by

$$F\begin{pmatrix} x \\ y \end{pmatrix} = \begin{pmatrix} \frac{x^2+y^2}{x+y} - \mu x \\ \frac{x^2+y^2}{x+y} - \mu y \end{pmatrix}, \text{ if } \begin{pmatrix} x \\ y \end{pmatrix} \neq 0, \text{ and } F(0) = 0.$$

Here $\mu > 0$ is a given and fixed parameter.

We observe that the function F is Lipschitz continuous on the bounded sets of

$[0, +\infty)^2$. In order to consider the above example one can use the following theorem.

Theorem 7.14 *Let $F : [0, \infty)^n \to \mathbb{R}^n$ be a Lipschitz continuous function on bounded sets. Assume that for each $M > 0$ there exists a $\lambda = \lambda(M) > 0$ such that*

$$F(x) + \lambda x \geq 0,$$

whenever $x \geq 0$ and $\|x\| \leq M$.

Then there exist a unique map $\tau : [0, +\infty)^n \to (0, +\infty]$ and a unique maximal continuous semiflow $U : D_\tau \to [0, +\infty)^n$, where

$$D_\tau := \{(t, x) \in [0, \infty) \times [0, +\infty)^n : 0 \leq t \leq \tau(x)\},$$

such for all $x \in [0, +\infty)^n$, the map $u(t) = U(t)x$ is the unique non-negative solution of the integral equation

$$u(t) = x + \int_0^t F(u(s))\mathrm{d}s, \text{ for all } t \in [0, \tau(x)).$$

The map U satisfies the maximal continuous semiflow properties

 (i) $U(0)x = x$ for all $x \in [0, +\infty)^n$;
 (ii) $\tau(U(t)x) = \tau(x) - t$ for all $x \in [0, +\infty)^n$ and $t \in [0, \tau(x))$;
 (iii) $U(t - s)U(s)x = U(t)x$ for all $x \in [0, +\infty)^n$ and $0 \leq s \leq t \leq \tau(x)$;
 (iv) *The map $(t, x) \mapsto U(t)x$ is continuous from D_τ to $\mathbb{R}^n$;*
 (v) *If $\tau(x) < +\infty$ then*
$$\lim_{t \to \tau(x)^-} \|U(t)x\| = +\infty.$$

Exercise 7.15 Prove the above theorem.

An infinite-dimensional example

As mentioned above, Theorem 7.1 can be extended to infinite-dimensional systems. We refer to Thieme [337], Magal [227], and Magal and Ruan [238] to quote a few. Below we present the statement of the positivity theorem for ordinary differential equations in ordered Banach spaces.

Theorem 7.16 *Let $(X, \|\cdot\|)$ be a partially ordered Banach space and $\geq$ be the partial order (see Definition 4.60). Let $F : X \to X$ be a map which is Lipschitz continuous on bounded sets of X. Assume that for each $M > 0$ we can find a $\lambda = \lambda(M) > 0$ such that*

$$x \geq 0 \text{ and } \|x\| \leq M \Rightarrow F(x) + \lambda x \geq 0.$$

Then each solution of the ordinary differential equation

$$u'(t) = F(u(t)) \text{ for } t \geq 0 \text{ and } u(0) = x$$

starting from a non-negative initial value $x \geq 0$ is positive up to its maximal time of existence $\tau(x)$, namely

$$u(t) \geq 0 \text{ for all } t \in [0, \tau(x)).$$

Chapter 8
Monotone Semiflows

8.1 Comparison Principles for Scalar Equations

Let $f : \mathbb{R} \to \mathbb{R}$ be a C^1 map. Consider the ordinary differential equation

$$\begin{cases} u'(t) = f(u(t)), \text{ for all } t \geq 0, \\ u(0) = x \in \mathbb{R}. \end{cases}$$

From Chapter 5, we know that there exists a unique maximal semiflow $U(t, x)$ combined with a blow-up time $\tau(x)$ such that $u(t) := U(t, x)$ is the unique solution of the fixed-point problem

$$u(t) = x + \int_0^t f(u(s)) \mathrm{d}s \text{ for all } t \in [0, \tau(x)),$$

and

$$\lim_{t \to \tau(x)} |u(t)| = +\infty, \text{ whenever } \tau(x) < +\infty.$$

In this chapter, we will be interested in the comparison property for semiflows. This type of property can be proved by using very simple arguments for the one-dimensional case.

Lemma 8.1 *Assume that $f : \mathbb{R} \to \mathbb{R}$ is a C^1-map. Then the following comparison principle holds*

$$x < y \Longrightarrow U(t, x) < U(t, y), \text{ for all } 0 \leq t < \min\big(\tau(x), \tau(y)\big).$$

Proof Let $x < y$ be given. Assume by contradiction that we can find $0 \leq t_0 < \min\big(\tau(x), \tau(y)\big)$ such that

$$U(t_0, x) = U(t_0, y) \text{ and } U(t, x) < U(t, y) \text{ for all } t \in (0, t_0).$$

Set $v_1(t) := U(t_0 - t, x)$ and $v_2(t) := U(t_0 - t, y)$ for each $t \in [0, t_0]$. Then we have

$$v_1(0) = v_2(0)$$

and

$$v_1'(t) = -f(v_1(t)) \text{ and } v_2'(t) = -f(v_2(t)) \text{ for all } t \in [0, t_0].$$

Since the equation $v'(t) = -f(v(t))$ admits at most one solution with initial value $v(0) = v_1(0) = v_2(0)$, we have $v_1(t) = v_2(t)$ for all $t \in [0, t_0]$ and therefore $x = v_1(t_0) = v_2(t_0) = y$. This is a contradiction.   □

The following lemma says that if the solutions with positive initial values remain positive for all times, then the solution starting from a larger initial value will blow-up first.

Lemma 8.2 *Assume that $f \in C^1(\mathbb{R})$ and $f(0) \geq 0$. Then it holds that*

$$0 \leq x < y \Rightarrow \tau(y) \leq \tau(x).$$

Proof Let $0 \leq x < y$ be given. Assume that $\tau(x) < \tau(y)$. Since $f(0) \geq 0$, we have

$$0 \leq U(t, x) < U(t, y), \text{ for all } t \in [0, \tau(x)).$$

This implies that $\tau(x) < +\infty$, and we must have

$$\lim_{t \to \tau(x)} U(t, x) = +\infty.$$

But $\tau(x) < \tau(y)$ also implies that $t \mapsto U(t, y)$ belongs to $C([0, \tau(x)], \mathbb{R})$. So we obtain

$$+\infty = \lim_{t \to \tau(x)} U(t, x) \leq \limsup_{t \to \tau(x)} U(t, y) < +\infty,$$

which is a contradiction.   □

Exercise 8.3 Let $f \in C^1(\mathbb{R})$ be given and assume that (as in the logistic equation) there exists a $\kappa > 0$ such that

$$f(0) = f(\kappa) = 0 \text{ and } f(x) > 0 \text{ for all } x \in (0, \kappa).$$

Consider the ordinary differential equation

$$\begin{cases} u'(t) = f(u(t)) \text{ for all } t \geq 0, \\ u(0) = x \in [0, \kappa]. \end{cases}$$

1. Prove that, for each $x_0 \in (0, \kappa]$, we have

$$\lim_{t \to +\infty} u(t) = \kappa.$$

2. By using a similar argument, show that for each $x_0 \in [0, \kappa)$, we have

$$\lim_{t \to -\infty} u(t) = 0.$$

Hint: consider reversing the time (i.e. replace $u(t)$ by $v(t) = u(-t)$).

Remark 8.4 Under the conditions of Exercise 8.3, we can show that the points in $(0, \kappa)$ all belong to a unique heteroclinic orbit joining 0 to κ.

Example 8.5 (Strong Allee effect) A population may go extinct because the number of individuals is too small. This was the case for the bears of the Pyrenées, where the males and females were unable to meet and therefore could not reproduce. This phenomenon is called the *Allee effect* [3, 4]. The term "Allee's principle" was introduced in the 1950s, a time when the field of ecology was heavily focused on the role of competition among and within species.

In order to describe this mechanism people consider the strong Allee effect

$$u'(t) = \lambda u(t)(u(t) - \varepsilon)(1 - u(t)/\kappa),$$

with a positive initial value

$$u(0) = x \geq 0.$$

We assume that the parameters satisfy

$$\lambda > 0 \text{ and } 0 < \varepsilon < \kappa.$$

Characterization of the Allee effects

Consider a scalar equation of the form

$$N'(t) = (\beta(N) - \mu(N)) N(t). \tag{8.1}$$

The birth and the death rate are respectively given by

$$\beta(N) = -aN^2 + bN + c \text{ and } \mu(N) = dN + e,$$

where $a, b, c, d, e \geq 0$ are given parameters.
By summing-up the two terms in (8.1) we obtain

$$N' = N(-aN^2 + (b - d)N - (e - c)).$$

Therefore, by choosing

$$e - c > 0$$

and $b - d$ large enough, we obtain

$$\Delta = (b - d)^2 - 4a(e - c) > 0,$$

a strong Allee effect.

Example 8.6 (Weak Allee effect) In order to describe the fact that the speed of growth is sub-linear, one may introduce the so-called *weak Allee effect*. Namely, we consider a population growing as

$$u'(t) = \lambda u(t)^\alpha (1 - u(t)/\kappa),$$

with
$$\alpha > 1.$$
It is called a weak Allee effect because the derivative of the right-hand side at zero is null.

It may be consistent to introduce an Allee effect in some epidemic models (see Hilker, Langlais, and Malchow [151]). The resulting systems may undergo a complex dynamic. One may combine the Allee effect with the spatial motion of individuals. This leads to some delicate analysis for the so-called bistable nonlinearity of reaction-diffusion equations. We refer to [1, 14, 107, 115, 306] for more results and references on this topic.

8.2 Gronwall's Lemma

We continue this chapter with Gronwall's Lemma [130]. Because this result can be very useful when obtaining estimates, and since it can be proved by using a comparison argument, it serves as a good introduction to monotone ordinary differential equations and comparison arguments. There are many variants of Gronwall's Lemma, of which we introduce only the most commonly used in the present section.

8.2.1 Differential form of Gronwall's lemma

Let $u \in C^1([0, \tau], \mathbb{R})$. Assume that u satisfies the following differential inequality
$$\frac{du(t)}{dt} \leq \alpha u(t) + \beta \text{ for all } t \in [0, \tau],$$
where $\alpha \in \mathbb{R}$ and $\beta \in \mathbb{R}$.

We remark that this inequality can be rewritten as
$$\frac{du(t)}{dt} \leq \alpha u(t) + \beta$$
$$\Leftrightarrow \frac{du(t)}{dt} - \alpha u(t) \leq \beta$$
$$\Leftrightarrow e^{\alpha t} \frac{d}{dt}(e^{-\alpha t} u(t)) \leq \beta$$
$$\Leftrightarrow \frac{d}{dt}(e^{-\alpha t} u(t)) \leq \beta e^{-\alpha t},$$

and by integrating both sides of this last inequality between 0 and t we obtain
$$e^{-\alpha t} u(t) - e^{-\alpha 0} u(0) \leq \int_0^t e^{-\alpha l} \beta dl.$$

Thus, we obtain the following lemma, which is the differential form of Gronwall's lemma.

Lemma 8.7 (Gronwall, differential form) *Let $\alpha, \beta \in \mathbb{R}$ be given. Assume that $u \in C^1([0, \tau], \mathbb{R})$ satisfies the following inequality*

$$\frac{du(t)}{dt} \le \alpha u(t) + \beta \text{ for all } t \in [0, \tau].$$

Then u satisfies

$$u(t) \le e^{\alpha t} u(0) + \int_0^t e^{\alpha(t-l)} \beta dl, \text{ for all } t \in [0, \tau].$$

8.2.2 Integral form of Gronwall's lemma

Let $u \in C([0, \tau], \mathbb{R})$ satisfying

$$u(t) \le \alpha + \beta \int_0^t u(s) ds, \text{ for all } t \in [0, \tau], \tag{8.2}$$

for some $\alpha \in \mathbb{R}$ and $\beta \ge 0$.

By setting

$$N(t) = \int_0^t u(s) ds \text{ for all } t \in [0, \tau],$$

we obtain

$$N'(t) \le \alpha + \beta N(t) \text{ for all } t \in [0, \tau],$$

and by using the differential form of Gronwall's lemma we deduce that

$$N(t) \le \int_0^t e^{\beta(t-l)} \alpha dl, \text{ for all } t \in [0, \tau].$$

Since $\beta \ge 0$ we obtain

$$u(t) \le \alpha + \beta N(t) \le \alpha + \beta \int_0^t e^{\beta(t-l)} \alpha dl = \alpha e^{\beta t},$$

and we obtain the integral form of Gronwall's Lemma.

Lemma 8.8 (Gronwall, integral form) *Let $\alpha \in \mathbb{R}$ and $\beta \ge 0$ be given. Let $u \in C([0, \tau], \mathbb{R})$ such that*

$$u(t) \le \alpha + \beta \int_0^t u(s) ds \text{ for all } t \in [0, \tau].$$

Then, it holds that

$$u(t) \le \alpha e^{\beta t} \text{ for all } t \in [0, \tau].$$

An alternative proof using a comparison argument. Consider the map Γ : $C([0, \tau], \mathbb{R}) \to C([0, \tau], \mathbb{R})$ defined by

$$\Gamma(u)(t) = \alpha + \beta \int_0^t u(s)\mathrm{d}s \text{ for all } t \in [0, \tau].$$

Then (8.2) can be rewritten as

$$u \leq \Gamma(u) \Leftrightarrow u(t) \leq \Gamma(u)(t) \text{ for all } t \in [0, \tau].$$

Since $\beta \geq 0$ the map Γ is monotone non-decreasing, that is,

$$u \leq v \Rightarrow \Gamma(u) \leq \Gamma(v).$$

This implies that

$$u \leq \Gamma(u) \Rightarrow u \leq \Gamma(u) \leq \Gamma^2(u)$$

and by induction we find that for each integer $n \geq 1$,

$$u \leq \Gamma(u) \leq \Gamma^2(u) \leq \cdots \leq \Gamma^n(u).$$

We know that the operator Γ is also the fixed-point operator of the linear scalar ordinary differential equation $u'(t) = \beta u(t)$. Therefore by using the fixed-point argument in Chapter 2 we have

$$\lim_{n \to +\infty} \Gamma^n(u) = v,$$

where $v \in C([0, \tau], \mathbb{R})$ satisfies

$$v = \Gamma(v) \Leftrightarrow v(t) = \alpha + \beta \int_0^t v(s)\mathrm{d}s \text{ for all } t \in [0, \tau],$$

or equivalently,

$$\begin{cases} v'(t) = \beta v(t) \text{ for all } t \in [0, \tau], \\ v(0) = \alpha. \end{cases}$$

We deduce that

$$v(t) = \alpha e^{\beta t} \text{ for all } t \in [0, \tau],$$

and the result follows.

Exercise 8.9 Let $\alpha, \gamma \in \mathbb{R}$ and $\beta \geq 0$ be given. Let $u \in C([0, \tau], \mathbb{R})$ and assume that

$$u(t) \leq \alpha e^{\gamma t} + \int_0^t \beta e^{\gamma(t-s)} u(s)\mathrm{d}s \text{ for all } t \in [0, \tau].$$

Extend the arguments of the two proofs above to deduce that

$$u(t) \leq \alpha e^{(\gamma+\beta)t} \text{ for all } t \in [0, \tau].$$

8.2.3 Ordinary differential equations with Lipschitz continuous right-hand side

As a consequence of Gronwall's lemma, we are in the position to prove the following global existence result.

Corollary 8.10 *Let $F : \mathbb{R}^n \to \mathbb{R}^n$ be a locally Lipschitz continuous map (that is, a map that is Lipschitz continuous on bounded sets of $\mathbb{R}^n$), and assume that*

$$\|F(x)\| \le \alpha\|x\| + \beta \text{ for all } x \in \mathbb{R}^n,$$

for some $\alpha \ge 0$ and $\beta \ge 0$.

Then there exists a (globally defined) unique continuous semiflow $\{U(t)\}_{t \ge 0}$ on $\mathbb{R}^n$ such that for each $x \in \mathbb{R}^n$, $u(t) := U(t)x$ is the unique solution of

$$\begin{cases} u'(t) = F(u(t)) \text{ for all } t \ge 0, \\ u(0) = x. \end{cases}$$

Moreover we have

$$\|U(t)x\| \le e^{\alpha t}\|x\| + \int_0^t e^{\alpha(t-s)}\beta ds \text{ for all } t \ge 0.$$

Proof Let $x \in \mathbb{R}^n$ be given. We know that there exist $\tau(x) \le +\infty$ and a continuous function $t \mapsto u(t)$ from $[0, \tau(x))$ into $\mathbb{R}^n$ such that

$$u(t) = x + \int_0^t F(u(s))ds \text{ for all } t \in [0, \tau(x)),$$

and

$$\lim_{t \to \tau(x)^-} \|u(t)\| = +\infty \text{ if } \tau(x) < +\infty.$$

We have

$$\|u(t)\| \le \|x\| + \int_0^t \|F(u(s))\|ds \text{ for all } t \in [0, \tau(x)),$$

hence by using the assumption on F we deduce that

$$\|u(t)\| \le \|x\| + \int_0^t \alpha\|u(s)\| + \beta ds \text{ for all } t \in [0, \tau(x)).$$

Setting

$$X(t) := \int_0^t \alpha\|u(s)\| + \beta ds \text{ for all } t \in [0, \tau(x)),$$

we obtain (since $\alpha \ge 0$)

$$X'(t) = \alpha\|u(t)\| + \beta \le \alpha\|x\| + \alpha X(t) + \beta \text{ for all } t \in [0, \tau(x)).$$

Thus

$$X'(t) \leq [\alpha\|x\| + \beta] + \alpha X(t) \text{ for all } t \in [0, \tau(x)).$$

Now by applying the differential form of Gronwall's lemma, we obtain

$$X(t) \leq \int_0^t e^{\alpha(t-s)} [\alpha\|x\| + \beta]ds = \int_0^t e^{\alpha l} [\alpha\|x\| + \beta]dl \text{ for all } t \in [0, \tau(x)),$$

and

$$\|u(t)\| \leq \|x\| + \int_0^t e^{\alpha l} [\alpha\|x\| + \beta]dl, \text{ for all } t \in [0, \tau(x)).$$

This implies $\tau(x) = +\infty$ and the result follows.   □

Whenever the map F is Lipschitz continuous we obtain the following theorem, which can be regarded as a direct extension of the linear case described in Chapter 2.

Theorem 8.11 *Let $F : \mathbb{R}^n \to \mathbb{R}^n$ be a Lipschitz continuous map on $\mathbb{R}^n$. There exists a (global) unique semiflow $\{U(t)\}_{t \geq 0}$ on $\mathbb{R}^n$ such that for each $x \in \mathbb{R}^n$, $u(t) := U(t)x$ is the unique solution of the ordinary differential equation*

$$\begin{cases} u'(t) = F(u(t)) \text{ for all } t \geq 0 \\ u(0) = x. \end{cases}$$

Moreover, we have

$$\|U(t)x\| \leq e^{\|F\|_{\mathrm{Lip}}t}\|x\| + \int_0^t e^{\|F\|_{\mathrm{Lip}}(t-s)}\|F(0)\|ds, \text{ for all } t \geq 0$$

and

$$\|U(t)x - U(t)y\| \leq e^{\|F\|_{\mathrm{Lip}}t}\|x - y\| \text{ for all } t \geq 0,$$

where

$$\|F\|_{\mathrm{Lip}} := \sup_{x,y \in \mathbb{R}^n : x \neq y} \frac{\|F(x) - F(y)\|}{\|x - y\|}.$$

Proof Observe that

$$\|F(x)\| = \|F(x) - F(0)\| + \|F(0)\| \leq \|F\|_{\mathrm{Lip}}\|x - 0\| + \|F(0)\|.$$

Then by applying Corollary 8.10, the first part of the result follows.

To prove the second part of the theorem, we observe that

$$U(t)x - U(t)y = x - y + \int_0^t F(U(s)x) - F(U(s)y)ds \text{ for all } t \geq 0.$$

Therefore

$$\|U(t)x - U(t)y\| \leq \|x - y\| + \int_0^t \|F(U(s)x) - F(U(s)y)\|ds, \text{ for all } t \geq 0,$$

and by using the fact that F is Lipschitz continuous we obtain

$$\|U(t)x - U(t)y\| \le \|x - y\| + \|F\|_{\text{Lip}} \int_0^t \|U(s)x - U(s)y\|ds, \text{ for all } t \ge 0.$$

The result follows by using the integral form of Gronwall's lemma.   □

Exercise 8.12 Consider the map $F : [0, +\infty)^n \to \mathbb{R}^n$ defined by $F(0) = 0$ and

$$F(x) = \frac{B(x, x)}{\|x\|_1} \text{ if } x > 0,$$

where $B : \mathbb{R}^n \times \mathbb{R}^n \to \mathbb{R}^n$ is a bilinear map satisfying

$$B(x, x) \ge 0 \text{ for all } x \ge 0$$

and

$$\|x\|_1 = \sum_{i=1}^n |x_i|.$$

Consider the ordinary differential equation

$$U'(t) = F(U(t)) - U(t) \text{ for all } t \ge 0$$

with initial distribution $U(0) = U_0 \ge 0$. (Observe that it is not clear that F can be extended to a Lipschitz continuous map on the whole space $\mathbb{R}^n$.)

1. Prove that F is Lipschitz continuous. Hint: observe that

$$\frac{B(x, x)}{\|x\|_1} - \frac{B(y, y)}{\|y\|_1} = \|x\|_1^{-1} B(x, x-y) + \left[\|x\|_1^{-1} - \|y\|_1^{-1}\right] B(x, y) + \|y\|_1^{-1} B(x-y, y).$$

2. Prove the global existence and uniqueness of non-negative solutions.
3. Prove that the system generates a continuous semiflow on $\mathbb{R}_+^n$.

8.2.4 Non-autonomous form of Gronwall's Lemma

Recall that

$$W^{1,\infty}(0, \tau) := \{u \in L^\infty(0, \tau) : u' \in L^\infty(0, \tau)\}.$$

This space is called a *Sobolev space*. The notion of derivative used in the definition of this space is the derivative *in the sense of distributions*, that is,

$$\int_0^\tau \varphi'(s)u(s)ds = -\int_0^\tau \varphi(s)u'(s)ds,$$

whenever $\varphi \in C_c^\infty(0, \tau)$ (i.e. φ is of class C^∞ and has a compact support in $(0, \tau)$).
It turns out that this notion of differentiable function is equivalent to saying that

$$u(t) = c + \int_0^t u'(s)ds \text{ for almost every } t \in [0, \tau],$$

where the last integral is a Lebesgue integral. Therefore by using this representation, u can be regarded as a continuous function. We refer to the book of Brezis [38] for more results on Sobolev spaces. By using the notion of absolutely continuous function, one can also prove that $u(t)$ is differentiable almost everywhere on $[0, \tau]$ with $u' \in L^\infty(0, \tau)$. We refer for instance to the book of Rudin [304] for a proof of this result.

The point of this section is to extend the previous inequalities to the case where α and β depend on the variable t, namely, we consider inequalities of the form

$$u'(t) \leq \alpha(t)u(t) + \beta(t) \text{ for almost every } t \in [0, \tau],$$

where $\alpha, \beta \in L^1(0, \tau)$.

Then for almost every $t \in [0, \tau]$ we have

$$\frac{d}{dt}\left[e^{-\int_0^t \alpha(l)dl}u(t)\right] = -\alpha(t)e^{-\int_0^t \alpha(l)dl}u(t) + e^{-\int_0^t \alpha(l)dl}u'(t).$$

Therefore

$$\frac{d}{dt}\left[e^{-\int_0^t \alpha(l)dl}u(t)\right] \leq \beta(t)e^{-\int_0^t \alpha(l)dl}$$

and by integrating we obtain

$$e^{-\int_0^t \alpha(l)dl}u(t) - u(0) \leq \int_0^t \beta(s)e^{-\int_0^s \alpha(l)dl}ds.$$

Thus

$$u(t) \leq e^{\int_0^t \alpha(l)dl}u(0) + \int_0^t e^{\int_s^t \alpha(l)dl}\beta(s)ds, \text{ for all } t \in [0, \tau].$$

Lemma 8.13 (Non-autonomous Gronwall's lemma) *Let $\alpha, \beta \in L^1(0, \tau)$. Let $u \in W^{1,\infty}((0, \tau), \mathbb{R})$ and assume that*

$$u'(t) \leq \alpha(t)u(t) + \beta(t) \text{ for almost every } t \in [0, \tau].$$

Then

$$u(t) \leq e^{\int_0^t \alpha(l)dl}u(0) + \int_0^t e^{\int_s^t \alpha(l)dl}\beta(s)ds, \text{ for all } t \in [0, \tau].$$

8.2.5 Henry's lemma

In the context of parabolic equations, Henry [149, Lemma 7.1.1, p. 188] proved the following important extension of Gronwall's lemma.

Lemma 8.14 (Henry) *Let $\tau > 0$, $\alpha \geq 0$ and $\beta \geq 0$. Assume that $u \in C([0, \tau], \mathbb{R})$ is a non-negative function satisfying*

$$u(t) \leq \alpha t^{\chi-1} + \beta \int_0^t (t - \sigma)^{\gamma-1}u(\sigma)d\sigma \text{ for all } t \in (0, \tau],$$

for some constants

$$\chi > 0 \ and \ \gamma > 0.$$

Then there exists a constant $\delta > 0$ such that

$$u(t) \le \delta t^{\chi-1} \ for \ all \ t \in [0, \tau].$$

Proof For $\eta > 0$ and $\zeta > 0$ we define

$$B(\eta, \zeta) := \int_0^1 (1-r)^{\eta-1} r^{\zeta-1} dr.$$

Applying twice the inequality satisfied by u, we get

$$u(t) \le \alpha t^{\chi-1} + \beta \int_0^t (t-\sigma)^{\gamma-1} u(\sigma) d\sigma$$

$$\le \alpha t^{\chi-1} + \beta \int_0^t (t-\sigma)^{\gamma-1} \alpha \sigma^{\chi-1} d\sigma$$

$$+ \beta^2 \int_0^t (t-\sigma_1)^{\gamma-1} \int_0^{\sigma_1} (\sigma_1 - \sigma_2)^{\gamma-1} u(\sigma_2) d\sigma_2 d\sigma_1. \qquad (8.3)$$

By using the change of variable $\sigma = tr$, we rewrite the first integral term of (8.3) as

$$\int_0^t (t-\sigma)^{\gamma-1} \alpha \sigma^{\chi-1} d\sigma = \alpha \int_0^1 (t-tr)^{\gamma-1} (tr)^{\chi-1} t dr = \alpha t^{\gamma+\chi-1} B(\gamma, \chi).$$

Next by using Fubini's theorem in the last term of the inequality (8.3), we obtain

$$\int_0^t (t-\sigma_1)^{\gamma-1} \int_0^{\sigma_1} (\sigma_1 - \sigma_2)^{\gamma-1} u(\sigma_2) d\sigma_2 d\sigma_1$$

$$= \int_0^t \int_{\sigma_2}^t (t-\sigma_1)^{\gamma-1} (\sigma_1 - \sigma_2)^{\gamma-1} u(\sigma_2) d\sigma_1 d\sigma_2$$

and

$$\int_{\sigma_2}^t (t-\sigma_1)^{\gamma-1} (\sigma_1 - \sigma_2)^{\gamma-1} d\sigma_1 = \int_0^{t-\sigma_2} (t-\sigma_2-l)^{\gamma-1} l^{\gamma-1} dl$$

$$= (t-\sigma_2)^{2(\gamma-1)+1} \int_0^1 (1-r)^{\gamma-1} r^{\gamma-1} dr.$$

Hence

$$\int_{\sigma_2}^t (t-\sigma_1)^{\gamma-1} (\sigma_1 - \sigma_2)^{\gamma-1} d\sigma_1 = (t-\sigma_2)^{2\gamma-1} B(\gamma, \gamma).$$

Therefore we obtain

$$u(t) \le \left[1 + \beta t^\gamma B(\gamma, \chi)\right] \alpha t^{\chi-1} + \beta^2 B(\gamma, \gamma) \int_0^t (t-\sigma)^{2\gamma-1} u(\sigma) d\sigma.$$

By fixing $\alpha_1 = \alpha + \beta \tau^\gamma B(\gamma, \chi) > 0$ and $\beta_1 = \beta^2 B(\gamma, \gamma)$ we obtain

$$u(t) \leq \alpha_1 t^{\chi-1} + \beta_1 \int_0^t (t - \sigma)^{2\gamma-1} u(\sigma) d\sigma.$$

By induction, we deduce that for each integer $n \geq 1$ we can find $\alpha_n > 0$ and $\beta_n > 0$ such that

$$u(t) \leq \alpha_n t^{\chi-1} + \beta_n \int_0^t (t - \sigma)^{2n\gamma-1} u(\sigma) d\sigma.$$

Therefore by choosing an integer $n > 0$ such that $2n\gamma > 1$, this yields

$$u(t) \leq \alpha_n t^{\chi-1} + \hat{\beta}_n \int_0^t u(\sigma) d\sigma,$$

with $\hat{\beta}_n := \beta_n \tau^{2n\gamma-1}$.

Setting

$$U(t) := \int_0^t u(\sigma) d\sigma,$$

we have

$$U'(t) \leq \hat{\beta}_n U(t) + \alpha_n t^{\chi-1}.$$

Thus

$$U(t) \leq \int_0^t e^{\hat{\beta}_n (t-s)} \alpha_n s^{\chi-a} ds \leq \alpha_n e^{\alpha_n \hat{\beta}_n \tau} \int_0^t s^{\chi-1} ds = \alpha_n e^{\alpha_n \hat{\beta}_n \tau} \frac{t^\chi}{\chi}.$$

The result follows.   □

8.2.6 Osgood's lemma

The following lemma can be regarded as a nonlinear version of Gronwall's lemma. This result gives an alternative criterion to show the uniqueness of solutions for an ordinary differential equation when the right-hand side is not Lipschitz continuous. We refer to the book of Hartman [145, Corollary 6.2, p. 33].

Lemma 8.15 (Osgood) *Let $\tau > 0$, $\alpha \geq 0$ and $\beta \in C([0, \tau], [0, +\infty))$ be given. Let $\chi \in C([0, +\infty), [0, +\infty))$ be a non-decreasing function satisfying*

$$\chi(0) = 0 \text{ and } \chi(x) > 0 \text{ for all } x > 0.$$

Assume that $u \in C([0, \tau], [0, +\infty))$ satisfies the following inequality

$$u(t) \leq \alpha + \int_0^t \beta(s) \chi(u(s)) ds \text{ for all } t \in [0, \tau].$$

If $\alpha > 0$ then the following inequality holds

$$\int_{\alpha}^{u(t)} \frac{1}{\chi(\sigma)} d\sigma \leq \int_{0}^{t} \beta(\sigma) d\sigma \text{ for all } t \in [0, \tau].$$

If $\alpha = 0$ then we have

$$\int_{0}^{\varepsilon} \frac{1}{\chi(\sigma)} d\sigma = \infty \text{ for all } \varepsilon > 0 \Rightarrow u(t) = 0 \text{ for all } t \in [0, \tau].$$

Proof Assume first that $\alpha > 0$. Define

$$U(t) = \int_{0}^{t} \beta(s) \chi(u(s)) ds.$$

Then we have

$$U'(t) = \beta(t) \chi(u(t)) \leq \beta(t) \chi(\alpha + U(t))$$

and since $\alpha > 0$ we obtain

$$\frac{U'(t)}{\chi(\alpha + U(t))} \leq \beta(t).$$

By integrating this inequality, we obtain

$$\int_{0}^{t} \frac{U'(\sigma)}{\chi(\alpha + U(\sigma))} d\sigma \leq \int_{0}^{t} \beta(\sigma) d\sigma.$$

We use the change of variable $r = \alpha + U(\sigma)$ to obtain

$$\int_{\alpha}^{\alpha + U(t)} \frac{1}{\chi(r)} dr \leq \int_{0}^{t} \beta(\sigma) d\sigma, \text{ for all } t \in [0, \tau],$$

and since $u(t) \leq \alpha + U(t)$ we deduce the first statement in the lemma.

Next we consider the case where $\alpha = 0$ and assume by contradiction that there exists a $t^* \in (0, \tau]$ such that $u(t^*) > 0$. Then

$$u(t) \leq \int_{0}^{t} \beta(s) \chi(u(s)) ds \text{ for all } t \in [0, \tau],$$

and this implies that

$$u(t) \leq \alpha + \int_{0}^{t} \beta(s) \chi(u(s)) ds \text{ for all } t \in [0, \tau],$$

for each $\alpha > 0$. Proceeding as above we obtain for each $\alpha < u(t^*)$

$$\int_{\alpha}^{u(t^*)} \frac{1}{\chi(\sigma)} d\sigma \leq \int_{0}^{t} \beta(\sigma) d\sigma,$$

and we get a contradiction by choosing α sufficiently small. □

Example 8.16 (Lifetime of a blow-up solution) Osgood's lemma can be used to estimate the lifetime of solutions in the presence of a blow-up. Consider for instance a nonlinearity $f \in C^1([0, +\infty), [0, +\infty))$ such that

$$f(u) \leq \beta u^2.$$

Then it is known that there exists a function $\tau(x) \in (0, +\infty]$ such that, for all $x \geq 0$, there is a unique solution $u(t)$ of the equation

$$\begin{cases} u'(t) = f(u(t)), \\ u(0) = x, \end{cases}$$

which is defined on $[0, \tau(x))$, and

$$\lim_{t \to \tau(x)^-} u(t) = +\infty \text{ if } \tau(x) < +\infty.$$

Integrating the equation satisfied by u we find that

$$u(t) \leq u(0) + \int_0^t f(u(s)) ds \leq u(0) + \int_0^t \beta u(s)^2 ds \text{ for all } t \in [0, \tau(x)).$$

Therefore by applying Osgood's Lemma, we have

$$\int_{u(0)}^{u(t)} \frac{1}{\sigma^2} d\sigma \leq \int_0^t \beta ds = \beta t,$$

$$\frac{1}{2} \left(\frac{-1}{u(t)} + \frac{1}{x} \right) \leq \beta t,$$

so that finally

$$u(t) \leq \frac{x}{1 - 2x\beta t}.$$

Therefore, we end-up with a lower estimate of the lifetime of u

$$\tau(x) \geq \frac{1}{2\beta x}.$$

Exercise 8.17 Apply the Osgood criterion to prove the uniqueness of the solution in the following example

$$U'(t) = \begin{cases} 0, & \text{if } U(0) = 0, \\ U(t) \ln(|U(t)|), & \text{if } U(0) \neq 0. \end{cases}$$

Solution If $U(0) \neq 0$ then the uniqueness of the solution follows from the standard theory of locally Lipschitz continuous equations. What we need to show is that there cannot exist a solution $U(t)$ not identically equal to 0 and such that $U(t) \to 0$ when $t \to 0$. Suppose by contradiction that there exists such a solution $U(t)$ defined for all $t \in [0, \tau)$. Integrating the equation satisfied by U and $-U$, we get

$$U(t) = 0 + \int_0^t U(s) \ln(|U(s)|)ds \leq \int_0^t |U(s)| \, |\ln(|U(s)|)|ds, \quad \forall t \in [0, \tau),$$

$$-U(t) = 0 + \int_0^t -U(s) \ln(|U(s)|)ds \leq \int_0^t |U(s)| \, |\ln(|U(s)|)|ds, \quad \forall t \in [0, \tau),$$

so that

$$|U(t)| \leq \int_0^t |U(s)| \, |\ln(|U(s)|)|ds, \text{ for all } t \in [0, \tau).$$

We remark that $\int_0^\varepsilon \frac{1}{\sigma |\ln(\sigma)|} d\sigma$ is a Bertrand integral which is divergent, that is,

$$\int_0^\varepsilon \frac{1}{\sigma |\ln(\sigma)|} d\sigma = +\infty \text{ for all } \varepsilon > 0, \tag{8.4}$$

so that Osgood's lemma implies that $|U(t)| = 0$ for all $t \in [0, \tau]$. This is a contradiction.

To prove (8.4) we change the variable $\ln(\sigma) = s$ in $\int_{\varepsilon_1}^\varepsilon \frac{1}{\sigma |\ln(\sigma)|} d\sigma$,

$$\int_{\varepsilon_1}^\varepsilon \frac{1}{\sigma |\ln(\sigma)|} d\sigma = \int_{\ln(\varepsilon_1)}^{\ln(\varepsilon)} \frac{1}{|s|} ds$$

and let $\varepsilon_1 \to 0$.

Remark 8.18 (A counterexample for the uniqueness of the solution) If $f(u) = \sqrt{u}$ then one can check that

$$u(t) := \left(\sqrt{u_0} + \frac{t}{2} \right)^2$$

is a solution of the ordinary differential equation

$$\begin{cases} u'(t) = f(u(t)), \\ u(0) = u_0, \end{cases}$$

for all $u_0 \geq 0$. In particular, there are two solutions corresponding to the initial condition $u_0 = 0$: $u(t) = \frac{t^2}{4}$ and $u(t) = 0$.

8.3 Monotone Semiflows

In this section we will assume that the semiflow U is positive (see Chapter 7 for more results), that is,

$$x \geq 0 \Rightarrow U(t)x \geq 0 \text{ for all } t \in [0, \tau(x)),$$

and we will focus on the following property.

Definition 8.19 We will say that a maximal semiflow $U : D_\tau \to \mathbb{R}^n$ is *monotone* on $\mathbb{R}_+^n$ if

$$0 \le x \le y \Rightarrow 0 \le U(t)x \le U(t)y \text{ for all } t \in \left[0, \min\left(\tau(x), \tau(y)\right)\right).$$

From now on we assume that the positive cone $\mathbb{R}_+^n$ is *normal*, that is,

$$0 \le x \le y \Rightarrow \|x\| \le \|y\|,$$

or (equivalently) that the norm on $\mathbb{R}^n$ is monotone. One can choose for example

$$\|x\|_1 = \sum_{i=1}^{n} |x_i|.$$

Lemma 8.20 *If U is a positive monotone semiflow on $\mathbb{R}_+^n$, then for each $x, y \in \mathbb{R}^n$,*

$$0 \le x \le y \Rightarrow \tau(y) \le \tau(x).$$

Proof We have

$$0 \le U(t)x \le U(t)y \text{ for all } t \in \left[0, \min\left(\tau(x), \tau(y)\right)\right),$$

and since the norm is monotone, we have

$$\|U(t)x\| \le \|U(t)y\| \text{ for all } t \in \left[0, \min\left(\tau(x), \tau(y)\right)\right).$$

Assume for instance that $\tau(x) < \tau(y)$. Then we have

$$+\infty = \lim_{\substack{t \to \tau(x) \\ t < \tau(x)}} \|U(t)x\| \le \lim_{\substack{t \to \tau(x) \\ t < \tau(x)}} \|U(t)y\| < +\infty,$$

which is a contradiction. $\qquad\qquad\qquad\qquad\qquad\qquad\qquad\qquad\qquad\qquad\quad\square$

Lemma 8.21 *Let $A \in C([0, \tau], M_n(\mathbb{R}))$ be given for some $\tau > 0$. For each $s \in [0, \tau]$ and each $x \in \mathbb{R}^n$ consider the unique solution $t \mapsto U(t, s)x$ of the non-autonomous ordinary differential equation*

$$\begin{cases} \dfrac{\partial U(t, s)x}{\partial t} = A(t)U(t, s)x \text{ for all } t \in [s, \tau], \\ U(s, s)x = x \in \mathbb{R}^n. \end{cases}$$

Then the two following properties are equivalent.

(i) *For each $x \in \mathbb{R}^n$,*

$$x \ge 0 \Rightarrow U(t, s)x \ge 0, \text{ for all } t, s \in [0, \tau] \text{ with } t \ge s.$$

(ii) *For each $t \in [0, \tau]$, the off-diagonal elements of $A(t)$ are non-negative.*

Remark 8.22 Since $t \to A(t)$, assertion (ii) is equivalent to the existence of a $\lambda > 0$ such that

$$A(t) + \lambda I \geq 0 \text{ for all } t \in [0, \tau].$$

Proof Proof of (i)$\Leftarrow$(ii). Assume that (ii) is satisfied, then there exists a $\lambda_0 > 0$ such that $A(t) + \lambda_0 I \geq 0$ for all $t \in [0, \tau]$. We have

$$\frac{\partial U}{\partial t}(t, s)x = -\lambda_0 U(t, s)x + \left[A(t) + \lambda_0 I\right] U(t, s)x,$$

and by using the non-autonomous variation of constant formula we obtain

$$U(t, s)x = e^{-\lambda_0(t-s)}x + \int_s^t e^{-\lambda_0(t-l)} \left[A(l) + \lambda_0 I\right] U(l, s)x \, dl.$$

Now by using the fixed-point method, (i) follows.

Proof of (i)$\Rightarrow$(ii). Let $s \in [0, \tau)$. Assume that

$$U(\varepsilon + s, s)x \geq 0 \text{ for all } \varepsilon \in [0, \tau - s] \text{ and } x \geq 0.$$

Let $x^* \geq 0$ be given. Then we have

$$\langle x^*, U(\varepsilon + s, s)x \rangle = \langle x^*, x \rangle + \int_s^{\varepsilon+s} \langle x^*, A(l)U(l, s)x \rangle dl.$$

If $\langle x^*, x \rangle = 0 \ (\Leftrightarrow x^* \perp x)$ then by dividing by ε we obtain

$$0 \leq \frac{\langle x^*, U(\varepsilon + s, s)x \rangle}{\varepsilon} = \frac{1}{\varepsilon} \int_s^{\varepsilon+s} \langle x^*, A(l)U(l, s)x \rangle dl,$$

and by taking the limit as ε approaches 0, we obtain

$$0 \leq \langle x^*, A(s)x \rangle.$$

We deduce that for each $x^* \geq 0$ and $x \geq 0$, one has

$$\langle x^*, x \rangle = 0 \Rightarrow \langle x^*, A(s)x \rangle \geq 0 \text{ for all } s \in [0, \tau).$$

Choosing $x^* = e_i$ and $x = e_j$ with $i \neq j$ (where e_i is the i-th element of the canonical basis), since

$$\langle e_i, A(s)e_j \rangle = A_{ij}(s) \geq 0 \text{ for all } s \in [0, \tau),$$

we deduce that

$$i \neq j \Rightarrow A_{ij}(s) \geq 0 \text{ for all } s \in [0, \tau).$$

Therefore all the off-diagonal elements of $A(s)$ are non-negative. $\qquad \square$

The first main result of this section is the following theorem.

Theorem 8.23 (Positive and monotone semiflow) *Let $F \in C^1(\mathbb{R}^n)$ be given. Let $U : D_\tau \to \mathbb{R}^n$ be the maximal semiflow generated by*

$$\begin{cases} U'(t)x = F(U(t)x), \\ U(0)x = x \in \mathbb{R}^n. \end{cases}$$

Then the following properties are equivalent.

(i) *U is positive and monotone on $\mathbb{R}_+^n$.*

(ii) *$F(0) \geq 0$ and $\dfrac{\partial F_i}{\partial x_j}(x) \geq 0$ whenever $x \geq 0$ and $i \neq j$.*

(iii) *For each $M > 0$, there exists a $\lambda = \lambda(M) > 0$ such that for each $x, y \in B_{\mathbb{R}^n}(0, M)$,*

$$0 \leq x \leq y \Rightarrow (\lambda I + F)(x) \leq (\lambda I + F)(y).$$

That is, $x \mapsto (\lambda I + F)(x)$ is non-negative and monotone non-decreasing on $B_{\mathbb{R}^n}(0, M) \cap \mathbb{R}_+^n$.

Remark 8.24 In practice we will use the property (ii) to show the monotony of a semiflow. A map $F \in C^1(\mathbb{R}^n)$ is *quasi-monotone* on $\mathbb{R}_+^n$ if

$$\frac{\partial F_i}{\partial x_j}(x) \geq 0 \text{ whenever } x \geq 0 \text{ and } i \neq j.$$

Proof Proof of (i)$\Rightarrow$(ii). Since the semiflow is positive, we know from Chapter 7 that we must have $F(0) \geq 0$. Moreover, for each $x, y \geq 0$ and each $t \in [0, \tau(x))$, since the semiflow is monotone we must have

$$\lim_{\varepsilon \to 0^+} \frac{U(t)(x + \varepsilon y) - U(t)x}{\varepsilon} \geq 0,$$

and we obtain

$$V(t, 0)y := \partial_x U(t)(x)(y) \geq 0, \text{ for all } x, y \geq 0 \text{ and } t \in [s, \tau(x)).$$

Similarly by replacing x by $U(s)x$ (for some $s \in [0, \tau(x))$) we must have

$$V(t, s)y = \partial_x U(t)(U(s)x)(y) \geq 0 \text{ for all } x, y \geq 0 \text{ and } t \in [s, \tau(x)).$$

From Chapter 6 we know that for each $s \in [0, \tau(x))$, the map $t \mapsto V(t, s)y$ is the unique solution of the non-autonomous ordinary differential equation

$$\partial_t V(t, s)y = DF(U(t + s)x)V(t, s)y \text{ for all } t \in [s, \tau(x)), V(s, s)y = y.$$

By using Lemma 8.21 (with $A(t) = DF(U(t + s)x)$) we deduce that for each $x \in \mathbb{R}_+^n$ there exists a $\lambda > 0$ such that

$$DF(x) + \lambda I \geq 0,$$

and (ii) follows.

Proof of (ii)$\Rightarrow$(iii). Since the map $x \mapsto DF(x)$ is continuous, we deduce that for each $M > 0$ there exists a $\lambda > 0$ such that

$$DF(x) + \lambda I \geq 0,$$

whenever $x \geq 0$ and $\|x\| \leq M$.

Let $y \geq x \geq 0$. We have (see Lemma 5.3)

$$F(y) - F(x) = \int_0^1 DF(sy + (1-s)x)(y-x)\mathrm{d}s.$$

Therefore

$$(\lambda I + F)(y) - (\lambda I + F)(x) = \lambda(y-x) + F(y) - F(x)$$
$$= \int_0^1 (\lambda I + DF)\big[sy + (1-s)x\big](y-x)\mathrm{d}s \geq 0,$$

and (iii) follows.

Proof of (iii)$\Rightarrow$(i). Let $M > 0$ be given and $x \in \mathbb{R}^n$ satisfy $\|x\| \leq M$. We choose $\lambda_0 := \lambda(2M)$ so that, for all $x, y \in B(0, 2M)$,

$$0 \leq x \leq y \Rightarrow (\lambda_0 I + F)(x) \leq (\lambda_0 I + F)(y).$$

Define

$$E := \{u \in C([0,\tau], \mathbb{R}^n) \, : \, u(t) \geq 0 \text{ and } \|u(t)\| \leq 2M \text{ for all } t \in [0,\tau]\}.$$

Recall that $t \mapsto u(t)$ is a solution of

$$\begin{cases} u'(t) = F(u(t)) \text{ for all } t \in [0,\tau], \\ u(0) = x \end{cases}$$

if and only if

$$u(t) = \mathrm{e}^{-\lambda t}x + \int_0^t \mathrm{e}^{-\lambda(t-s)}(\lambda I + F)(u(s))\mathrm{d}s \text{ for all } t \in [0,\tau].$$

Therefore, it is natural to consider the fixed-point operator

$$\Psi_x(u)(t) = \mathrm{e}^{-\lambda t}x + \int_0^t \mathrm{e}^{-\lambda(t-s)}(\lambda I + F)(u(s))\mathrm{d}s,$$

whenever $x \in B_{\mathbb{R}^n}(0, M) \cap \mathbb{R}_+^n$, $u \in E$ and $\lambda \geq \lambda_0$.

We observe that $(u, x) \mapsto \Psi_x(u)$ is a monotone non-decreasing map from $E \times B(0, M) \cap \mathbb{R}_+^n$ into $C([0,\tau], \mathbb{R}^n)$ and

$$\Psi_x(0) \geq 0$$

whenever $x \geq 0$.

Let $x \in B_{\mathbb{R}^n}(0, M) \cap \mathbb{R}^n_+$, $u \in E$ and $\lambda \geq \lambda_0$. For each $t \in [0, \tau]$ we have

$$\|\Psi_x(u)(t)\| \leq e^{-\lambda t}M + \int_0^t e^{-\lambda(t-s)}\|(\lambda I + F)(u(s)) - (\lambda I + F)(0)\|ds$$

$$+ \int_0^t e^{-\lambda(t-s)}\|(\lambda I + F)(0)\|ds$$

$$\leq M + \tau\big[(\lambda + k(2M))2M + \|F(0)\|\big],$$

where $k(2M)$ denotes the Lipschitz constant of F on the ball $B_{\mathbb{R}^n}(0, 2M)$, and when $\tau > 0$ is sufficiently small

$$\tau\big[((\lambda + k(2M))2M + \|F(0)\|\big] < M, \tag{8.5}$$

and then

$$\Psi_x(E) \subset E.$$

Moreover, under the condition (8.5) the map Ψ_x is K-Lipschitz with $K := \tau(\lambda + k(2M)) < \frac{1}{2}$.

Let $x, y \in B_{\mathbb{R}^n}(0, M)$ with $y \geq x$. Set

$$u_0(t) = x \text{ and } v_0(t) = y \text{ for all } t \in [0, \tau].$$

By using the monotone properties of Ψ we obtain

$$\Psi_x(u_0)(t) \leq \Psi_y(v_0)(t) \text{ for all } t \in [0, \tau],$$

and

$$\Psi_x^2(u_0)(t) = \Psi_x(\Psi_x(u_0))(t) \leq \Psi_x(\Psi_y(v_0))(t) \leq \Psi_y(\Psi_y(v_0))(t)$$

so that

$$\Psi_x^2(u_0)(t) \leq \Psi_y^2(v_0)(t) \text{ for all } t \in [0, \tau].$$

By induction we obtain for each $n \geq 1$

$$\Psi_x^m(u_0)(t) \leq \Psi_y^m(v_0)(t) \text{ for all } t \in [0, \tau],$$

and by taking the limit when m goes to $+\infty$ on both sides, we obtain

$$U(t)x = \lim_{m \to +\infty} \Psi_x^m(u_0)(t) \leq \lim_{m \to +\infty} \Psi_y^m(v_0)(t) = U(t)y \text{ for all } t \in [0, \tau].$$

The proof is complete. $\square$

Corollary 8.25 *Let $F \in C^1(\mathbb{R}^n)$. Let $U : D_\tau \to \mathbb{R}^n$ be the maximal semiflow generated by*

$$\begin{cases} U'(t)x = F(U(t)x), \\ U(0)x = x \in \mathbb{R}^n. \end{cases}$$

Assume that U is positive and monotone on $\mathbb{R}^n_+$.

Then we have the following properties.

(i) *If $F(x) \geq 0$ then the map $t \to U(t)x$ is non-decreasing on $[0, \tau(x))$ (i.e. $t \leq s \Rightarrow U(t)x \leq U(s)x$).*

(ii) *If $F(x) \leq 0$ then the map $t \to U(t)x$ is non-increasing on $[0, \tau(x))$ (i.e. $t \leq s \Rightarrow U(t)x \geq U(s)x$).*

Proof We observe that $U(t + h)x = U(t)U(h)x$. Then differentiating with respect to h and evaluating at $h = 0$ we have

$$\partial_t U(t)x = \partial_x U(t)(x)(\partial_t U(0)x) = \partial_x U(t)(x)(F(x)).$$

Moreover since the semiflow is monotone we have

$$\partial_x U(t)(x) \geq 0_{M_n(\mathbb{R})} \text{ for all } t \geq 0 \text{ and } x \geq 0.$$

The result follows. $\qquad \square$

Corollary 8.26 *Let $F \in C^1(\mathbb{R}^n)$. Let $U : D_\tau \to \mathbb{R}^n$ be the maximal semiflow generated by*

$$\begin{cases} U'(t)x = F(U(t)x) \\ U(0)x = x \in \mathbb{R}^n. \end{cases}$$

Assume that U is positive and monotone on $\mathbb{R}^n_+$.

Then we have the following properties.

(i) *If $F(x) \leq 0$ then there is an equilibrium $\bar{y} \geq 0$ (i.e. $F(\bar{y}) = 0$) such that*

$$\lim_{t \to +\infty} U(t)x = \bar{y}.$$

(ii) *If $F(x) \geq 0$ then the map $t \mapsto U(t)x$ is bounded if and only if there exists an equilibrium $\bar{x} \geq x$. Moreover, in that case there is an equilibrium $\bar{y} \leq \bar{x}$ such that*

$$\lim_{t \to +\infty} U(t)x = \bar{y}.$$

Proof If $F(x) \leq 0$, the map $t \mapsto U(t)x$ is non-increasing and non-negative and we can find $\bar{x} \geq 0$ such that

$$\bar{x} = \lim_{t \to +\infty} U(t)x.$$

We have

$$U(s + t)x = U(s)U(t)x.$$

Thus

$$\bar{x} = \lim_{t \to +\infty} U(t + s)x = U(s)\left(\lim_{t \to +\infty} U(t)x\right) = U(s)\bar{x}.$$

Hence

$$U(s)\bar{x} = \bar{x}, \text{ for all } s \geq 0.$$

When $F(0) \geq 0$ and $t \mapsto U(t)x$ is bounded, the proof is similar. $\qquad \square$

8.4 Comparison Principle

Similarly to Gronwall's Lemma, we can write a differential and integral form of the comparison principle. There are many different formulations of the comparison principle. We start with an integral form formulation.

Theorem 8.27 (Comparison principle, integral form) *Let $F \in C^1(\mathbb{R}^n)$. Let $U : D_\tau \to \mathbb{R}^n$ be the maximal semiflow (where $\tau(x)$ is the maximal time of existence of the solution starting from x) generated by*

$$\begin{cases} U'(t)x = F(U(t)x), \forall t \in [0, \tau(x)), \\ U(0)x = x. \end{cases}$$

Assume that U is positive and monotone on $\mathbb{R}^n_+$. Then we have the following properties.

(i) **(Sub-solution)** *Let $x \geq 0$ and $v \in C([0, \sigma], \mathbb{R}^n)$ (with $\sigma > 0$), and $v \geq 0$. Assume that*

$$v(t) \leq e^{-\lambda t}x + \int_0^t e^{-\lambda(t-s)}(\lambda I + F)(v(s))ds$$

for each $\lambda > 0$ sufficiently large and each $t \in [0, \sigma]$. Then

$$v(t) \leq U(t)x \text{ for all } t \in [0, \sigma] \cap [0, \tau(x)).$$

(ii) **(Super-solution)** *Let $x \geq 0$ and $w \in C([0, \sigma], \mathbb{R}^n)$ (with $\sigma > 0$), and $w \geq 0$. Assume that*

$$w(t) \geq e^{-\lambda t}x + \int_0^t e^{-\lambda(t-s)}(\lambda I + F)(w(s))ds$$

for each $\lambda > 0$ sufficiently large and for each $t \in [0, \sigma]$. Then

$$w(t) \geq U(t)x \text{ for all } t \in [0, \sigma] \cap [0, \tau(x)).$$

Proof For each $\lambda > 0$ sufficiently large we have

$$v(t) \leq e^{-\lambda t}x + \int_0^t e^{-\lambda(t-s)}(\lambda I + F)(v(s))ds =: \Psi_x(v(t)).$$

Therefore by using similar arguments as in the proof of Theorem 8.23 we have for all $t \in [0, \tau]$ with τ sufficiently small and λ sufficiently large,

$$v \leq \Psi_x(v) \leq \cdots \leq \Psi_x^m(v) \xrightarrow[m \to +\infty]{} U(t)x.$$

(i) follows. The proof of (ii) is similar.   □

Next we present a differential form of the comparison principle.

Theorem 8.28 (Comparison principle, differential form) *Let $F \in C^1(\mathbb{R}^n)$. Let $U : D_\tau \to \mathbb{R}^n$ be the maximal (where $\tau(x)$ is the maximal time of existence of the solution starting from x) semiflow generated by*

$$\begin{cases} U'(t)x = F(U(t)x), \forall t \in [0, \tau(x)), \\ U(0)x = x \in \mathbb{R}^n. \end{cases}$$

Assume that U is positive and monotone on $\mathbb{R}^n_+$. Then the following properties hold

(i) *(Sub-solution) Let $x \geq 0$ and $v \in C^1([0, \sigma], \mathbb{R}^n)$ (with $\sigma > 0$), and $v \geq 0$. Assume that*

$$\begin{cases} v'(t) \leq F(v(t)) \text{ for all } t \in [0, \sigma], \\ v(0) \leq x. \end{cases}$$

Then

$$v(t) \leq U(t)x \text{ for all } t \in [0, \sigma] \cap [0, \tau(x)).$$

(ii) *(Super-solution) Let $x \geq 0$ and $w \in C^1([0, \sigma], \mathbb{R}^n)$ (with $\sigma > 0$), and $w \geq 0$. Assume that*

$$\begin{cases} w'(t) \geq F(w(t)) \text{ for all } t \in [0, \sigma], \\ w(0) \geq x. \end{cases}$$

Then

$$w(t) \geq U(t)x \text{ for all } t \in [0, \sigma] \cap [0, \tau(x)).$$

Proof We only proof (ii), the proof for (i) being similar. Let $\lambda \in \mathbb{R}$. Assume (ii), then for each $t \in [0, \sigma]$,

$$w'(t) \geq F(w(t)) \Leftrightarrow w'(t) \geq -\lambda w(t) + (F + \lambda I)(w(t))$$

$$\Leftrightarrow e^{\lambda t}(w'(t) + \lambda w(t)) \geq e^{\lambda t}(F + \lambda I)(w(t))$$

hence

$$\left(e^{\lambda t} w(t)\right)' \geq e^{\lambda t}(F + \lambda I)(w(t)).$$

By integrating both sides of the above inequality between 0 and t, we obtain

$$e^{\lambda t} w(t) - w(0) \geq \int_0^t e^{\lambda s}(F + \lambda I)(w(s)) ds,$$

therefore

$$w(t) \geq e^{-\lambda t} w(0) + \int_0^t e^{-\lambda(t-s)}(F + \lambda I)(w(s)) ds$$

and since $w(0) \geq x$, we obtain for $t \in [0, \sigma]$,

$$w(t) \geq e^{-\lambda t} x + \int_0^t e^{-\lambda(t-s)}(F + \lambda I)(w(s)) ds.$$

The result follows from Theorem 8.27. $\qquad\qquad\qquad\qquad\qquad\qquad\qquad\qquad\square$

Exercise 8.29 Let $f \in C^1(\mathbb{R})$ be given with $f(0) \geq 0$. Consider the scalar ordinary differential equation

$$\begin{cases} u'(t) = f(u(t)), \\ u(0) = x \geq 0. \end{cases} \qquad (8.6)$$

1. Assume that there exist three constants $x^* > 0$, $\beta > 0$ and $\lambda \in \mathbb{R}$ such that

$$f(x) \leq \beta x + \lambda \text{ for all } x > x^*.$$

By using the comparison principle, prove that for each $x \geq 0$ the solution of equation (8.6) exists for all positive time (i.e. $\tau(x) = +\infty$).

2. Assume that there are four constants $x^* > 0$, $\beta > 0$, $\lambda \in \mathbb{R}$ and $\gamma \in \mathbb{R}$ such that

$$f(x) \geq \beta x^2 + \lambda x + \gamma, \text{ for all } x > x^*.$$

By using the comparison principle, show that for each $x \geq 0$ sufficiently large the solution of (8.6) blows-up in finite time (i.e. $\tau(x) < +\infty$).

8.5 Competitive and Cooperative Systems: Lotka–Volterra Equations

To illustrate the notion of the competitive and cooperative Lotka–Volterra model we refer to [215, 216, 217, 351, 352].

8.5.1 The Lotka–Volterra model with two species

The model is written as

$$\begin{cases} u_1' = u_1 \left(\lambda_1 + \alpha_{11} u_1 + \alpha_{12} u_2 \right), \\ u_2' = u_2 \left(\lambda_2 + \alpha_{21} u_1 + \alpha_{22} u_2 \right), \end{cases} \qquad (8.7)$$

where $u_i(t)$ ($i = 1, 2$) denotes the number of individuals in the species i at time t. The parameter $\lambda_i \in \mathbb{R}$ ($i = 1, 2$) is the growth rate of the species i, and $\alpha_{ii} \leq 0$ describes the intra-specific growth limitations for the species i. The coefficient α_{ij} (with $i \neq j$) corresponds either to a term of inter-specific competition when $\alpha_{ij} \leq 0$, or to a term of inter-specific cooperation when $\alpha_{ij} \geq 0$.

Definition 8.30 System (8.7) is said to be *cooperative* if and only if

$$\alpha_{12} \geq 0 \text{ and } \alpha_{21} \geq 0.$$

This means that all the inter-specific interactions are cooperative.

System (8.7) is said to be *competitive* if and only if

$$\alpha_{12} \leq 0 \text{ and } \alpha_{21} \leq 0.$$

This means that all the inter-specific interactions are competitive.

8.5.2 The Lotka–Volterra model with multiple species

The model is written as

$$
\begin{cases}
u_1' = u_1 \left(\lambda_1 + \alpha_{11} u_1 + \cdots + \alpha_{1n} u_n \right), \\
u_2' = u_2 \left(\lambda_2 + \alpha_{21} u_1 + \cdots + \alpha_{2n} u_n \right), \\
\vdots \\
u_n' = u_n \left(\lambda_n + \alpha_{n1} u_1 + \cdots + \alpha_{nn} u_n \right),
\end{cases}
\tag{8.8}
$$

where $u_i(t)$ $(i = 1, \ldots, n)$ denotes the number of individuals in the species i at time t. The parameter $\lambda_i \in \mathbb{R}$ $(i = 1, \ldots, n)$ is the growth rate of the species i, and $\alpha_{ii} \leq 0$ describes the intra-specific growth limitations for the species i. The coefficient α_{ij} (with $i \neq j$) corresponds either to a term of inter-specific competition whenever $\alpha_{ij} \leq 0$, or to a term of inter-specific cooperation whenever $\alpha_{ij} \geq 0$.

Definition 8.31 The system (8.8) is said to be *cooperative* if and only if

$$
\alpha_{ij} \geq 0, \forall i \neq j.
$$

The system (8.8) is said to be *competitive* if and only if

$$
\alpha_{ij} \leq 0, \forall i \neq j.
$$

Definition 8.32 Consider the system

$$
\begin{cases}
u_1' = F_1(u_1, u_2, \ldots, u_n), \\
u_2' = F_2(u_1, u_2, \ldots, u_n), \\
\vdots \\
u_n' = F_n(u_1, u_2, \ldots, u_n).
\end{cases}
\tag{8.9}
$$

The system (8.9) is *cooperative* if and only if

$$
\partial_{x_i} F_j(x) \geq 0, \quad \forall i \neq j, \forall x \geq 0.
\tag{8.10}
$$

The system (8.9) is *competitive* if and only if

$$
\partial_{x_i} F_j(x) \leq 0, \quad \forall i \neq j, \forall x \geq 0.
\tag{8.11}
$$

Remark 8.33 A system $u' = F(u(t))$ is competitive if and only if the system $v'(t) = -F(v(t))$ is cooperative. This means that a competitive system is nothing but a cooperative system when we reverse the time (i.e. $v(t) = u(-t)$).

8.6 Applications to Diffusive Equations

8.6.1 Logistic equations and diffusion between two cities with local limitations in space

We investigate the system

$$\begin{cases} u_1'(t) = \gamma\left[u_2(t) - u_1(t)\right] + \lambda_1 u_1(t) - \kappa_1^{-1} u_1(t)^2, \\ u_2'(t) = \gamma\left[u_1(t) - u_2(t)\right] + \lambda_2 u_2(t) - \kappa_2^{-1} u_2(t)^2, \end{cases} \qquad (8.12)$$

where $\lambda_1 \in \mathbb{R}$ is the growth rate of group 1 and $\lambda_2 \in \mathbb{R}$ is the growth rate of group 2. The parameter $\kappa_1 > 0$ (respectively $\kappa_2 > 0$) describes the growth limitation in group 1 (respectively 2). The parameter $\gamma > 0$ is the rate at which individuals from group 1 (respectively 2) are leaving to the other group 2 (respectively 1). For the movement of individuals, we consider a two-patch model with symmetric transfer rates.

By setting $U(t) = (u_1(t), u_2(t))^T$, the system (8.12) can be written in the more condensed form

$$U'(t) = F\big(U(t)\big), \forall t \geq 0, \text{ and } U(0)x = x \geq 0,$$

where

$$F(u) = F\begin{pmatrix} u_1 \\ u_2 \end{pmatrix} = \begin{pmatrix} \gamma[u_2 - u_1] + \lambda_1 u_1 - \kappa_1^{-1} u_1^2 \\ \gamma[u_1 - u_2] + \lambda_2 u_2 - \kappa_2^{-1} u_2^2 \end{pmatrix} = \begin{pmatrix} F_1(U) \\ F_2(U) \end{pmatrix}.$$

Positivity

The positivity follows by using the criterion proved in Chapter 7. Namely for each $M > 0$ we can find a $\lambda = \lambda(M) > 0$ such that

$$F(u) + \lambda u \geq 0, \forall u \in [0, M\mathbb{1}] := \left\{ U \in \mathbb{R}^2 : 0 \leq U \leq M\mathbb{1} \right\},$$

where

$$\mathbb{1} = (1, 1)^T.$$

Remark 8.34 (An alternative proof of the positivity) We have

$$u_i' \geq (\lambda_i - \gamma)u_i - \kappa_i^{-1} u_i^2.$$

Therefore by using the comparison principle, we deduce that each component $u_i(t)$ is bounded from below by the solution of the logistic equation

$$v_i' = (\lambda_i - \gamma)v_i - \kappa_i^{-1} v_i^2,$$

and the positivity follows. We can also deduce that the species i will persist whenever $\lambda_i - \gamma > 0$.

Monotone semiflow

We have $F(0) = 0_{\mathbb{R}^2}$ and the Jacobian matrix of F is

$$\partial F(U) = \begin{pmatrix} \lambda_1 - \gamma - 2\kappa_1^{-1}u_1 & \gamma \\ \gamma & \lambda_2 - \gamma - 2\kappa_2^{-1}u_2 \end{pmatrix}.$$

Since the off-diagonal entries of $\partial F(U)$ are non-negative for all $U \in \mathbb{R}^2$ with $U \geq 0$, a direct application of Theorem 8.23 shows that the differential system (8.12) generates a unique maximal semiflow which is positive and monotone.

Remark 8.35 The off-diagonal terms in the Jacobian matrix correspond to the fluxes from group 1 (respectively 2) to group 2 (respectively 1) and are equal to $\gamma > 0$.

The linearized equation at 0

The behavior of the system close to 0 will be characterized by the sign of the dominant eigenvalue of the Jacobian matrix of F at $u = 0$. In particular, the lower solutions will start from a multiple of the associated positive eigenvector. We have

$$\partial F(0) = \begin{pmatrix} \lambda_1 - \gamma & \gamma \\ \gamma & \lambda_2 - \gamma \end{pmatrix}.$$

The characteristic equation is

$$(\lambda_1 - \gamma - \Lambda)(\lambda_2 - \gamma - \Lambda) - \gamma^2 = 0$$
$$\Leftrightarrow \Lambda^2 - [\lambda_1 + \lambda_2 - 2\gamma]\Lambda + (\lambda_1 - \gamma)(\lambda_2 - \gamma) - \gamma^2 = 0. \qquad (8.13)$$

The discriminant is

$$\Delta = [\lambda_1 + \lambda_2 - 2\gamma]^2 - 4[\lambda_1\lambda_2 - \gamma(\lambda_1 + \lambda_2)].$$

Hence by developing this formula we obtain

$$\Delta = (\lambda_1 + \lambda_2)^2 - 4\gamma(\lambda_1 + \lambda_2) + 4\gamma^2 - 4\lambda_1\lambda_2 + 4\gamma(\lambda_1 + \lambda_2).$$

After simplification and since $\gamma > 0$, we obtain

$$\Delta = (\lambda_1 - \lambda_2)^2 + 4\gamma^2 > 0. \qquad (8.14)$$

Let Λ be the maximal eigenvalue (or dominant eigenvalue) of $\partial F(0)$, that is,

$$\Lambda := \frac{1}{2}\left([\lambda_1 + \lambda_2 - 2\gamma] + \sqrt{\Delta}\right). \qquad (8.15)$$

Right eigenvector: The corresponding eigenvector $\mathbb{V}$ satisfies

$$\begin{pmatrix} \lambda_1 - \gamma & \gamma \\ \gamma & \lambda_2 - \gamma \end{pmatrix} \begin{pmatrix} \mathbb{V}_1 \\ \mathbb{V}_2 \end{pmatrix} = \Lambda \begin{pmatrix} \mathbb{V}_1 \\ \mathbb{V}_2 \end{pmatrix} \Leftrightarrow \begin{cases} [\Lambda - (\lambda_1 - \gamma)]\, \mathbb{V}_1 = \gamma \mathbb{V}_2, \\ [\Lambda - (\lambda_2 - \gamma)]\, \mathbb{V}_2 = \gamma \mathbb{V}_1. \end{cases}$$

We observe that (independently of the sign of Λ) we always have

$$\Lambda - (\lambda_1 - \gamma) = \frac{1}{2}\left([\lambda_2 - \lambda_1] + \sqrt{\Delta}\right) > 0 \text{ and}$$

$$\Lambda - (\lambda_2 - \gamma) = \frac{1}{2}\left([\lambda_1 - \lambda_2] + \sqrt{\Delta}\right) > 0. \tag{8.16}$$

Therefore, the sign of $\mathbb{V}_1$ is the same as the sign of $\mathbb{V}_2$. In other words, the eigenspace associated with Λ is spanned by a positive vector.

Global asymptotic stability of the trivial equilibrium when $\Lambda \le 0$

Assume that $\Lambda \le 0$. Then we can find a left eigenvector $\mathbb{W} \gg 0$ (i.e. $\mathbb{W}_1 > 0$ and $\mathbb{W}_2 > 0$) of $\partial F(0)$ associated to Λ. That is,

$$\mathbb{W}^T \partial F(0) = \Lambda \mathbb{W}^T.$$

Therefore

$$\mathbb{W}^T u(t)' = \mathbb{W}^T \partial F(0) u(t) - \mathbb{W}_1\, \kappa_1^{-1} u_1(t)^2 - \mathbb{W}_2\, \kappa_2^{-1} u_2(t)^2.$$

It follows that the quantity $V(u(t)) = \mathbb{W}^T u(t)$ is strictly decreasing as long as $u(t) \ne 0$. Since $\mathbb{W}_1 > 0$ and $\mathbb{W}_2 > 0$ we deduce the following proposition.

Proposition 8.36 (Global stability of 0**)** *Assume that* $\Lambda \le 0$. *Then the trivial equilibrium* 0 *is globally asymptotically stable.*

Proof This proof is left as an exercise. *Hint:* Set $x(t) = \mathbb{W}^T u(t)$ and observe that $x(t)' \le \Lambda x(t)$. $\qquad\square$

Dissipativity

To prove the dissipativity of (8.12) we use a family of upper solutions starting from

$$\overline{U}_\alpha = \alpha \mathbb{1}.$$

We choose such an initial value in order to get rid of the γ terms in (8.12) at $t = 0$.
   Indeed, we have

$$F(\alpha \mathbb{1}) = \alpha \begin{pmatrix} \lambda_1 - \kappa_1^{-1}\alpha \\ \lambda_2 - \kappa_2^{-1}\alpha \end{pmatrix}.$$

By choosing $\alpha^+ := \max(\lambda_1 \kappa_1, \lambda_2 \kappa_2) > 0$ we deduce that

$$F(\alpha \mathbb{1}) \ll 0, \forall \alpha > \alpha^+. \tag{8.17}$$

Therefore by applying Corollary 8.25 and using the fact that 0 is an equilibrium we deduce the following.

Lemma 8.37 (Upper solutions) *For each $\alpha > \max(\alpha^+, 0)$, the interval $[0, \alpha \mathbb{1}] = \left\{ x \in \mathbb{R}^2 : 0 \leq x \leq \alpha \mathbb{1} \right\}$ is positively invariant for the semiflow generated by (8.12). That is,*

$$U(t)\,[0, \alpha \mathbb{1}] \subset [0, \alpha \mathbb{1}]\,, \forall t \geq 0.$$

Moreover the solution $t \to u(t) = U(t)\,(\alpha \mathbb{1})$ starting from $\alpha \mathbb{1}$ converges to the largest equilibrium of (8.12) in the interval $[0, \alpha \mathbb{1}]$ (this equilibrium can be 0).

Lower solutions

Assume that $\Lambda > 0$. We can also compute a right eigenvector $\mathbb{V} \gg 0$ (i.e. $\mathbb{V}_1 > 0$ and $\mathbb{V}_2 > 0$) of $\partial F(0)$ associated with Λ. We can choose for example

$$\mathbb{V} := \begin{pmatrix} \gamma \\ \Lambda - (\lambda_1 - \gamma) \end{pmatrix} \tag{8.18}$$

or

$$\mathbb{V} := \begin{pmatrix} \Lambda - (\lambda_2 - \gamma) \\ \gamma \end{pmatrix}. \tag{8.19}$$

We then have

$$F(\alpha \mathbb{V}) = \alpha \begin{pmatrix} (\Lambda - \kappa_1^{-1} \alpha \mathbb{V}_1)\,\mathbb{V}_1 \\ (\Lambda - \kappa_2^{-1} \alpha \mathbb{V}_2)\,\mathbb{V}_2 \end{pmatrix}.$$

Therefore if $\Lambda > 0$ we obtain

$$F(\alpha \mathbb{V}) \gg 0, \quad \forall \alpha \in (0, \alpha^-), \tag{8.20}$$

with

$$\alpha^- := \min \left(\frac{\Lambda \kappa_1}{\mathbb{V}_1}, \frac{\Lambda \kappa_2}{\mathbb{V}_2} \right) > 0. \tag{8.21}$$

By a direct application of Corollary 8.25 we obtain the following result.

Lemma 8.38 (Lower solutions) *Assume that $\Lambda > 0$. For each $\alpha \in (0, \alpha^-)$, the interval $[\alpha \mathbb{V}, +\infty) = \left\{ x \in \mathbb{R}^2 : x \geq \alpha \mathbb{V} \right\}$ is positively invariant for the semiflow generated by (8.12). Moreover, the solution $t \to u(t) = U(t)\,(\alpha \mathbb{V})$ starting from $\alpha \mathbb{V}$ converges to the smallest equilibrium of (8.12) in the interval $[\alpha^- \mathbb{V}, \alpha^+ \mathbb{1}]$.*

Equilibrium

It follows from Proposition 8.36 that there cannot exist a positive equilibrium when $\Lambda \leq 0$. When $\Lambda > 0$, Lemma 8.37 and 8.38 show that there exists a positive equilibrium and any solution starting from a non-negative and nontrivial initial value $U(0)$ converges to such an equilibrium. Here we show that there exists a *unique* positive equilibrium which attracts any non-negative and non-trivial initial value.

Proposition 8.39 (Uniqueness of the positive equilibrium) *Assume $\Lambda > 0$. There exists a unique positive equilibrium for (8.12), which attracts any non-negative and non-zero initial value.*

Proof Assume by contradiction that there exist two non-negative equilibria $U := (u_1, u_2)^T \neq 0_{\mathbb{R}^2}$ and $V := (v_1, v_2)^T \neq 0_{\mathbb{R}^2}$, that is,

$$F(U) = F(V) = 0_{\mathbb{R}^2}.$$

First we show that U and V are both positive, that is, $U \gg 0$ and $V \gg 0$. Indeed by considering the first equation of the system

$$\begin{cases} 0 = \gamma[u_2 - u_1] + \lambda_1 u_1 - \kappa_1^{-1} u_1^2 \\ 0 = \gamma[u_1 - u_2] + \lambda_2 u_2 - \kappa_2^{-1} u_2^2, \end{cases} \tag{8.22}$$

we deduce that $u_1 = 0$ implies $u_2 = 0$. Similarly the second equation of (8.22) shows that $u_2 = 0$ implies $u_1 = 0$. Therefore, since U is not zero, both components of U are positive (i.e. $U \gg 0$). A similar argument shows that $V \gg 0$.

Next we show that U and V are ordered, that is, $U \leq V$. To do so we use the fact that F is strictly sub-homogeneous, that is,

$$\eta F(U) \ll F(\eta U) \text{ for all } \eta \in (0, 1).$$

Define

$$\eta^* := \sup\{\eta > 0 : \eta U \leq V\}$$

and assume by contradiction that $\eta^* < 1$. Then

$$0_{\mathbb{R}^2} = \eta^* F(U) \ll F(\eta^* U). \tag{8.23}$$

On the other hand, there must be an $i \in \{1, 2\}$ such that $\eta^* u_i = v_i$. Otherwise we would get a contradiction with the definition of η^*, namely, we could find $\tilde{\eta} > \eta$ such that $\tilde{\eta} u_i \leq v_i$. Then, letting $j \neq i$ and recalling that $\eta^* u_i \leq v_j$ by definition of η^*, we have

$$\begin{aligned} F_i(\eta^* U) &= \gamma(\eta^* u_j - \eta^* u_i) + \lambda_i(\eta^* u_i) - \kappa_i^{-1}(\eta^* u_i)^2 \\ &= \gamma(\eta^* u_j) - \gamma v_j + \gamma(v_j - v_i) + \lambda_i v_i - \kappa_i^{-1} v_i^2 \\ &\leq F_i(V) = 0, \end{aligned}$$

which contradicts (8.23).

We conclude that $\eta \geq 1$. Therefore, U and V can be compared with

$$U \leq V.$$

By exchanging the roles of U and V, we also have $V \leq U$, which shows that $U = V$. Therefore there cannot exist more than one positive equilibrium. This completes the proof of Proposition 8.39. $\square$

Remark 8.40 The argument used to prove the uniqueness of the equilibrium in the previous proposition is borrowed from Krasnoselskii [189]. It is an important tool in the study of monotone systems.

Invariant subregion in $\mathbb{R}_+^2$

We have seen in the previous sections that there exist positive subregions of $\mathbb{R}_+^2$, starting with $\mathbb{R}_+^2$ itself. Thanks to the upper solution of Lemma 8.37, the interval $[0, \alpha\mathbb{1}]$ is an invariant subregion of $\mathbb{R}_+^2$ for α sufficiently large (more precisely, for $\alpha \geq \alpha^+$). Then, in Lemma 8.38 we have shown that $[\alpha\mathbb{V}, +\infty)$ is invariant for $\alpha \in (0, \alpha^-]$ and, therefore, so is $[\alpha^-\mathbb{V}, \alpha^+\mathbb{1}]$.

Let us consider the case where $\lambda_1 = \lambda_2 =: \lambda$ and $\kappa_1 = \kappa_2 =: \kappa$. Then (8.12) becomes

$$\begin{cases} u_1'(t) = \gamma[u_2(t) - u_1(t)] + \lambda u_1(t) - \kappa^{-1}u_1(t)^2 \\ u_2'(t) = \gamma[u_1(t) - u_2(t)] + \lambda u_2(t) - \kappa^{-1}u_2(t)^2. \end{cases} \tag{8.24}$$

In this case one can check that the solution starting from an initial condition $u_0\mathbb{1}$ stays aligned with the vector $\mathbb{1}$. Indeed, if the function $u(t)$ is a solution to the scalar ODE

$$\begin{cases} u'(t) = \lambda u(t)(1 - \kappa^{-1}u(t)), \\ u(0) = u_0, \end{cases}$$

then the vector function $U(t) := u(t)\mathbb{1}$ solves (8.24) with initial condition $U(0) := u_0\mathbb{1}$. Thus the vector space spanned by $\mathbb{1}$ is an invariant subregion of $\mathbb{R}_+^2$.

Exercise 8.41 Extend the above results to the following two-patch model

$$\begin{cases} u_1'(t) = \gamma_2 u_2(t) - \gamma_1 u_1(t) + \lambda_1 u_1(t) - \kappa_1^{-1}u_1(t)^2 \\ u_2'(t) = \gamma_1 u_1(t) - \gamma_2 u_2(t) + \lambda_2 u_2(t) - \kappa_2^{-1}u_2(t)^2 \end{cases} \tag{8.25}$$

with $\gamma_1 > 0$ is the leaving rate from patch 1 and $\gamma_2 > 0$ is leaving rate from patch 2.

8.6.2 *N*-dimensional logistic equations with diffusion: local limitations in space

Consider the system

$$\begin{cases} U'(t) = \gamma DU(t) + \lambda U(t) - \kappa^{-1}U(t)^2 \\ U(0) = U_0 \geq 0, \end{cases} \tag{8.26}$$

where $U_i(t)$ is the number of individuals in the i-th compartment, $\lambda := (\beta - \mu)$ is the growth rate of individuals and the matrix describes the spatial motion of individuals between the $N \geq 3$ compartments

$$D = \begin{pmatrix} -1 & 1 & 0 & \cdots & \cdots & \cdots & 0 \\ 1 & -2 & 1 & & & & \vdots \\ 0 & 1 & -2 & 1 & & & \vdots \\ \vdots & & & & & & 0 \\ \vdots & & & & & & \\ & & & & & -2 & 1 \\ 0 & \cdots & \cdots & \cdots & 0 & 1 & -1 \end{pmatrix}$$

$U(t)^2$ is the column vector formed by the square of the components of $U(t)$ and

$$F(U) := \gamma D U + \lambda U - \kappa^{-1} U^2 = (F_1(U), F_2(U), \ldots, F_N(U))^T.$$

The system can be rewritten component by component as follows

$$
\begin{aligned}
U_1'(t) &= \gamma \left[U_2(t) - U_1(t) \right] + \lambda U_1(t) - \kappa^{-1} U_1(t)^2 = F_1(U), \\
U_2'(t) &= \gamma \left[U_3 + U_1 \right] - 2\gamma U_2 + \lambda U_2(t) - \kappa^{-1} U_2(t)^2 = F_2(U), \\
&\vdots \\
U_i'(t) &= \gamma \left[U_{i+1} + U_{i-1} \right] - 2\gamma U_i + \lambda U_i(t) - \kappa^{-1} U_i(t)^2 = F_i(U), \\
&\vdots \\
U_{N-1}'(t) &= \gamma \left[U_N + U_{N-2} \right] - 2\gamma U_{N-1} + \lambda U_{N-1}(t) - \kappa^{-1} U_{N-1}(t)^2 = F_{N-1}(U), \\
U_N'(t) &= \gamma \left[U_{N-1} - U_N(t) \right] + \lambda U_N(t) - \kappa^{-1} U_N(t)^2 = F_N(U),
\end{aligned}
$$

$$(8.27)$$

where $i \in \{2, \ldots, N-1\}$ and γ^{-1} is the average time spent in the i-th compartment.

Most of the arguments from Section 8.6.1 can be adapted to the case of an N-component system.

Positivity

We can use a criterion from Chapter 7. More precisely, for each $M > 0$ we can find a $\Lambda = \Lambda(M) > 0$ such that

$$F(u) + \Lambda u \geq 0 \quad \text{for all } u \in [0, M\mathbb{1}],$$

where

$$\mathbb{1} = (1, 1, \ldots, 1)^T$$

is the N-component vector with all entries equal to 1. Actually we can take

$$\Lambda(M) = \kappa^{-1} M - \min(\lambda, 0) + 2\gamma.$$

Monotone semiflow

We have $F(0) = 0_{\mathbb{R}^N}$ and the Jacobian of F is

$$\partial F(U) = \gamma D + \lambda I - 2\kappa^{-1} \mathrm{diag}\,(U_1, U_2, \ldots, U_N)\,. \tag{8.28}$$

Since the off-diagonal entries of $\partial F(U)$ are non-negative for all $U \in \mathbb{R}_+^N$, a direct application of Theorem 8.23 shows that the differential system (8.26) generates a unique semiflow which is positive and monotone.

The linearized equation at 0

The behavior of the system close to 0 can be characterized by the sign of the dominant eigenvalue of the Jacobian matrix of F at $u = 0$. In the case of equation (8.26), we admit that this eigenvalue is equal to λ and corresponds to the right eigenvector $\mathbb{1}$. The fact that $(\lambda, \mathbb{1})$ is an eigenpair for $\partial F(0)$ can be checked from (8.28). The fact that λ is the dominant eigenvalue of $\partial F(0)$ is a consequence of the Perron–Frobenius Theorem in Chapter 4.

Global asymptotic stability of $0_{\mathbb{R}^N}$ when $\lambda \leq 0$

Assume $\lambda \leq 0$. Then since $\partial F(0) = \gamma D + \lambda I$ is symmetric, $\mathbb{1}$ is a left eigenvector of $\partial F(0)$ associated with λ,

$$\mathbb{1}^T \partial F(0) = \lambda \mathbb{1}^T\,.$$

Therefore

$$\mathbb{1}^T U'(t) = \lambda \mathbb{1}^T U(t) - \kappa^{-1} \mathbb{1}^T U(t)^2\,.$$

It follows that the quantity $V(u(t)) := \mathbb{1}^T U(t) = \sum_{i=1}^N U_i$ is strictly decreasing as long as $U(t) \neq 0$. Since $\mathbb{1} \gg 0$ we deduce the following proposition.

Proposition 8.42 (Global stability of $0_{\mathbb{R}^N}$) *Assume that $\lambda \leq 0$. Then the trivial equilibrium 0 is globally asymptotically stable.*

Proof The result has been proved already, and we now provide an alternative proof. Let us assume first that $\lambda < 0$. Define $\overline{U}(t) := M e^{\lambda t} \mathbb{1}$. Then $\overline{U}(t)$ is a super-solution in the sense that it satisfies the differential inequality

$$\frac{d\overline{U}(t)}{dt} = \lambda M e^{\lambda t} \mathbb{1} = \lambda \overline{U}(t) = (\gamma D + \lambda I)\,\overline{U}(t)$$
$$\geq (\gamma D + \lambda I)\,\overline{U}(t) - \kappa^{-1}\overline{U}(t)^2 = F\big(\overline{U}(t)\big)\,.$$

Therefore by Theorem 8.28 (ii) we have

$$x \leq M\mathbb{1} \Rightarrow U(t)x \leq \overline{U}(t) = M e^{\lambda t} \mathbb{1}, \forall t \geq 0\,.$$

Hence $\overline{U}(t)$ is a super-solution in the sense of Theorem 8.28 (ii). In particular, for each initial condition $U_0 \in \mathbb{R}_+^N$, we can choose $M = \|U_0\|_\infty$ (so that $\overline{U}(0) = \|U_0\|_\infty \mathbb{1} \geq x$) and by a direct application of Theorem 8.28 we find that

$$U(t) \leq \|U_0\|_\infty e^{\lambda t} \mathbb{1}, \text{ therefore } \lim_{t \to +\infty} U(t) = 0_{\mathbb{R}^N}\,.$$

If $\lambda = 0$, we observe that the function

$$\overline{U}(t) := \frac{U_0}{1 + \kappa^{-1} U_0 t} \mathbb{1}$$

solves the differential system

$$\frac{\mathrm{d}\overline{U}(t)}{\mathrm{d}t} = -\kappa^{-1}\overline{U}(t)^2 = \frac{\gamma}{2} D\overline{U}(t) - \kappa^{-1}\overline{U}(t)^2$$

$$\geq F\big(\overline{U}(t)\big).$$

Therefore we obtain from Theorem 8.28 that for all $U_0 \geq 0$

$$U(t) \leq \frac{\|U_0\|_\infty}{1 + \kappa^{-1}\|U_0\|_\infty t} \mathbb{1},$$

so that $\lim_{t \to +\infty} U(t) = 0_{\mathbb{R}^N}$. $\square$

Dissipativity

In order to prove the dissipativity of (8.26) we use a family of upper solutions starting from

$$\overline{U}_\alpha := \alpha \mathbb{1}.$$

Indeed, since $\alpha D \mathbb{1} = 0$, we have

$$F(\alpha \mathbb{1}) = \alpha D \mathbb{1} + \lambda \alpha \mathbb{1} - \alpha^2 \kappa^{-1} \mathbb{1} = \alpha(\lambda - \kappa^{-1}\alpha)\mathbb{1},$$

so that by choosing $\overline{\alpha} := \lambda \kappa$, we deduce that

$$F(\alpha \mathbb{1}) \ll 0 \text{ for all } \alpha > \overline{\alpha}.$$

Therefore by applying Corollary 8.25 and using the fact that $0_{\mathbb{R}^N}$ is an equilibrium we deduce the following.

Lemma 8.43 (Upper solutions) *For each $\alpha > \max(\overline{\alpha}, 0)$, the interval $[0, \alpha \mathbb{1}] = \{U \in \mathbb{R}^N : 0 \leq U \leq \alpha \mathbb{1}\}$ is positively invariant for the semiflow generated by (8.26). Moreover, the solution $t \to U(t)(\alpha \mathbb{1})$ starting from $\alpha \mathbb{1}$ converges to the largest equilibrium of (8.26) in the interval $[0, \alpha \mathbb{1}]$ (this equilibrium can be 0).*

Lower solutions

Assume that $\lambda > 0$. Since $\mathbb{1}$ is an eigenvector of D, we have that for all $\alpha \in (0, \overline{\alpha})$

$$F(\alpha \mathbb{1}) = \alpha(\lambda - \kappa^{-1}\alpha)\mathbb{1} \gg 0 \text{ for all } \alpha \in (0, \overline{\alpha}),$$

where $\overline{\alpha} := \lambda \kappa$. Therefore applying Corollary 8.25 we have the following result.

Lemma 8.44 (Lower solutions) *Assume that $\lambda > 0$. For each $\alpha \in (0, \overline{\alpha})$, the interval $[\alpha\mathbb{1}, +\infty)$ is positively invariant for the semiflow generated by (8.26). Moreover, the solution $t \mapsto U(t)$ starting from $U(0) = \alpha\mathbb{1}$ converges to the smallest equilibrium of (8.26) in the interval $[\alpha\mathbb{1}, +\infty)$.*

Equilibrium

It follows from Proposition 8.42 that there cannot exist a positive equilibrium when $\lambda \leq 0$. When $\lambda > 0$, Lemma 8.43 and Lemma 8.44 show that there exists a positive equilibrium such that any solution starting from a non-negative and non-trivial initial value $U(0)$ converges to such an equilibrium. Here we show the uniqueness of the positive equilibrium, which consequently attracts any non-negative and non-trivial initial value.

Proposition 8.45 (Uniqueness of the positive equilibrium) *Assume $\lambda > 0$. Then $\overline{\alpha}\mathbb{1}$ is the unique positive equilibrium of (8.26), which attracts any non-negative and non-zero initial value.*

Proof Let us first remark that the solution of (8.26) starting from an initial condition $U(0) = U_0\mathbb{1}$ for $U_0 > 0$ always stays in the vector space spanned by $\mathbb{1}$, that is, $\text{Vect}\,\mathbb{1}$ is a positively invariant subregion of $\mathbb{R}_+^N$. Actually we have an explicit solution for the solutions of (8.26) when $U(0) = U_0\mathbb{1}$, which is

$$U^*(t, U_0) := \frac{\lambda\kappa U_0 e^{\lambda t}}{\lambda\kappa + U_0(e^{\lambda t} - 1)}\mathbb{1} \text{ if } U_0 \neq \lambda\kappa \text{ and } U^*(t, \lambda\kappa) := \lambda\kappa.$$

Next, we show that a solution that starts from the boundary of the positive cone will immediately enter the interior of the cone. Let $U_0 = (U_1(0), \ldots, U_N(0))^T \in \mathbb{R}^N$ be a non-negative non-trivial vector. Assume that there exists a $j \in \{1, \ldots, N\}$ such that $U_j = 0$. Then select $j_0 \in \{1, \ldots, N\}$ such that $U_{j_0} = 0$ and $U_{j_0+1} + U_{j_0-1} > 0$, and according to (8.26) we have

$$U'_{j_0}(0) = \frac{\gamma}{2}\left(U_{j_0+1} + U_{j_0-1}\right) > 0$$

and therefore U_{j_0} is positive on $(0, \tau)$ for some $\tau > 0$. By induction we can prove that $U_j(t) > 0$ on an interval $(0, \tau)$ for all $j \in \{1, \ldots, N\}$ and some $\tau > 0$. Therefore, we can restrict the analysis to initial conditions that start from a $U_0 = (U_1(0), \ldots, U_N(0))^T$ with $U_i(0) > 0$ for all $i \in \{1, \ldots, N\}$.

Finally, we construct a pair of upper and lower solutions which allow us to prove the convergence of $U(t)$ to the positive equilibrium. Let $U_0 := (U_1(0), \ldots, U_N(0))^T$ with $U_i(0) > 0$ for all $i \in \{1, \ldots, N\}$ be given. Define

$$\underline{U}_0 := \min(U_1(0), \ldots, U_N(0)) > 0 \text{ and } \overline{U}_0 := \max(U_1(0), \ldots, U_N(0)).$$

Then we have

$$\underline{U}_0\mathbb{1} \leq U_0 = U(0) \leq \overline{U}_0\mathbb{1},$$

and therefore by the comparison principle (Theorem 8.28) we have

$$U^*(t, \underline{U}_0) \le U(t) \le U^*(t, \overline{U}_0) \text{ for all } t \ge 0.$$

Since

$$\lim_{t \to +\infty} U^*(t, \underline{U}_0) = \lim_{t \to +\infty} U^*(t, \overline{U}_0) = \lambda \kappa \mathbb{1},$$

we have shown that $U(t) \to \lambda \kappa \mathbb{1}$ when $t \to +\infty$. This completes the proof of Proposition 8.45.

Invariant subregions of $\mathbb{R}_+^N$

We have seen in the previous sections that there exist positive subregions of $\mathbb{R}_+^N$, starting with $\mathbb{R}_+^N$ itself. Thanks to the upper solution of Lemma 8.43, the interval $[0, \alpha \mathbb{1}]$ is an invariant subregion of $\mathbb{R}_+^N$ for α sufficiently large (more precisely, for $\alpha \ge \overline{\alpha}$). Then, in Lemma 8.44 we have shown that $[\overline{\alpha} \mathbb{1}, +\infty)$ is invariant for $\alpha \in (0, \overline{\alpha}]$. Finally, the vector space spanned by $\mathbb{1}$ is an invariant subregion of $\mathbb{R}_+^N$.

8.6.3 N-dimensional systems with arbitrary growth rates

The analysis of the previous subsection can be adapted in a much more general framework. More precisely, let $M = (m_{ij})_{1 \le i,j \le N}$ be a square matrix of size N with non-negative off-diagonal entries, which is irreducible in the sense that for all partitions I, J of $\{1, \ldots, N\}$ (i.e. $I \cup J = \{1, \ldots, N\}$ and $I \cap J = \emptyset$) there are $i \in I$ and $j \in J$ such that $m_{ij} > 0$.

Let $f_1, \ldots, f_N : \mathbb{R}_+ \to \mathbb{R}_+$ be positive, locally Lipschitz continuous and sub-1-homogeneous functions, that is,

$$f_i(\lambda x) \le \lambda f_i(x) \text{ for all } \lambda \in (0, 1) \text{ and } x \ge 0 \text{ and } i \in \{1, \ldots, N\}.$$

We investigate the problem

$$U'(t) = MU(t) - F(U(t))U(t), \tag{8.29}$$

where $F(U)U$ is defined as

$$F(U)U := (f_1(U_1)U_1, \ldots, f_N(U_N)U_N)^T.$$

We define the *spectral bound* of M as

$$\Lambda := \sup\{\lambda : \lambda \in \sigma(M)\}.$$

Theorem 8.46 *If $\Lambda \le 0$ then $0_{\mathbb{R}^N}$ is the only non-negative equilibrium of (8.29). If $\Lambda > 0$ then there exists a positive equilibrium which attracts every non-negative non-trivial initial condition of (8.29).*

Exercise 8.47 (For advanced readers) Prove Theorem 8.46. The case $\Lambda \leq 0$ can be done by using an explicit super-solution. Here we detail some of the important steps of the proof when $\Lambda > 0$.

1. Use the Perron–Frobenius theorem to show that there is a unique (up to multiplication by a positive scalar) $\Phi \in \mathbb{R}^N$, $\Phi \geq 0$, satisfying

$$M\Phi = \Lambda\Phi.$$

   Notice that $\eta\Phi$ is a sub-solution to (8.29) for sufficiently small $\eta > 0$.
2. Show that every orbit is bounded. Deduce that for all $U_0 \in \mathbb{R}^N$ with $U_0 \geq 0$ the corresponding solution to (8.29) satisfies

$$\lim_{t \to +\infty} U(t) = \bar{U}.$$

3. Show that there exists a unique equilibrium to (8.29). One can use an argument similar to the one found in the proof of Proposition 8.39. The interested reader may have a look at [189, Theorem 6.3, p. 188].

8.7 Remarks and Notes

Monotone dynamics consist of both monotone semiflows (continuous-time systems) and monotone mappings (discrete-time systems). Autonomous (or non-autonomous) monotone systems occur in ordinary differential equations, delay differential equations, parabolic equations, abstract non-densely defined Cauchy problems, random dynamical systems, control systems, etc. Schneider and Vidyasagar [308] introduced the quasi-monotone condition for autonomous finite-dimensional linear systems. This has been extended by Volkmann [349] to nonlinear infinite-dimensional systems and we refer to the works of Hirsch and Smith [156], Walter [355], Uhl [345] for more results and references. Monotonicity methods and comparison arguments are largely developed in ordinary differential equations, delay differential equations, and partial differential equations. We refer for instance to Smoller [330], Smith [326], Zhao [388, 389], Hirsch and Smith [156], and Chueshov [61] for more results and references on this subject. Here we have only selected a few topics and a few references.

Monotone dynamical systems

Monotone ordinary differential equations

We refer to Smoller [330], Smith [326], Zhao [388], Hirsch and Smith [156] for more results on monotone ordinary differential equations. In Section 8.6, we have analyzed logistic equations with diffusion in detail, which are examples of autonomous monotone ordinary differential equations.

Monotone theory for delay differential equations

As already mentioned, the theory developed in this chapter can also be extended and applied to delay differential equations. We refer to Hirsch and Smith [156] for results on monotone theory for differential equations with bounded delays. For systems of delay differential equations with unbounded and infinite delay, we refer for instance to Wu [373] and to Krisztin and Wu [192] for the neutral delay differential equations.

Monotone abstract non-densely defined Cauchy problems

A recent extension of the monotone theory to non-densely defined Cauchy problems has been obtained in Magal, Seydi and Wang [239]. Several examples of differential equations, such as delay differential equations [102, 206], parabolic equations with nonlinear and non-local boundary conditions [57, 98, 100] can be put into the abstract non-densely defined Cauchy problems. More results and examples of abstract non-densely defined Cauchy problems can be found in Magal and Ruan [233, 236]. Thus, the theory of monotone semiflows, the comparison principle, and invariance of solutions for abstract non-densely defined Cauchy problems obtained in [239] will have a wide range of applicability. In particular, they provide an application to age-structured population dynamics models (see the book of Webb [363] and Magal and Ruan [236] for more results on this topic), where a monotone semiflow theory and some comparison principles for age-structured models are consequently obtained. As a special case, the Kermack and McKendrick model with age of infection can be handled, as will be seen below in this section.

Monotone mappings

A continuous map $T : X \to X$ on an ordered metric space X is monotone if

$$x \leq y \Rightarrow Tx \leq Ty.$$

Monotone maps play an important role in the study of periodic solutions to periodic quasi monotone systems of ordinary differential equations (see, e.g., the monographs of Krasnoselskii [189, 190] and the papers [5, 142, 260, 321, 322, 335, 362]). Furthermore, monotone maps frequently arise as mathematical models (see, e.g., [335, 366], and the references therein). For instance, the following system is a discrete Lotka–Volterra competition model:

$$(u_{n+1}, v_{n+1}) = T(u_n, v_n) := (u_n \exp[r(1 - u_n - bv_n)], v_n \exp[s(1 - cu_n - v_n)]) .$$

We refer to Smith [325] for more results on this Lotka–Volterra competition model.

Monotone random dynamical systems

Monotonicity methods as well as comparison arguments have mainly been used to study one-dimensional random or stochastic differential equations (see, e.g., [195]). The book of Chueshov [62] proposes a systematic treatment of the basic ideas and methods for monotone random dynamical systems with infinite-dimensional phase space. This book focuses on the qualitative behavior of monotone random dynamical systems and its applications on finite cooperative random and stochastic ordinary differential equations, that occur in the field of ecology, epidemiology, economics, and biochemistry (see Smith [326]). For results on monotone methods and comparison arguments to random and stochastic parabolic partial differential equations and non-autonomous parabolic equations, we refer for instance to the papers by Chueshov (see, e.g.,[59, 60]) and the paper by Shen and Yi [315].

Various examples

Monotone systems occur in many fields, including ecological systems, chemistry, economic models, epidemiology, and biological models. Population dynamics is an important subject in mathematical biology, and a central aim is to study the long-term behavior of the associated models. Monotonicity methods and comparison principles are the main tools in the investigation of the global dynamics of such systems. The theory of monotone dynamical systems has been widely used in population dynamics. There is a long history of the application of monotone methods and comparison arguments (see, e.g., [62, 326] and the literature quoted there).

The chemostat system

The chemostat is a laboratory device that is a dynamic system with continuous material inputs and outputs. The continuous turnover follows the input and removal of nutrients. The specific death, predation, or emigration which always occurs in nature is equivalent to the washout of organisms. The apparatus consists of three connected vessels: the feed bottle, the culture vessel, and the collection vessel. The culture vessel, where the "action" takes place, contains a mixture of nutrients and organisms. The following model is a classical chemostat model

$$\begin{cases} S'(t) = D(S^0 - S) - \dfrac{1}{\gamma} \dfrac{rSN}{a+S} \\ N'(t) = \dfrac{rSN}{a+S} - DN. \end{cases}$$

Here $S(t)$ denotes the concentration of the nutrient in the culture vessel at time t, $N(t)$ denotes the concentration of the organism at time t. The constant S^0 represents the concentration of the input nutrient while D is the dilution (or washout) rate. It is defined as $D = F/V$, where V denotes the volume of the culture vessel and F denotes the volumetric flow rate. Finally, $\dfrac{rSN}{a+S}$ corresponds to the consumption term, where r is the maximal growth rate, a is the Michaelis–Menten (or half-saturation) constant, while γ is a "yield" constant reflecting the conversion of nutrients to organisms. Note that D and S^0 are environmental parameters, and r, a and γ are biological parameters.

The book of Smith and Waltman [329] is devoted to the theoretical description of ecological models based on the chemostat. The theory of the chemostat (and/or dynamics of microbial competition) is a very good example of the application of monotone systems. We refer to the books of Waltman [357] and Hsu and Waltman [164], and references therein for more references and results on this subject. We also refer to the book of Perthame [276] for more results about chemostats.

Lotka–Volterra equations

Competitive and cooperative Lotka–Volterra systems are also a very important class of monotone systems. This covers many different formulations, including autonomous ordinary differential equations, non-autonomous ordinary differential equations, partial differential equations and so on. We refer for instance to [68, 158, 218, 383, 384, 385, 386, 392] and the references cited therein.

Application to the Kermack and McKendrick model

We now present an important monotone property of the Kermack–McKendrick model that will be used in Chapter 12 to construct various algorithms. The Kermack–McKendrick model takes the following form

$$\begin{cases} S'(t) = -\nu S(t)I(t), \\ I'(t) = \nu S(t)I(t) - \gamma I(t), \\ R'(t) = \gamma I(t), \end{cases} \tag{8.30}$$

supplemented with the initial values

$$S(0) = S_0 \geq 0 \text{ and } I(0) = I_0 \text{ and } R(0) = R_0.$$

The Kermack and McKendrick system is not monotone in itself. Nevertheless, it becomes monotone by considering the cumulative number of I, that is, the quantity $CI(t)$ given by

$$CI(t) = \int_0^t I(s)\mathrm{d}s, \ t \geq 0. \tag{8.31}$$

Indeed, integrating the S-equation yields

$$S(t) = S_0 \exp\left(-\nu CI(t)\right), \forall t \geq 0.$$

So that the I-equation can be rewritten as

$$I'(t) = S_0 \exp\left(-\nu CI(t)\right) \nu CI'(t) - \gamma I(t). \tag{8.32}$$

By integrating the I-equation we obtain

$$CI'(t) = I_0 + S_0 \left[1 - \exp\left(-vCI(t)\right)\right] - \gamma CI(t). \tag{8.33}$$

Now since the map

$$G(x) = I_0 + S_0 \left[1 - \exp\left(-vx\right)\right]$$

is monotone increasing and

$$G(0) = I_0 > 0,$$

we obtain the following result.

Theorem 8.48 *Assume that $S_0 > 0$ and $I_0 > 0$ are given. Let $t > 0$ be given and fixed. The quantity $CI(t)$ is increasing with respect to S_0, I_0, v and $-\gamma$. Moreover, $t \to CI(t)$ is strictly increasing and*

$$\lim_{t \to \infty} CI(t) = CI_\infty,$$

where $CI_\infty > 0$ is called the final size of the epidemic and $CI_\infty > 0$ is the unique positive solution of

$$I_0 + S_0 \left[1 - \exp\left(-vCI_\infty\right)\right] = \gamma CI_\infty.$$

Application to the Kendall model

The model introduced by Kendall in 1957 [175] is the following

$$\begin{cases} \partial_t s(t,x) = -vs(t,x)b(t,x), \\ \partial_t i(t,x) = \quad vs(t,x)b(t,x) - \eta i(t,x), \\ \partial_t r(t,x) = \eta i(t,x), \end{cases} \tag{8.34}$$

and

$$\varepsilon^2 b(t,x) - \partial_x^2 b(t,x) = \chi i(t,x). \tag{8.35}$$

The above system is supplemented with the initial distributions

$$s(0,x) = s_0(x) \in BC_+(\mathbb{R}), \ i(0,x) = i_0(x) \in BC_+(\mathbb{R}),$$
$$\text{and } r(0,x) = r_0(x) \in BC_+(\mathbb{R}),$$

where $BC_+(\mathbb{R})$ is the space of positive bounded continuous functions on $\mathbb{R}$.

In this model $s(t,x)$ is the distribution of susceptible at time t, $i(t,x)$ is the distribution of infectious at time t, and $r(t,x)$ is the distribution of recovered at time t. In this model, the individuals are not moving, because by summing the three equations of (8.34) we obtain

$$\partial_t \left(s(t,x) + i(t,x) + r(t,x)\right) = 0.$$

Here the spatial movement of the pathogen is described by equation (8.35). Indeed, the equation (8.35) expresses that the distribution of the pathogen is locally around the location of infectious (which released the pathogen). Indeed, the equation (8.35) is equivalent to

$$b(t,x) = \frac{\chi}{2\varepsilon} \int_{\mathbb{R}} e^{-\varepsilon|x-\sigma|} i(t,\sigma) d\sigma. \tag{8.36}$$

Remark 8.49 Kendall's original model does not specify the kernel $k(x) = \frac{\chi}{2\varepsilon} e^{-\varepsilon|x|}$ as we do here. The advantage of this special form is that it can be used on a bounded domain with suitable boundary conditions. Such models have been introduced for the influenza epidemic on the island of Puerto Rico by Magal et al. [231].

Define

$$I(t,x) = \int_0^t i(\sigma,x) d\sigma \text{ and } B(t,x) = \int_0^t b(\sigma,x) d\sigma.$$

Without loss of generality, we can assume that

$$\chi = \varepsilon^2.$$

The S-equation of (8.2) gives

$$s(t,x) = s_0(x) \exp\left(-\nu \int_0^t b(\sigma,x) d\sigma\right).$$

Therefore by integrating the I-equation in time, we obtain the following monotone equation

$$\partial_t I(t,x) = i_0(x) + s_0(x) \left[1 - \exp\left(-\nu B(t,x)\right)\right] - \eta I(t,x) \tag{8.37}$$

and the equation (8.35) becomes

$$\varepsilon^2 B(t,x) - \partial_x^2 B(t,x) = \varepsilon^2 B(t,x), \tag{8.38}$$

which is equivalent to

$$B(t,x) = \frac{\varepsilon}{2} \int_{\mathbb{R}} e^{-\varepsilon|x-\sigma|} I(t,\sigma) d\sigma. \tag{8.39}$$

The above procedure to transform the Kendall epidemic model into a single monotone system is originally due to Aronson [13]. We refer to Aronson [13], Diekmann [84] and Thieme [336] for more results about this class of equations. We also refer to the survey paper by Ruan [303] for more results about this subject.

Application to the Kermack and McKendrick model with age of infection

In this subsection, we derive a similar monotone property for the Kermack and McKendrick model with age of infection, denoted by $a > 0$. Let $\eta > 0, \beta \in L_+^\infty(0,\infty)$ and $\nu \in L_+^\infty(0,\infty)$ be given. Let us first consider the equation for the susceptible individuals that reads as

$$\begin{cases} S'(t) = -\eta S(t) \int_0^{+\infty} \beta(a)i(t,a)\mathrm{d}a, \\ S(0) = S_0 \geq 0. \end{cases} \tag{8.40}$$

By integrating the above S-equation, we obtain

$$S(t) = S_0 \exp\left(-\eta \int_0^t \int_0^{+\infty} \beta(a)i(s,a)\mathrm{d}a\mathrm{d}s\right), \quad \forall t \geq 0.$$

Next the equation for the density of the infected is the following

$$\begin{cases} \partial_t i(t,a) + \partial_a i(t,a) = -\nu(a)i(t,a), \text{ for } a \in (0,\infty), \\ i(t,0) = \eta S(t) \int_0^{+\infty} \beta(a)i(t,a)\mathrm{d}a, \\ i(0,\cdot) = i_0 \in L^1_+((0,+\infty),\mathbb{R}). \end{cases} \tag{8.41}$$

Now consider the function

$$CI(t,a) = \int_0^t i(s,a)\mathrm{d}s.$$

Integrating the i-equation, we obtain (at least formally)

$$\begin{cases} \partial_t CI(t,a) + \partial_a CI(t,a) = i_0(a) - \nu(a)CI(t,a), \text{ for } a \in (0,\infty), \\ CI(t,0) = \int_0^t S_0 \exp\left(-\eta \int_0^s \int_0^{+\infty} \beta(a)i(\sigma,a)\mathrm{d}a\mathrm{d}\sigma\right) \eta \int_0^{+\infty} \beta(a)i(s,a)\mathrm{d}a\,\mathrm{d}s, \\ CI(0,\cdot) = 0 \in L^1_+((0,+\infty),\mathbb{R}). \end{cases}$$

By integrating the boundary condition and by applying Fubini's theorem, we obtain

$$\begin{cases} \partial_t CI(t,a) + \partial_a CI(t,a) = i_0(a) - \nu(a)CI(t,a), \text{ for } a \in (0,\infty), \\ CI(t,0) = S_0 \left[1 - \exp\left(-\eta \int_0^{+\infty} \beta(a)CI(\sigma,a)\mathrm{d}a\mathrm{d}\sigma\right)\right], \\ CI(0,\cdot) = 0 \in L^1_+((0,+\infty),\mathbb{R}). \end{cases} \tag{8.42}$$

Now since the functional $G : L^1_+(0,\infty) \to [0,\infty)$ given by

$$G(CI) = S_0 \left[1 - \exp\left(-\eta \int_0^{+\infty} \beta(a)CI(a)\mathrm{d}a\mathrm{d}\sigma\right)\right]$$

is monotone increasing, and

$$G(0_{L^1}) = 0_{\mathbb{R}},$$

we can apply the result in Magal, Seydi and Wang [239], and this yields the following (new) result on the Kermack and McKendrick model with age of infection.

Theorem 8.50 Assume that $S_0 > 0$ and $i_0 = i_0(a) \in L^1_+(0,\infty) \setminus \{0\}$. Let $t > 0$ be given and fixed. Then the distribution $a \to CI(t,a)$ is monotone increasing with respect to S_0, $a \to i_0(a)$ and η and $a \to -\nu(a)$.

Moreover, the map $t \to CI(t,a)$ is increasing in time and

$$\lim_{t \to \infty} CI(t,a) = CI_\infty(a), \text{ in } L^1(0,\infty),$$

where $a \to CI_\infty(a) > 0$ is the so-called final size age distribution of the epidemic and $a \to CI_\infty(a) > 0$ is the unique positive solution of the system

$$\begin{cases} \partial_a CI_\infty(a) = i_0(a) - \nu(a)CI_\infty(a), \; for \; a \in (0, \infty), \\ CI_\infty(0) = S_0 \left[1 - \exp\left(-\eta \int_0^{+\infty} \beta(a)CI_\infty(a)\mathrm{d}a\right) \right]. \end{cases}$$

Remark 8.51 We can calculate the distribution $a \to CI_\infty(a)$ a little further. Indeed the first equation of (8.42) gives

$$CI_\infty(a) = \Pi(a)CI_\infty(0) + \int_0^a \frac{\Pi(a)}{\Pi(s)}i_0(s)\mathrm{d}s \text{ with } \Pi(a) = \exp\left(-\int_0^a v(s)\mathrm{d}s\right).$$

By substituting this formula into the second equation of (8.42) we obtain the following scalar equation for the unknown $CI_\infty(0) > 0$

$$CI_\infty(0) = S_0\left[1 - \exp\left(-A \times CI_\infty(0) - B\right)\right],$$

wherein A and B are given by

$$A = \eta \int_0^{+\infty} \beta(a)\Pi(a)\mathrm{d}a \text{ and } B = \eta \int_0^{+\infty} \beta(a)\int_0^a \frac{\Pi(a)}{\Pi(s)}i_0(s)\mathrm{d}s\mathrm{d}a.$$

Volterra's formulation of the Kermack and McKendrick model with age of infection

To explain the partial differential equation formulation of the Kermack–McKendrick model with age of infection, we can use Volterra's integral formulation. Let $a > 0$ denote the time since an individual has become infected by the pathogen. Then the model of Kermack and McKendrick with age of infection can be rewritten as follows. The number of susceptible individuals $S(t)$ satisfies the following equation

$$S'(t) = -v\,S(t) \int_0^\infty \beta(a)i(t,a)\mathrm{d}a, \text{ for } t \geq 0, \text{ with } S(0) = S_0 \geq 0.$$

Now recall that the function $a \to \beta(a) \in L_+^\infty(0,\infty)$ is the fraction of infectious individuals (capable of transmitting the pathogen to the susceptible) with infection age a, and let $a \to \Pi(a)$ be the probability for individuals to remain infected after infection age a,

$$\Pi(a) = \exp\left(-\int_0^a v(\sigma)\mathrm{d}\sigma\right).$$

Next define

$$B(t) = \int_0^\infty \beta(a)i(t,a)\mathrm{d}a,$$

so that the distribution of the infected population $a \to i(t,a)$ at time t satisfies

$$i(t,a) = \begin{cases} \dfrac{\Pi(a)}{\Pi(a-t)}i_0(a-t), & \text{if } a > t, \\ \Pi(a)\,v\,S(t-a)\,B(t-a), & \text{if } t > a, \end{cases} \tag{8.43}$$

where $a \to i_0(a) \in L_+^1(0,\infty)$ denotes the initial distribution of the population of the infected.

Using (8.43), we deduce that $t \rightarrow B(t) \in C([0, \infty), \mathbb{R})$ becomes the unique non-negative solution of the following Volterra integral equation for $t \geq 0$,

$$B(t) = \left[\int_t^\infty \beta(a) \frac{\Pi(a)}{\Pi(a-t)} i_0(a-t) \mathrm{d}a + \int_0^t \beta(a) \Pi(a) \, v \, S(t-a) \, B(t-a) \mathrm{d}a \right].$$

Moreover, by applying the variation of constant formula to the S-equation, the map $t \rightarrow S(t)$ is given by

$$S(t) = \mathrm{e}^{-\int_0^t v \, B(\sigma) \mathrm{d}\sigma} S_0.$$

To conclude, one may alternatively use Volterra's integral formulation to prove some results about monotonicity for age-structured models, as in Magal, Seydi and Wang [239].

Part III
Applications to Epidemic Models

Chapter 9

Understanding and Predicting Unreported Cases in the 2019-nCov Epidemic Outbreak in Wuhan, China, and the Importance of Major Public Health Interventions

This chapter is based on the papers by Liu et al. [207, 210].

9.1 Introduction

An epidemic outbreak of a new human coronavirus, termed the novel coronavirus COVID-19, has occurred in Wuhan, China. The first cases occurred in early December 2019, and by January 29, 2020, more than 7000 cases had been reported in China.[1] Early reports advise that COVID-19 transmission may occur from an infectious individual, who is not yet symptomatic [301]. Such asymptomatic infectious cases are not reported to medical authorities. For epidemic influenza outbreaks, reported cases are typically only a fraction of the total number of symptomatic infectious individuals. For the current epidemic in Wuhan, intensive efforts by Chinese public health authorities have likely reduced the number of unreported cases.

Our objective in this chapter is to present a mathematical model which reproduces the number of unreported cases for the COVID-19 epidemic in Wuhan thanks to a parameter identification method that uses actual reported cases data. This method was originally developed in [207]. For this epidemic, a modeling approach has been developed in [334], which did not consider unreported cases. This method continues the work in [241] and [99] of the fundamental problem of parameter identification in mathematical epidemic models. We address the following fundamental issues concerning this epidemic: How will the epidemic evolve in Wuhan concerning the number of reported cases and unreported cases? How will the number of unreported cases influence the severity of the epidemic? How will public health measures, such as isolation, quarantine, and public closings, mitigate the final size of the epidemic?

---

[1] Chinese Center for Disease Control and Prevention. http://www.chinacdc.cn/jkzt/crb/zl/szkb_11803/jszl_11809/. Accessed June 9, 2021.

9.2 The Model and Data

The model consists of the following system of ordinary differential equations:

$$\begin{cases} S'(t) = -\tau S(t)[I(t) + U(t)], \\ I'(t) = \tau S(t)[I(t) + U(t)] - \nu I(t) \\ R'(t) = \nu_1 I(t) - \eta R(t) \\ U'(t) = \nu_2 I(t) - \eta U(t). \end{cases} \tag{9.1}$$

Here $t \geq t_0$ is time in days, t_0 is the beginning date of the epidemic, $S(t)$ is the number of individuals susceptible to infection at time t, $I(t)$ is the number of asymptomatic infectious individuals at time t, $R(t)$ is the number of reported symptomatic infectious individuals (i.e. symptomatic infectious with severe symptoms) at time t, and $U(t)$ is the number of unreported symptomatic infectious individuals (i.e. symptomatic infectious with mild symptoms) at time t. This system is supplemented by initial data

$$S(t_0) = S_0 > 0, \; I(t_0) = I_0 > 0, \; R(t_0) = 0 \text{ and } U(t_0) = U_0 \geq 0. \tag{9.2}$$

A flow chart of the model is presented in Figure 9.1

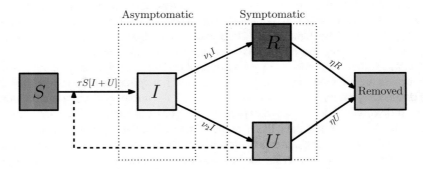

Fig. 9.1: *Flux diagram*

The parameters of the model are listed in Table 9.1.

Symbol	Interpretation	Method
t_0	Time at which the epidemic started	fitted
S_0	Number of susceptible at time t_0	fixed
I_0	Number of asymptomatic infectious at time t_0	fitted
U_0	Number of unreported symptomatic infectious at time t_0	fitted
τ	Transmission rate	fitted
$1/\nu$	Average time during which asymptomatic infectious are asymptomatic	fixed
f	Fraction of asymptomatic infectious that become reported symptomatic infectious	fixed
$\nu_1 = f\,\nu$	Rate at which asymptomatic infectious become reported symptomatic	fitted
$\nu_2 = (1-f)\,\nu$	Rate at which asymptomatic infectious become unreported symptomatic	fitted
$1/\eta$	Average time symptomatic infectious have symptoms	fixed

Table 9.1: *Parameters of the model.*

We use three sets of reported data to model the epidemic in Wuhan: First, data from the Chinese CDC for all of China (Table 9.2), second, data from the Wuhan Municipal Health Commission for Hubei Province (Table 9.3), and third, data from the Wuhan Municipal Health Commission for Wuhan Municipality (Table 9.4). These data vary but represent the epidemic transmission in Wuhan, from which almost all the cases originated in the larger regions.

Date January	20	21	22	23	24	25	26	27	28	29
Confirmed cases (cumulated) for China	291	440	571	830	1287	1975	2744	4515	5974	7711
Mortality cases (cumulated) for China		9	17	25	41	56	80	106	132	170

Table 9.2: *Reported case data Jan. 20, 2020 – Jan. 29, 2020, reported for all of China by the Chinese CDC.*

Date January	23	24	25	26	27	28	29	30	31
Confirmed cases (cumulated) for Hubei	549	729	1052	1423	2714	3554	4586	5806	7153
Mortality cases (cumulated) for Hubei	24	39	52	76	100	125	162	204	249

Table 9.3: *Reported case data Jan. 23, 2020 – Jan. 31, 2020, reported for Hubei Province by the Wuhan Municipal Health Commission.*

Date	January	23	24	25	26	27	28	29	30	31
Confirmed cases (cumulated) for Wuhan		495	572	618	698	1590	1905	2261	2639	3215
Mortality cases (cumulated) for Wuhan		23	38	45	63	85	104	129	159	192

Table 9.4: *Reported case data Jan. 23, 2020 – Jan. 31, 2020, reported for Wuhan Municipality by the Wuhan Municipal Health Commission.*

9.3 Comparison of the Model (9.1) with the Data

For influenza disease outbreaks, the parameters τ, v, v_1, v_2, η, as well as the initial conditions $S(t_0)$, $I(t_0)$, and $U(t_0)$, are usually unknown. Our goal is to identify them from specific time data of reported symptomatic infectious cases. To identify the unreported asymptomatic infectious cases, we assume that the cumulative reported symptomatic infectious cases at time t consist of a constant fraction along time of the total number of symptomatic infectious cases up to time t. In other words, we assume that the removal rate v takes the following form: $v = v_1 + v_2$, where v_1 is the removal rate of reported symptomatic infectious individuals, and v_2 is the removal rate of unreported symptomatic infectious individuals due to all other causes, such as mild symptom, or other reasons.

The cumulative number of reported symptomatic infectious cases at time t, denoted by $CR(t)$, is

$$CR(t) = v_1 \int_{t_0}^{t} I(s)\mathrm{d}s. \tag{9.3}$$

Our method is the following: We assume that $CR(t)$ has the following special form:

$$CR(t) = \chi_1 \exp(\chi_2 t) - \chi_3. \tag{9.4}$$

We evaluate χ_1, χ_2, χ_3 using the reported cases data in Table 9.2, Table 9.3 and Table 9.4. We obtain the model starting time of the epidemic t_0 from (9.4):

$$CR(t_0) = 0 \Leftrightarrow \chi_1 \exp(\chi_2 t_0) - \chi_3 = 0 \implies t_0 = \frac{1}{\chi_2}(\ln(\chi_3) - \ln(\chi_1)).$$

We fix $S_0 = 11.081 \times 10^6$, which corresponds to the total population of Wuhan. We assume that the variation in $S(t)$ is small during the period considered, and we fix v, η, f. By using the method described below, we can estimate the parameters v_1, v_2, τ and the initial conditions U_0 and I_0 from the cumulative reported cases $CR(t)$ given (9.4). We then construct numerical simulations and compare them with data.

The evaluation of χ_1, χ_2 and χ_3 and t_0, using the cumulative reported symptomatic infectious cases in Table 9.2, Table 9.3 and Table 9.4, is shown in Table 9.5 and in Figure 9.2.

Name of the parameter	χ_1	χ_2	χ_3	t_0
From Table 9.2 for China	0.16	0.38	1.1	5.12
From Table 9.3 for Hubei	0.23	0.34	0.1	−2.45
From Table 9.4 for Wuhan	0.36	0.28	0.1	−4.52

Table 9.5: *Estimation of the parameters χ_1, χ_2, χ_3 and t_0 by using the cumulated reported cases in Table 9.2, Table 9.3 and Table 9.4.*

Remark 9.1 According to Table 9.2, Table 9.3 and Table 9.4, the time $t = 0$ will correspond to December 31. So in Table 9.5, the value $t_0 = 5.12$ means that the starting time of the epidemic is January 5, the value $t_0 = -2.45$ means that the starting time of the epidemic is December 28, and $t_0 = -4.52$ means that the starting time of the epidemic is December 26.

Remark 9.2 As long as the number of reported cases follows (9.1), we can predict the future values of $CR(t)$. For $\chi_1 = 0.16$, $\chi_2 = 0.38$ and $\chi_3 = 1.1$, we obtain

Jan 30	Jan 31	Feb 1	Feb 2	Feb 3	Feb 4	Feb 5	Feb 6
8510	12390	18050	26290	38290	55770	81240	118320

The actual number of reported cases for China are $8,163$ confirmed for January 30, $11,791$ confirmed for January 30, and $14,380$ confirmed for February 1. So the exponential formula (9.4) overestimates the number reported after day 30.

From now on, we fix the fraction f of symptomatic infectious cases that are reported. We assume that between 80% and 100% of infectious cases are reported. Thus, f varies between 0.8 and 1. We assume $1/\nu$, the average time during which the patients are asymptomatic infectious, varies between 1 day and 7 days. We assume that $1/\eta$, the average time during which a patient is symptomatic infectious, varies between 1 day and 7 days. So, we fix f, ν, η. Since f and ν are known, we can compute

$$\nu_1 = f\nu \text{ and } \nu_2 = (1 - f)\nu.$$

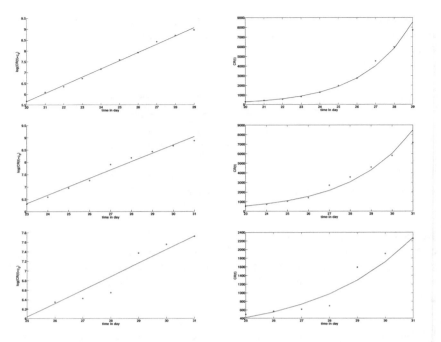

Fig. 9.2: *In the left side figures, the dots correspond to $t \to \ln(CR(t) + \chi_3)$, and in the right side figures, the dots correspond to $t \to CR(t)$, where $CR(t)$ is taken from the cumulated confirmed cases in Table 9.2 (top), in Table 9.3 (middle) and in Table 9.4 (bottom). The straight line in the left side figures corresponds to $t \to \ln(\chi_1) + \chi_2 t$. We first estimate the value of χ_3 and then use a least square method to evaluate χ_1 and χ_2. We observe that the data for China in Table 9.2 and Hubei in Table 9.3 provides a good fit for $CR(t)$ in (9.4), while the data for Wuhan in Table 9.4 does not provide a good fit for $CR(t)$ in (9.4).*

9.3.1 Identification of I_0, U_0 and τ

The identification procedure can be divided into three steps. We recall that the parameters f, ν, and S_0 are assumed to be known.

Step 1: Since f and ν we know that

$$\nu_1 = f\nu \text{ and } \nu_2 = (1 - f)\nu.$$

Step 2: By using equation (9.3) we obtain

$$CR'(t) = \nu_1 I(t) \Leftrightarrow \chi_1 \chi_2 \exp(\chi_2 t) = \nu_1 I(t) \tag{9.5}$$

and

$$\frac{\exp(\chi_2 t)}{\exp(\chi_2 t_0)} = \frac{I(t)}{I(t_0)},$$

and therefore

$$I(t) = I_0 \exp\left(\chi_2\left(t - t_0\right)\right). \tag{9.6}$$

Moreover, by using (9.5) at $t = t_0$, we have

$$I_0 = \frac{\chi_1 \chi_2 \exp\left(\chi_2 t_0\right)}{f\,\nu} = \frac{\chi_3 \chi_2}{f\,\nu}.$$

Step 3: To evaluate the parameters of the model we replace $S(t)$ by $S_0 = 11.081 \times 10^6$ in the right-hand side of (9.1) (which is equivalent to neglecting the variation of susceptibles due to the epidemic, which is consistent with the fact that $t \to CR(t)$ grows exponentially). Therefore, it remains to estimate τ and η in the following system:

$$\begin{cases} I'(t) = \tau S_0[I(t) + U(t)] - \nu I(t) \\ U'(t) = \nu_2 I(t) - \eta U(t). \end{cases} \tag{9.7}$$

By using the first equation we obtain

$$U(t) = \frac{1}{\tau S_0}\left[I'(t) + \nu I(t)\right] - I(t),$$

and therefore by using (9.6) we must have

$$I(t) = I_0 \exp\left(\chi_2\left(t - t_0\right)\right) \text{ and } U(t) = U_0 \exp\left(\chi_2\left(t - t_0\right)\right),$$

so by substituting these expressions into (9.7) we obtain

$$\begin{cases} \chi_2 I_0 = \tau S_0[I_0 + U_0] - \nu I_0 \\ \chi_2 U_0 = \nu_2 I_0 - \eta U_0. \end{cases} \tag{9.8}$$

Remark 9.3 Here we fix τ in such a way that the value χ_2 becomes the dominant eigenvalue of the linearized equation (9.14) and (I_0, U_0) is the positive eigenvector associated to this dominant eigenvalue χ_2. thus, we apply implicitly the Perron–Frobenius theorem. Moreover, the exponentially growing solution $(I(t), U(t))$ that we consider (which starts very close to $(0, 0)$) follows the direction of the positive eigenvector associated with the dominant eigenvalue χ_2.

By dividing the first equation of (9.8) by I_0 we obtain

$$\chi_2 = \tau S_0\left[1 + \frac{U_0}{I_0}\right] - \nu$$

and hence

$$\frac{U_0}{I_0} = \frac{\chi_2 + \nu}{\tau S_0} - 1. \tag{9.9}$$

By using the second equation of (9.8) we obtain

$$\frac{U_0}{I_0} = \frac{\nu_2}{\eta + \chi_2}. \tag{9.10}$$

By using (9.9) and (9.10) we obtain

$$\tau = \frac{\chi_2 + \nu}{S_0} \frac{\eta + \chi_2}{\nu_2 + \eta + \chi_2}.$$

(9.11)

By using (9.10) we can compute

$$U_0 = \frac{\nu_2}{\eta + \chi_2} I_0 = \frac{(1-f)\nu}{\eta + \chi_2} I_0.$$

$$I_0 = \frac{\chi_1 \chi_2 \exp(\chi_2 t_0)}{f \nu} = \frac{\chi_3 \chi_2}{f \nu},$$

(9.12)

$$\tau = \frac{\chi_2 + \nu}{S_0} \frac{\eta + \chi_2}{\nu_2 + \eta + \chi_2},$$

and

$$U_0 = \frac{\nu_2}{\eta + \chi_2} I_0 = \frac{(1-f)\nu}{\eta + \chi_2} I_0.$$

(9.13)

9.3.2 Computation of the basic reproductive number $\mathcal{R}_0$

In this section we apply results in Diekmann, Heesterbeek and Metz [88] and van den Driessche and Watmough [93]. The linearized equation of the infectious part of the system is given by

$$\begin{cases} I'(t) = \tau S_0 [I(t) + U(t)] - \nu I(t), \\ U'(t) = \nu_2 I(t) - \eta U(t). \end{cases}$$

(9.14)

The corresponding matrix is

$$A = \begin{bmatrix} \tau S_0 - \nu & \tau S_0 \\ \nu_2 & -\eta \end{bmatrix}$$

and the matrix A can be rewritten as

$$A = V - S$$

where

$$V = \begin{bmatrix} \tau S_0 & \tau S_0 \\ \nu_2 & 0 \end{bmatrix} \text{ and } S = \begin{bmatrix} \nu & 0 \\ 0 & \eta \end{bmatrix}.$$

Therefore, the next-generation matrix is

$$VS^{-1} = \begin{bmatrix} \dfrac{\tau S_0}{\nu} & \dfrac{\tau S_0}{\eta} \\ \dfrac{\nu_2}{\nu} & 0 \end{bmatrix},$$

which is a Leslie matrix, and the basic reproductive number becomes

$$\mathcal{R}_0 = \frac{\tau S_0}{\nu} \left(1 + \frac{\nu_2}{\eta}\right).$$

By using (9.11) we obtain

$$\mathcal{R}_0 = \frac{\chi_2 + \nu}{S_0} \frac{\eta + \chi_2}{\nu_2 + \eta + \chi_2} \frac{S_0}{\nu} \left(1 + \frac{\nu_2}{\eta}\right)$$

and by using $\nu_2 = (1 - f)\nu$ we obtain

$$\mathcal{R}_0 = \frac{\chi_2 + \nu}{\nu} \frac{\eta + \chi_2}{(1 - f)\nu + \eta + \chi_2} \left(1 + \frac{(1 - f)\nu}{\eta}\right). \tag{9.15}$$

9.4 Numerical Simulations

We can find multiple values of η, ν, and f which provide a good fit for the data. For the application of our model, η, ν, and f must vary in a reasonable range. For the coronavirus COVID-19 epidemic in Wuhan at its current stage, the values of η, ν, and f are not known. From the preliminary information, we use the values

$$f = 0.8, \ \eta = 1/7, \ \nu = 1/7.$$

By using the formula (9.15) for the basic reproduction number, we obtain from the data in Table 9.2 that $\mathcal{R}_0 = 4.13$. Using model (9.1) and the values in Table 9.5, we plot the graph of $t \rightarrow CR(t)$, $t \rightarrow U(t)$ and the data for the confirmed cumulated cases in Figure 9.3, according to Table 9.2 for China, Table 9.3 for Hubei and Table 9.4 for Wuhan. We observe from these figures that the data for China and Hubei fit the model (9.1), but the data for Wuhan do not fit the model (9.1) because the model (9.4) is not a good model for the data for Wuhan in Table 9.4. The data for Wuhan do not fit an exponential function.

In what follows, we plot the graphs of $t \rightarrow CR(t)$, $t \rightarrow U(t)$, and $t \rightarrow R(t)$ for Wuhan by using model (9.1). We define the turning point t_p as the time at which the red curve (i.e., the curve of the non-cumulated reported infectious cases) reaches its maximum value. For example, in the figure below, the turning point t_p is day 54, which corresponds to February 23 for Wuhan.

In the following, we take into account the fact that very strong isolation measures have been imposed for all of China since January 23. Specifically, since January 23, families in China are required to stay at home.

In order to take into account such a public intervention, we assume that the transmission of COVID-19 from infectious to susceptible individuals stopped after January 25.

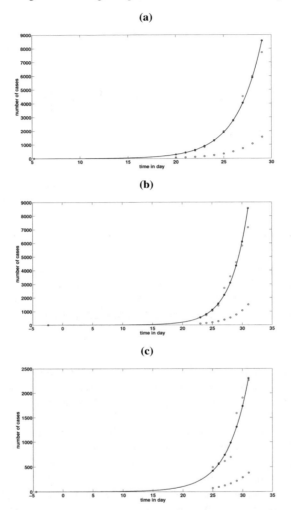

Fig. 9.3: *In these figures we use $f = 0.8$, $\eta = 1/7$, $v = 1/7$ and $S_0 = 11.081 \times 10^6$. The remaining parameters are derived by using (9.12)–(9.13). In Figure (a), we plot the number of $t \to CR(t)$ (black solid line) and $t \to U(t)$ (blue dotted) and the data (red dotted) corresponding to the confirmed cumulated case for all of China in Table 9.2. We use $\chi_1 = 0.16$, $\chi_2 = 0.38$, $\chi_3 = 1.1$, $t_0 = 5.12$ and $S_0 = 11.081 \times 10^6$, which give $\tau = 4.44 \times 10^{-8}$, $I_0 = 3.62$, $U_0 = 0.2$ and $\mathcal{R}_0 = 4.13$. In Figure (b), we plot the number of $t \to CR(t)$ (black solid line) and $t \to U(t)$ (blue dotted) and the data (red dotted) corresponding to the confirmed cumulated case for Hubei province in Table 9.3. We use $\chi_1 = 0.23$, $\chi_2 = 0.34$, $\chi_3 = 0.1$ and $t_0 = -2.45$ and $S_0 = 11.081 \times 10^6$, which give $\tau = 4.11 \times 10^{-8}$ $I_0 = 0.3$, $U_0 = 0.02$ and $\mathcal{R}_0 = 3.82$. In Figure (c), we plot the number of $t \to CR(t)$ (black solid line) and $t \to U(t)$ (blue dotted) and the data (red dotted) corresponding to the confirmed cumulated cases for Wuhan in Table 9.4. We use $\chi_1 = 0.36$, $\chi_2 = 0.28$, $\chi_3 = 0.1$ and $t_0 = -4.52$ and $S_0 = 11.08 \times 10^6$, which give $\tau = 3.6 \times 10^{-8}$, $I_0 = 0.25$, $U_0 = 0.02$ and $\mathcal{R}_0 = 3.35$.*

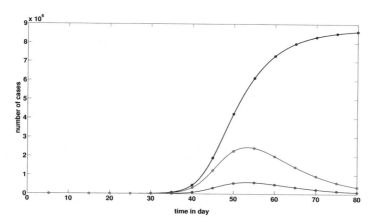

Fig. 9.4: *In this figure we plot the graphs of $t \to CR(t)$ (black solid line), $t \to U(t)$ (blue solid line) and $t \to R(t)$ (red solid line). We use $f = 0.8$, $\eta = 1/7$, $v = 1/7$, and $S_0 = 11.081 \times 10^6$. The remaining parameters are derived by using (9.12)–(9.13). We obtain $\tau = 4.44 \times 10^{-8}$, $I_0 = 3.62$ and $U_0 = 0.2$. The cumulated number of reported cases goes up to 8.5 million people and the turning point is day 54. So the turning point is February 23 (i.e. 54 − 31).*

Therefore, we consider the following model: for $t \geq t_0$

$$\begin{cases} S'(t) = -\tau(t)S(t)[I(t) + U(t)], \\ I'(t) = \tau(t)S(t)[I(t) + U(t)] - vI(t) \\ R'(t) = v_1 I(t) - \eta R(t) \\ U'(t) = v_2 I(t) - \eta U(t) \end{cases} \tag{9.16}$$

where

$$\tau(t) = \begin{cases} 4.44 \times 10^{-8}, & \text{for } t \in [t_0, 25], \\ 0, & \text{for } t > 25. \end{cases} \tag{9.17}$$

The figure takes into account the public health measures, such as isolation, quarantine, and public closings, which correspond to model (9.16) and (9.17). By comparison of Figure 9.5-(a) with Figure 9.4, we note that these measures greatly mitigate the final size of the epidemic, and shift the turning point about 24 days before the turning point without these measures.

9.5 Discussion

An epidemic outbreak of a new human coronavirus COVID-19 has occurred in Wuhan, China. For this outbreak, the unreported cases and the disease transmission rate are not known. To recover these values from reported medical data, we present the mathematical model (9.1) for outbreak diseases.

(a)

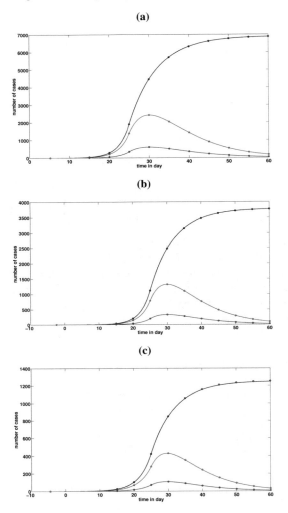

(b)

(c)

Fig. 9.5: *In this figure we plot the graphs of t → CR(t) (black solid line), t → U(t) (blue solid line) and t → R(t) (red solid line). We use again f = 0.8, η = 1/7, ν = 1/7, and S_0 = 11.081 × 10^6. In Figure (a), we use χ_1 = 0.16, χ_2 = 0.38, χ_3 = 1.1, t_0 = 5.12 for the parameter values for China, which give τ = 4.44 × 10^{-8} for t ∈ [t_0, 25] and τ = 0 for t > 25, I_0 = 3.62, U_0 = 0.2. In Figure (b), we use χ_1 = 0.23, χ_2 = 0.34, χ_3 = 0.1 and t_0 = −2.45, for the parameter values obtained from the data for Hubei province, which give τ = 4.11 × 10^{-8} for t ∈ [t_0, 25] and τ = 0 for t > 25, I_0 = 0.3, U_0 = 0.02. In Figure (c), we use χ_1 = 0.36, χ_2 = 0.28, χ_3 = 0.1, and t_0 = −4.52 for the parameter values obtained from the data for Wuhan, which give τ = 3.6 × 10^{-8} for t ∈ [t_0, 25] and τ = 0 for t > 25, I_0 = 0.25, U_0 = 0.02. The cumulated number of reported cases goes up to 7000 in Figure (a), 4000 in Figure (b) and 1400 in Figure (c), and the turning point is around January 30 in Figures (a), (b) and (c).*

By the knowledge of the cumulative reported symptomatic infectious cases, and assuming (1) the fraction f of asymptomatic infections that become reported symptomatic infectious cases, (2) the average time $1/\nu$ asymptomatic infectious are asymptomatic, and (3) the average time $1/\eta$ symptomatic infectious remain infectious, we estimate the epidemiological parameters in the model (9.1). We then make numerical simulations of the model (9.1) to predict forward in time the severity of the epidemic. We observe that public health measures, such as isolation, quarantine, and public closings, greatly reduce the final size of the epidemic, and make the turning point much earlier than without these measures. We observe that the predictive capability of model (9.1) requires valid estimates of the parameters f, ν, and η, which depend on the input of medical and biological epidemiologists. Our results can contribute to the prevention and control of the COVID-19 epidemic in Wuhan.

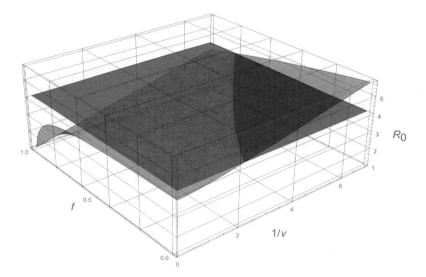

Fig. 9.6: *In this figure we use $1/\eta = 7$ days and we plot the basic reproductive number $\mathcal{R}_0$ as a function of f and $1/\nu$ using (9.15) with $\chi_2 = 0.38$, which corresponds to the data for China in Table 9.2. If both f and $1/\nu$ are sufficiently small, $\mathcal{R}_0 < 1$. The red plane is the value of $\mathcal{R}_0 = 4.13$.*

As a consequence of our study, we note that public health measures, such as isolation, quarantine, and public closings, greatly reduce the final size of this epidemic, and make the turning point much earlier than without these measures. With our method, we fix η, ν and f and get the same turning point for the three data sets in Table 9.2, Table 9.3 and Table 9.4. We choose $f = 0.8$, which means around 80% of cases are reported in the model since cases are very well documented in China. Thus, we only assume that a small fraction, 20% were not reported. This assumption may be confirmed later on.

We also vary the parameters η, ν, and f, and we do not observe a strong variation of the turning point. Nevertheless, the number of reported cases is very sensitive to the data sets, as shown in the figures. The formula (9.4) for $CR(t)$ is very descriptive until January 26 for the reported cases data for China and Hubei but is not reasonable for Wuhan data. This suggests that the turning point is very robust, while the number of cases is very sensitive. We can find multiple values of η, v, and f which provide a good fit for the data. This means that η, v, and f should also be evaluated using other methods. The values $1/\eta = 7$ days and $1/v = 7$ days are taken from information concerning earlier coronaviruses and are used now by medical authorities [301].

The predictive capability of models (9.1) and (9.16) requires valid estimates of the parameters f (fraction of asymptomatic infectious that become reported symptomatic infectious), the parameter $1/v$ (average time asymptomatic infectious are asymptomatic), and the parameter $1/\eta$ (average time symptomatic infectious remain infectious). In Figure 9.6, we graph $\mathcal{R}_0$ as a function of f and $1/v$ for the data in Table 9.2, to illustrate the importance of these values in the evolution of the epidemic. The accuracy of these values depends on the input of medical and biological epidemiologists.

In influenza epidemics, the fraction f of reported cases may be significantly increased by public health reporting measures, with greater efforts to identify all current cases. Our model reveals the impact of an increase in this fraction f in the value of $\mathcal{R}_0$, as evident in Figure 9.6 above, for the COVID-19 epidemic in Wuhan.

9.6 More Numerical Simulations

We assume that the exponentially increasing phase of the epidemic (as incorporated in τ_0) is intrinsic to the population of any subregion of China after it is has been established in the epidemic epicenter Wuhan. We also assume that the susceptible population $S(t)$ is not significantly reduced over the course of the epidemic. We set $\tau_0 = 4.51 \times 10^{-8}$, $t_0 = 5.0$, $I(t_0) = 3.3$, $U(t_0) = 0.18$, and $R(t_0) = 1.0$. We set $S(t_0)$ in (9.2) to $1,400,050,000$ (the population of mainland China). We set $\tau(t)$ in (9.16) to

$$\begin{cases} \tau(t) = \tau_0 \, S_0 \, / \, 1,400,050,000, \ 0 \le t \le 25, \\ \tau(t) = \tau_0 \, S_0 \, / 1,400,050,000 \, \exp\left(-\mu\left(t - 25\right)\right), \ 25 < t, \end{cases} \tag{9.18}$$

where $S_0 = 11,000,000$ (the population of Wuhan). We thus assume that the government imposed restriction measures became effective in reducing transmission on January 25.

In Figure 9.7, we plot the graphs of $CR(t)$, $CU(t)$, $R(t)$, and $U(t)$ from the numerical simulation for simulations based on six time intervals for known values of the cumulative reported cases data. For each of these time intervals, a value of μ is chosen so that the simulation for that time interval aligns with the cumulative reported cases data in that interval. In this way, we can predict the future values of the epidemic from early cumulative reported cases data.

In Figure 9.8, we plot the graphs of the reported cases $R(t)$, the unreported cases $U(t)$, and the infectious pre-symptomatic cases $I(t)$. The blue dots are obtained from the reported cases data (Table 9.2) for each day beginning on January 26, by subtracting from each day the value of the reported cases one week earlier.

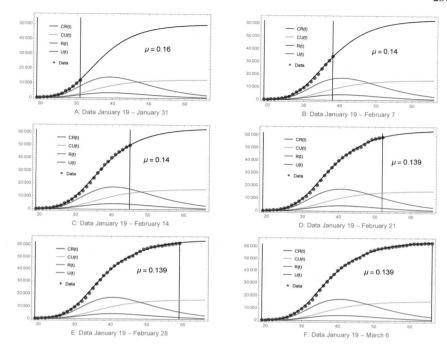

Fig. 9.7: *Graphs of* $CR(t)$, $CU(t)$, $U(t)$, $R(t)$. *The red dots are the reported cases data. The value of* μ *(indicated in each of the sub-figures) is estimated by fitting the model output for each time interval to the cumulative reported cases data for that time interval. The final size of cumulative cases is approximately (A)* $49,600$ *reported,* $12,400$ *unreported; (B) and (C)* $62,700$ *reported,* $15,700$ *unreported cases; and (D), (E), (F):* $63,500$ *reported,* $15,900$ *unreported.*

Our model transmission rate $\tau(t)$ can be modified to illustrate the effects of an earlier or later implementation of the major public policy interventions that occurred in this epidemic. The implementation one week earlier (25 is replaced by 18 in (9.18)) is graphed in Figure 9.9-A. All other parameters and the initial conditions remain the same. The total reported cases are approximately 4,500 and the total number of unreported cases is approximately 1,100. The implementation one week later (25 is replaced by 32 in (9.18)) is graphed in Figure 9.9-B. The total reported cases are approximately 820,000 and the total number of unreported cases is approximately 200,000. The timing of the institution of major social restrictions is critically important in mitigating the epidemic.

The number of unreported cases is of major importance in understanding the evolution of an epidemic and involves great difficulty in their estimation. The data from January 19 to February 15 for reported cases in Table 9.2, was only for confirmed tested cases. Between February 11 and February 15, additional clinically diagnosed case data, based on medical imaging showing signs of pneumonia, was also reported by the Chinese CDC. Since February 16, only tested case data has been reported by

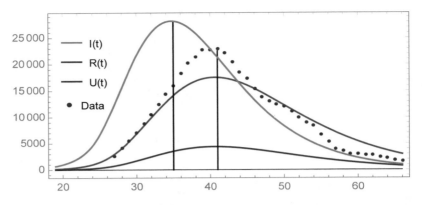

Fig. 9.8: *Graphs of R(t), U(t), I(t). The blue dots are the day by day weekly reported data. The turning point of the asymptomatic infectious cases I(t) is approximately day 35 = February 4. The turning point of the reported cases R(t) and the unreported cases U(t) is approximately day 41 = February 10. The turning point of the day-by-day weekly reported data is approximately day 41.*

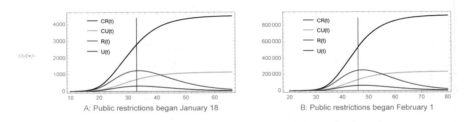

Fig. 9.9: *Graphs of CR(t), CU(t), U(t), R(t). A: The major public policy interventions were implemented one week earlier (January 18). B: The major public policy interventions were implemented one week later (February 1). The one week earlier turning point day is 33 = February 2. The one week later turning point is day 46 = February 15.*

the Chinese CDC because new NHC guidelines removed the clinically diagnosed category. Thus, after February 15, there is a gap in the reported cases data that we used up to February 15. The uncertainty of the number of unreported cases for this epidemic includes this gap but goes even further to include additional unreported cases.

We assumed previously that the fraction f of reported cases was $f = 0.8$ and the fraction of unreported cases was $1 - f = 0.2$. Our model formulation can be applied with varying values for the fraction f. In Figure 9.10, we provide illustrations with the fraction $f = 0.4$ (Figure 9.10-A) and $f = 0.6$ (Figure 9.10-B). For $f = 0.4$, the formula for the time-dependent transmission rate $\tau(t)$ in (9.18) involves new values for $\tau_0 = 4.08 \times 10^{-8}$ and $\mu = 0.148$. The initial conditions $I_0 = 6.65$ and

$U_0 = 1.09$ also have new values. The other parameters and initial conditions remain the same. For $f = 0.4$, the total reported cases is approximately $63, 100$ and the total unreported cases is approximately $94, 700$. For $f = 0.6$, the formula for the time-dependent transmission rate $\tau(t)$ in (9.18) involves new values for $\tau_0 = 4.28 \times 10^{-8}$ and $\mu = 0.144$. The initial conditions $I_0 = 4.43$ and $U_0 = 0.485$ also have new values. The other parameters and initial conditions remain the same. For $f = 0.6$, the total reported cases is approximately $63, 300$ and the total unreported cases is approximately $42, 200$. From these simulations, we see that estimation of the number of unreported cases has major importance in understanding the severity of this epidemic.

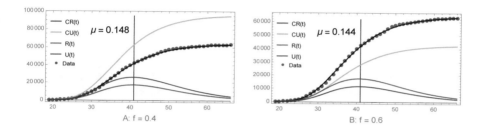

Fig. 9.10: *Graphs of $CR(t)$, $CU(t)$, $U(t)$, $R(t)$. The red dots are the cumulative reported case data from Table 9.2. A: $f = 0.4$. The basic reproductive number is $\mathcal{R}_0 = 5.03$. The final size of the epidemic is approximately $157, 800$ total cases. The turning point of the epidemic is approximately day $41 = $ February 10. B: $f = 0.6$. The basic reproductive number is $\mathcal{R}_0 = 4.62$. The final size of the epidemic is approximately $105, 500$ total cases. The turning point is approximately day $41 = $ February 10.*

The number of days an asymptomatic infected individual is infectious is uncertain. We simulate in Figure 9.11 the model with $\nu = 1/3$ (asymptomatic infected individuals are infectious on average 3 days before becoming symptomatic), and $\nu = 1/5$ (asymptomatic infected individuals are infectious on average 5 days before becoming symptomatic). For $\nu = 1/3$, $\tau_0 = 5.75 \times 10^{-8}$, $I_0 = 1.48$, $U_0 = 0.18$, $\mathcal{R}_0 = 2.78$, $\mu = 0.0765$, $N = 24$. For $\nu = 1/5$, $\tau_0 = 4.90 \times 10^{-8}$, $I_0 = 2.38$, $U_0 = 0.18$, $\mathcal{R}_0 = 3.45$, $\mu = 0.098$, $N = 24$. Because the asymptomatic infectious periods are shorter, the date N of the effective reduction of the transmission rate due to restriction measures is one day earlier.

In Figure 9.12, we illustrate the importance of the level of government-imposed public restrictions by altering the value of μ in formula (9.18). All other parameters and initial conditions are the same as in Figure 9.5. In Figure 9.12-A we set $\mu = 0.0$, corresponding to no restrictions. The final size of cumulative reported cases after 100 days is approximately $1,080,000,000$ cases, approximately $270,000,000$ unreported cases, and approximately $1,350,000,000$ total cases. The turning point is approximately day $65 = $ March 6. In Figure 9.12-B we set $\mu = 0.17$, corresponding to a higher level of restrictions than in Figure 9.5. The final size of cumulative reported cases after 70 days is approximately 45,300 cases, approximately 11,300 unreported cases, and approximately 56,600 total cases. The turning point is approximately day 38 = February 7. The level and timing of government restrictions on social distancing are very important in controlling the epidemic.

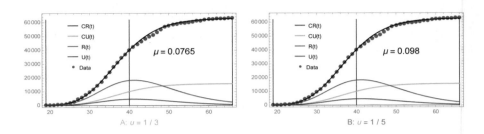

Fig. 9.11: *Graphs of $CR(t)$, $CU(t)$, $U(t)$, $R(t)$. The red dots are the cumulative reported cases data from Table 9.2. A: $v = 1/3$. B: $v = 1/5$. The turning point is approximately day 40 = February 9 for both cases. The final sizes of $CR(t)$ and $CU(t)$ are approximately the same as for $v = 1/7$ in both cases.*

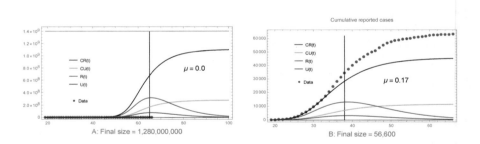

Fig. 9.12: *Graphs of $CR(t)$, $CU(t)$, $U(t)$, and $R(t)$. Case data from Table 9.2. A: $\mu = 0.0$. The orange horizontal line is the population of mainland China. B: $\mu = 0.17$. A significant reduction of cases occurs compared to the cumulative reported cases data (red dots).*

9.7 Further Discussion

We have developed a model of the COVID-19 epidemic in China that incorporates key features of this epidemic: (1) the importance of the timing and magnitude of the implementation of major government public restrictions designed to mitigate the severity of the epidemic; (2) the importance of both reported and unreported cases in interpreting the number of reported cases; and (3) the importance of asymptomatic infectious cases in disease transmission. In our model formulation, we divide infectious individuals into asymptomatic and symptomatic infectious individuals. The symptomatic infectious phase is also divided into reported and unreported cases. Our model formulation is based on our work [207], in which we developed a method to estimate epidemic parameters at an early stage of an epidemic when the number of cumulative cases grows exponentially. The general method in [207] was applied to the COVID-19 epidemic in Wuhan, China, to identify the constant transmission rate corresponding to the early exponential growth phase.

In this work, we use the constant transmission rate in the early exponential growth phase of the COVID-19 epidemic identified in [207]. We model the effects of the major government-imposed public restrictions in China, beginning on January 23, as a time-dependent exponentially decaying transmission rate after January 24. With this time-dependent exponentially decreasing transmission rate, we can fit, with increasing accuracy, our model simulations to the Chinese CDC reported cases data for all of China, forward in time from February 15, 2020.

Our model demonstrates the effects of implementing major government public policy measures. By varying the date of the implementation of these measures in our model, we show that had implementation occurred one week earlier, then a significant reduction in the total number of cases would have resulted. We show that if these measures had occurred one week later, then a significant increase in the total number of cases would have occurred. We also show that if these measures had been less restrictive on public movement, then a significant increase in the total size of the epidemic would have occurred. It is evident that control of a COVID-19 epidemic is very dependent on an early implementation and a high level of restrictions on public functions.

We varied the fraction $1 - f$ of unreported cases involved in the transmission dynamics. We showed that if this fraction is higher, then a significant increase in the number of total cases results. If it is lower, then a significant reduction occurs. It is evident that control of a COVID-19 epidemic is very dependent on identifying and isolating symptomatic unreported infectious cases. We also decreased the parameter ν (the reciprocal of the average period of asymptomatic infectiousness) and showed that the total number of cases is smaller. It is also possible to decrease η (the reciprocal of the average period of unreported symptomatic infectiousness), to obtain a similar result. Understanding these periods of infectiousness is important in understanding the total number of epidemic cases.

Our model was specific to the COVID-19 outbreak in China, but it applies to any outbreak location for a COVID-19 epidemic.

Chapter 10
The COVID-19 Outbreak in Japan: Unreported Age-Dependent Cases

This chapter is based on the paper by Griette et al. [126].

10.1 Introduction

COVID-19 disease caused by the severe acute respiratory syndrome coronavirus (SARS-CoV-2) first appeared in Wuhan, China, and the first cases were notified to the WHO on 31 December 2019.[1][2]

Beginning in Wuhan as an epidemic, it then spread very quickly and was characterized as a pandemic on 11 March 2020.[3] Symptoms of this disease include fever, shortness of breath, cough, and a non-negligible proportion of infected individuals may develop severe forms of the symptoms leading to their transfer to intensive care units and, in some cases, death, see e.g., Guan et al. [131] and Wei et al. [365]. Both symptomatic and asymptomatic individuals can be infectious [302, 365, 393], which makes the control of the disease particularly challenging.

The virus is characterized by its rapid progression among individuals, most often exponential in the first phase, but also a marked heterogeneity in populations and geographic areas [348, 390] and we also refer to a report from the WHO.[3] The number of reported cases worldwide exceeded 3 million as of 3 May 2020.[4] The heterogeneity of the number of cases and the severity according to the age groups, especially for

---

[1] WHO Timeline—COVID-19. Available at `https://www.who.int/news-room/detail/27-04-2020-who-timeline---covid-19` (accessed June 23, 2021).

[2] World Health Organization. Pneumonia of unknown cause—China. *Disease Outbreak News.* 5 January 2020. Available online: `https://www.who.int/csr/don/05-january-2020-pneumonia-of-unkown-cause-china/en/` (accessed on 21 May 2020).

[3] World Health Organization. Report of the WHO-China Joint Mission on Coronavirus Disease 2019 (COVID-19), 2020. Available online: `https://www.who.int/publications-detail/report-of-the-who-china-joint-mission-on-coronavirus-disease-2019-(covid-19)` (accessed June 23, 2021).

[4] World Health Organization. Coronavirus Disease 2019 (COVID-19): Situation Report, 104, 2020. Available online: `https://apps.who.int/iris/handle/10665/332058` (accessed on June 23, 2021).

children and elderly people, aroused the interest of several researchers [48, 219, 282, 317, 341]. Indeed, several studies have shown that the severity of the disease increases with the age and co-morbidity of hospitalized patients (see e.g., To et al. [341] and Zhou et al. [390]). Wu et al. [374] have shown that the risk of developing symptoms increases by 4% per year in adults aged between 30 and 60 years old while Davies et al. [72] found that there is a strong correlation between chronological age and the likelihood of developing symptoms. Since completely asymptomatic individuals can also be contagious, a higher probability of developing symptoms does not necessarily imply greater infectiousness: Zou et al. [393] found that, in some cases, the viral load in asymptomatic patients was similar to that in symptomatic patients. Moreover, while adults are more likely to develop symptoms, Jones et al. [170] found that the viral loads in infected children do not differ significantly from those of adults.

These findings suggest that a study of the dynamics of inter-generational spread is fundamental to better understand the spread of the coronavirus and most importantly to efficiently fight the COVID-19 pandemic. To this end, the distribution of contacts between age groups in society (work, school, home, and other locations) is an important factor to take into account when modeling the spread of the epidemic. To account for these facts, some mathematical models have been developed [18, 54, 72, 282, 317]. In Ayoub et al. [18] the authors studied the dependence of the COVID-19 epidemic on the demographic structures in several countries but did not focus on the contacts distribution of the populations. In [54, 72, 282, 317] a focus on the social contact patterns with respect to the chronological age has been made by using the contact matrices provided in Prem et al. [281]. While Ayoub et al. [18], Chikina and Pegden [54] and Davies et al. [72] included the example of Japan in their study, their approach is significantly different from ours. Indeed, Ayoub et al. [18] use a complex mathematical model to discuss the influence of the age structure on the infection in a variety of countries, mostly through the basic reproduction number $\mathcal{R}_0$. They use parameter values from the literature and from another study of the same group of authors [17], where the parameter identification is done by a nonlinear least-squares minimization. Chikina and Pegden [54] use an age-structured model to investigate age-targeted mitigation strategies. They rely on parameter values from the literature and discuss using age-structured temporal series to fit their model. Finally, Davies et al. [72] also discuss age-related effects in the control of the COVID epidemic, and use statistical inference to fit an age-structured SIR variant to data; the model is then used to discuss the efficiency of different control strategies. We provide a new, explicit computational solution for the parameter identification of an age-structured model. The model is based on the SIUR model developed in Liu et al. [207], which accounts for differentiated infectiousness for reported and unreported cases (contrary to, for instance, other SIR-type models). In particular, our method is significantly different from nonlinear least-squares minimization and does not involve statistical inference.

In this chapter, we focus on an epidemic model with unreported infectious symptomatic patients (i.e., with mild or no symptoms). Our goal is to investigate the age-structured data of the COVID-19 outbreak in Japan. In Section 10.2 we present the age-structured data and in Section 10.3 the mathematical models (with and without age structure). One of the difficulties in fitting the model to the data is that the growth rate of the epidemic is different in each age class, which leads us to adapt our early method presented in Liu et al. [207]. The new method is presented in Section 10.6. In Section 10.4 we present the comparison of the model with the data. In the last section, we discuss our results.

10.2 Data

Patient data in Japan have been made public since the early stages of the epidemic with the quarantine of the *Diamond Princess* in the Haven of Yokohama. We used data from the website covid19japan.com (https://covid19japan.com. Accessed 6 May 2020) which is based on reports from national and regional authorities. Patients are labeled "confirmed" when tested positive for COVID-19 by PCR. Interestingly, the age class of the patient is provided for 13,660 out of 13,970 confirmed patients (97.8% of the confirmed population) as of 29 April. The age distribution of the infected population is represented in Figure 10.1 compared to the total population per age class (data from the Statistics Bureau of Japan estimate for 1 October 2019). In Figure 10.2 we plot the number of reported cases per 10,000 people of the same age class (i.e., the number of infected patients divided by the population of the age class times 10,000). Both datasets are given in Table 10.1 and a statistical summary is provided by Table 10.2. Note that the high proportion of 20–60 year-old confirmed patients may indicate that the severity of the disease is lower for those age classes than for older patients, and therefore the disease transmits more easily in those age classes because of a higher number of asymptomatic individuals. Elderly infected individuals might transmit less because they are identified more easily. The cumulative number of deaths (Figure 10.3) is another argument in favor of this explanation. We also reconstructed the time evolution of the reported cases in Figures 10.4 and 10.5. Note that the steepest curves precisely concern the 20–60 year-olds, probably because they are economically active and therefore have a high contact rate with the population.

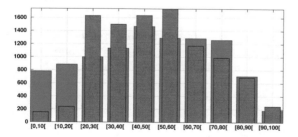

Fig. 10.1: *In this figure we plot in blue bars the age distribution of the Japanese population for 10,000 people and we plot in orange bars the age distribution of the number of reported cases of SARS-CoV-2 for 10,000 patient on 29 April (based on the total of 13,660 reported cases). We observe that 77% of the confirmed patients belong to the 20–60 years age class.*

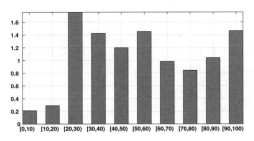

Fig. 10.2: *In this figure we plot the number of infected patients for each age class per 10,000 individuals of the same age class (i.e., the number of infected individuals divided by the population of the age class times 10,000). The figure shows that the individuals are more or less likely to becomes infected depending on their age class. The bars describe the susceptibility of people to SARS-CoV-2 depending on their age class.*

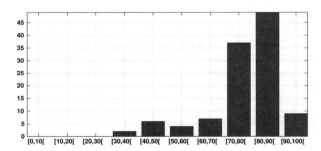

Fig. 10.3: *Cumulative number of SARS-CoV-2-induced deaths per age class (red bars). We observe that 83% of deaths occur in between 70 and 100 years old.*

Age group	[0, 10[	[10, 20[	[20, 30[	[30, 40[	[40, 50[	[50, 60[	[60, 70[	[70, 80[	[80, 90[	[90, 100[
Age class for 2019	9,859,515	11,171,044	12,627,964	14,303,042	18,519,755	16,277,853	16,231,582	15,926,926	8,939,954	2,309,313
Age class per 10,000 people	781	885	1000	1133	1467	1290	1286	1262	709	183
Confirmed Cases	211	327	2216	2034	2220	2355	1566	1289	857	304
Deaths	0	0	0	2	6	4	7	37	49	9

Table 10.1: *The age distribution of Japan is taken from the Statistics Bureau of Japan. For the number of cases and the number of deaths the data come from Prefectural Governments and Japan Ministry of Health, Labour and Welfare.*

Dataset	Japanese Population	Infected	Deceased
First Quartile	28	28	68
Median	48	44	75
Third Quartile	67	59	81

Table 10.2: *Statistical summary of the data from Table 10.1.*

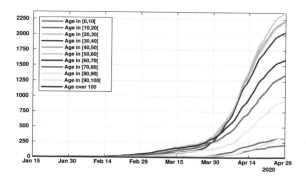

Fig. 10.4: *Time evolution of the cumulative number of reported cases of SARS-CoV-2 per age class. The vertical axis represents the total number of cumulative reported cases in each age class.*

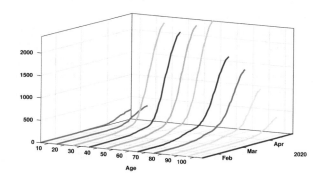

Fig. 10.5: *Time evolution of the cumulative number of reported cases of SARS-CoV-2 per age class. The vertical axis represents the total number of cumulative reported cases in each age class*

10.3 Methods

10.3.1 The SIUR model

The model consists of the following system of ordinary differential equations:

$$
\begin{cases}
S'(t) = -\tau(t)S(t)\dfrac{I(t) + U(t)}{N}, \\[2mm]
I'(t) = \tau(t)S(t)\dfrac{I(t) + U(t)}{N} - \nu I(t), \\[2mm]
R'(t) = \nu_1 I(t) - \eta R(t), \\[2mm]
U'(t) = \nu_2 I(t) - \eta U(t).
\end{cases}
\tag{10.1}
$$

This system is supplemented by initial data

$$S(t_0) = S_0 \geq 0, \ I(t_0) = I_0 \geq 0, \ R(t_0) \geq 0 \text{ and } U(t_0) = U_0 \geq 0. \tag{10.2}$$

Here $t \geq t_0$ is time in days, t_0 is the starting date of the epidemic in the model, $S(t)$ is the number of individuals susceptible to infection at time t, $I(t)$ is the number of asymptomatic infectious individuals at time t, $R(t)$ is the number of reported symptomatic infectious individuals at time t, and $U(t)$ is the number of unreported symptomatic infectious individuals at time t. A flow chart of the model is presented in Figure 10.6.

Asymptomatic infectious individuals $I(t)$ are infectious for an average period of $1/\nu$ days. Reported symptomatic individuals $R(t)$ are infectious for an average period of $1/\eta$ days, as are unreported symptomatic individuals $U(t)$. We assume that reported symptomatic infectious individuals $R(t)$ are reported and isolated immediately and cause no further infections. The asymptomatic individuals $I(t)$ can also be viewed as having a low-level symptomatic state. All infections are acquired from either $I(t)$ or $U(t)$ individuals. A summary of the parameters involved in the model is presented in Table 10.3.

Our study begins in the second phase of the epidemic, i.e., after the pathogen has succeeded in surviving in the population. During this second phase $\tau(t) \equiv \tau_0$ is constant. When strong government measures such as isolation, quarantine, and public closings are implemented, the third phase begins. The actual effects of these measures are complex, and we use a time-dependent decreasing transmission rate $\tau(t)$ to incorporate these effects. The formula for $\tau(t)$ is

$$\begin{cases} \tau(t) = \tau_0, \ 0 \leq t \leq D, \\ \tau(t) = \tau_0 \exp\left(-\mu\left(t - D\right)\right), \ D < t. \end{cases} \tag{10.3}$$

The date D is the first day of public intervention and μ characterizes the intensity of the public intervention.

A similar model has been used to describe the epidemics in mainland China, South Korea, Italy, and other countries, and give reasonable trajectories for the evolution of the epidemic based on actual data [124, 207, 208, 209, 210, 211]. Compared with these models, we added a scaling with respect to the total population size N, for consistency with the age-structured model (10.12). This only changes the value of the parameter τ and does not impact the qualitative or quantitative behavior of the model.

10.3.2 Comparison of the model (10.1) with the data

At the early stages of the epidemic, the infectious components of the model $I(t)$, $U(t)$ and $R(t)$ must be exponentially growing. Therefore, we can assume that

$$I(t) = I_0 \exp\left(\chi_2\left(t - t_0\right)\right).$$

The cumulative number of reported symptomatic infectious cases at time t, denoted by $CR(t)$, is

Symbol	Interpretation	Method
t_0	Time at which the epidemic started	fitted
S_0	Number of susceptible at time t_0	fixed
I_0	Number of asymptomatic infectious at time t_0	fitted
U_0	Number of unreported symptomatic infectious at time t_0	fitted
$\tau(t)$	Transmission rate at time t	fitted
D	The first day of public intervention	fitted
μ	Intensity of the public intervention	fitted
$1/\nu$	Average time during which asymptomatic infectious are asymptomatic	fixed
f	Fraction of asymptomatic infectious that become reported symptomatic infectious	fixed
$\nu_1 = f\,\nu$	Rate at which asymptomatic infectious become reported symptomatic	fixed
$\nu_2 = (1-f)\,\nu$	Rate at which asymptomatic infectious become unreported symptomatic	fixed
$1/\eta$	Average time symptomatic infectious have symptoms	fixed

Table 10.3: *Parameters of the model.*

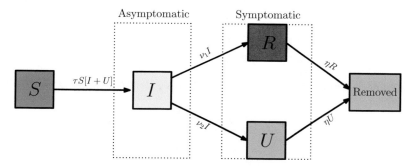

Fig. 10.6: *Compartments and flow chart of the model.*

$$CR(t) = \nu_1 \int_{t_0}^{t} I(s)\mathrm{d}s. \qquad (10.4)$$

Since $I(t)$ is an exponential function and $CR(t_0) = 0$, it is natural to assume that $CR(t)$ has the following special form:

$$CR(t) = \chi_1 \exp(\chi_2 t) - \chi_3. \qquad (10.5)$$

As in the early articles [207, 208, 209, 210, 211], we fix $\chi_3 = 1$ and we evaluate the parameters χ_1 and χ_2 by using an exponential fit to

$$\chi_1 \exp(\chi_2 t) \simeq CR_{data}(t).$$

We use only early data for this part, from day $t = d_1$ until day $t = d_2$, because we want to catch the exponential growth of the early epidemic and avoid the influence of saturation arising at later stages.

Remark 10.1 The estimated parameters χ_1 and χ_2 will vary if we change the interval $[d_1, d_2]$.

Once χ_1, χ_2, χ_3 are known, we can compute the starting time of the epidemic t_0 from (10.5) as:

$$CR(t_0) = 0 \Leftrightarrow \chi_1 \exp(\chi_2 t_0) - \chi_3 = 0 \implies t_0 = \frac{1}{\chi_2} (\ln(\chi_3) - \ln(\chi_1)).$$

We fix $S_0 = 126.8 \times 10^6$, which corresponds to the total population of Japan. The quantities I_0, R_0, and U_0 correspond to the values taken by $I(t)$, $R(t)$ and $U(t)$ at $t = t_0$ (and in particular R_0 should not be confused with the basic reproduction number $\mathcal{R}_0$). We fix the fraction f of symptomatic infectious cases that are reported. We assume that between 80% and 100% of infectious cases are reported. Thus, f varies between 0.8 and 1. We assume that the average time during which the patients are asymptomatic infectious $1/\nu$ varies between 1 day and 7 days. We assume that the average time during which a patient is symptomatic infectious $1/\eta$ varies between 1 day and 7 days. In other words we fix the parameters f, ν, η. Since f and ν are known, we can compute

$$\nu_1 = f\nu \text{ and } \nu_2 = (1 - f)\nu. \tag{10.6}$$

Computing further (see below for more details), we should have

$$I_0 = \frac{\chi_1 \chi_2 \exp(\chi_2 t_0)}{f\nu} = \frac{\chi_3 \chi_2}{f\nu}, \tag{10.7}$$

$$\tau = N \frac{\chi_2 + \nu}{S_0} \frac{\eta + \chi_2}{\nu_2 + \eta + \chi_2}, \tag{10.8}$$

$$R_0 = \frac{\nu_1}{\eta + \chi_2} I_0 = \frac{f\nu}{\eta + \chi_2} I_0. \tag{10.9}$$

and

$$U_0 = \frac{\nu_2}{\eta + \chi_2} I_0 = \frac{(1 - f)\nu}{\eta + \chi_2} I_0. \tag{10.10}$$

By using the approach described in Diekmann et al. [88], van den Driessche and Watmough [93], the basic reproductive number for model (10.1) is given by

$$\mathcal{R}_0 = \frac{\tau S_0}{\nu N} \left(1 + \frac{\nu_2}{\eta}\right).$$

By using (10.8) we obtain

$$\mathcal{R}_0 = \frac{\chi_2 + \nu}{\nu} \frac{(\eta + \chi_2)}{\nu_2 + \eta + \chi_2} \left(1 + \frac{\nu_2}{\eta}\right). \tag{10.11}$$

10.3.3 The SIUR model with age structure

In what follows $N_1, \ldots, N_{10}$ will denote the number of individuals in the respective age classes $[0, 10[, \ldots, [90, 100[$. The model for the number of susceptible individuals $S_1(t), \ldots, S_{10}(t)$ in the respective age classes $[0, 10[, \ldots, [90, 100[$ is the following

$$\begin{cases} S_1'(t) = -\tau_1 S_1(t)\left[\phi_{1,1}\dfrac{(I_1(t) + U_1(t))}{N_1} + \cdots + \phi_{1,10}\dfrac{(I_{10}(t) + U_{10}(t))}{N_{10}}\right], \\ \quad\vdots \\ S_{10}'(t) = -\tau_{10} S_{10}(t)\left[\phi_{10,1}\dfrac{(I_1(t) + U_1(t))}{N_1} + \cdots + \phi_{10,10}\dfrac{(I_{10}(t) + U_{10}(t))}{N_{10}}\right]. \end{cases}$$
$$(10.12)$$

The model for the number of asymptomatic infectious individuals $I_1(t), \ldots, I_{10}(t)$ in the respective age classes $[0, 10[, \ldots, [90, 100[$ is the following

$$\begin{cases} I_1'(t) = \tau_1 S_1(t)\left[\phi_{1,1}\dfrac{(I_1(t) + U_1(t))}{N_1} + \cdots + \phi_{1,10}\dfrac{(I_{10}(t) + U_{10}(t))}{N_{10}}\right] - \nu I_1(t), \\ \quad\vdots \\ I_{10}'(t) = \tau_{10} S_{10}(t)\left[\phi_{10,1}\dfrac{(I_1(t) + U_1(t))}{N_1} + \cdots + \phi_{10,10}\dfrac{(I_{10}(t) + U_{10}(t))}{N_{10}}\right] - \nu I_{10}(t). \end{cases}$$
$$(10.13)$$

The model for the number of reported symptomatic infectious individuals $R_1(t), \ldots, R_{10}(t)$ in the respective age classes $[0, 10[, \ldots, [90, 100[$ is

$$\begin{cases} R_1'(t) = \nu_1^1 I_1(t) - \eta R_1(t), \\ \quad\vdots \\ R_{10}'(t) = \nu_1^{10} I_{10}(t) - \eta R_{10}(t). \end{cases}$$
$$(10.14)$$

Finally the model for the number of unreported symptomatic infectious individuals $U_1(t), \ldots, U_{10}(t)$ in the respective age classes $[0, 10[, \ldots, [90, 100[$ is the following

$$\begin{cases} U_1'(t) = \nu_2^1 I_1(t) - \eta U_1(t), \\ \quad\vdots \\ U_{10}'(t) = \nu_2^{10} I_{10}(t) - \eta U_{10}(t). \end{cases}$$
$$(10.15)$$

In each age class $[0, 10[, \ldots, [90, 100[$ we assume that there is a fraction $f_1, \ldots, f_{10}$ of asymptomatic infectious individual who become reported symptomatic infectious (i.e., with severe symptoms) and a fraction $(1 - f_1), \ldots, (1 - f_{10})$ who become unreported symptomatic infectious (i.e., with mild symptoms). Therefore we define

$$\nu_1^1 = \nu f_1 \text{ and } \nu_2^1 = \nu(1 - f_1),$$
$$\vdots$$
$$\nu_1^{10} = \nu f_{10} \text{ and } \nu_2^{10} = \nu(1 - f_{10}).$$
$$(10.16)$$

In this model $\tau_1, \ldots, \tau_{10}$ are the respective transmission rates for the age classes $[0, 10[, \ldots, [90, 100[$.

The matrix ϕ_{ij} represents the probability for an individual in class i to meet an individual in class j. In their survey, Prem and co-authors [281] present a way to reconstruct contact matrices from existing data and provide such contact matrices for a number of countries including Japan. Based on the data provided by Prem et al. [281] for Japan we construct the contact probability matrix ϕ. More precisely, we inferred contact data for the missing age classes $[80, 90[$ and $[90, 100[$. The precise method used to construct the contact matrix γ is detailed in Section 10.7. An analogous contact matrix for Japan has been proposed by Munasinghe, Asai and Nishiura [261]. The contact matrix γ we used is the following

$$[\gamma_{ij}] = \begin{bmatrix} 4.03 & 0.92 & 0.47 & 1.69 & 0.83 & 0.92 & 0.78 & 0.56 & 0.57 & 0.57 \\ 0.71 & 8.06 & 1.38 & 1.36 & 1.96 & 1.74 & 0.75 & 0.86 & 0.74 & 0.57 \\ 0.55 & 1.05 & 4.63 & 2.25 & 1.84 & 1.92 & 0.94 & 0.46 & 0.74 & 0.73 \\ 1.52 & 1.20 & 2.54 & 4.97 & 2.98 & 2.40 & 1.76 & 0.99 & 0.53 & 0.73 \\ 0.69 & 1.42 & 1.93 & 2.87 & 3.91 & 2.76 & 1.35 & 1.33 & 0.95 & 0.53 \\ 0.34 & 0.48 & 1.20 & 1.46 & 1.61 & 2.97 & 1.40 & 0.98 & 1.23 & 0.95 \\ 0.28 & 0.18 & 0.20 & 0.52 & 0.38 & 0.77 & 2.67 & 1.72 & 0.92 & 1.23 \\ 0.12 & 0.10 & 0.09 & 0.18 & 0.19 & 0.25 & 0.76 & 1.99 & 1.18 & 0.93 \\ 0.09 & 0.10 & 0.08 & 0.09 & 0.13 & 0.17 & 0.27 & 0.64 & 1.61 & 1.19 \\ 0.09 & 0.09 & 0.10 & 0.08 & 0.09 & 0.13 & 0.17 & 0.27 & 0.64 & 1.61 \end{bmatrix}, \qquad (10.17)$$

where the ith line of the matrix γ_{ij} is the average number of contacts made by an individual in age class i with an individual in age class j during one day. Notice that the higher number of contacts are achieved within the same age class. The matrix of conditional probability ϕ of contact between age classes is given by (10.18) and we plot a visual representation of this matrix in Figure 10.7.

$$[\phi_{ij}] = \begin{bmatrix} 0.35 & 0.08 & 0.04 & 0.14 & 0.07 & 0.08 & 0.06 & 0.04 & 0.05 & 0.05 \\ 0.03 & 0.44 & 0.07 & 0.07 & 0.10 & 0.09 & 0.04 & 0.04 & 0.04 & 0.03 \\ 0.03 & 0.06 & 0.30 & 0.14 & 0.12 & 0.12 & 0.06 & 0.03 & 0.04 & 0.04 \\ 0.07 & 0.06 & 0.12 & 0.25 & 0.15 & 0.12 & 0.08 & 0.05 & 0.02 & 0.03 \\ 0.03 & 0.07 & 0.10 & 0.16 & 0.22 & 0.15 & 0.07 & 0.07 & 0.05 & 0.03 \\ 0.02 & 0.03 & 0.09 & 0.11 & 0.12 & 0.23 & 0.11 & 0.07 & 0.09 & 0.07 \\ 0.03 & 0.02 & 0.02 & 0.05 & 0.04 & 0.08 & 0.30 & 0.19 & 0.10 & 0.13 \\ 0.02 & 0.01 & 0.01 & 0.03 & 0.03 & 0.04 & 0.13 & 0.34 & 0.20 & 0.16 \\ 0.02 & 0.02 & 0.01 & 0.02 & 0.02 & 0.03 & 0.06 & 0.14 & 0.36 & 0.27 \\ 0.02 & 0.02 & 0.03 & 0.02 & 0.02 & 0.03 & 0.05 & 0.08 & 0.19 & 0.48 \end{bmatrix}. \qquad (10.18)$$

10.4 Results

10.4.1 Model without age structure

The daily number of reported cases from the model can be obtained by computing the solution of the following equation:

$$DR'(t) = \nu_1 \, I(t) - DR(t), \text{ for } t \geq t_0 \text{ and } DR(t_0) = DR_0. \qquad (10.19)$$

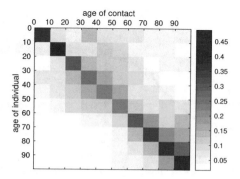

Fig. 10.7: *Graphical representation of the contact matrix ϕ. The intensity of blue in the cell (i, j) indicates the conditional probability that, given a contact between an individual of age group i and another individual, the latter belongs to the age class j. The matrix was reconstructed from the data of Prem et al. [281], with the method described in Section 10.7.*

In Figures, 10.8 and 10.9 we employ the method presented previously in Liu et al. [211] to fit the data for Japan without age structure.

The model to compute the cumulative number of death from the reported individuals is the following

$$D'(t) = \eta_D \, p \, R(t), \text{ for } t \geq t_0 \text{ and } D(t_0) = 0, \tag{10.20}$$

where η_D is the death rate of reported infectious symptomatic individuals and p is the case fatality rate (namely the fraction of death per reported infectious individuals).

In the simulation we chose $1/\eta_D = 6$ days and the case fatality rate $p = 0.286$ is computed by using the cumulative number of confirmed cases and the cumulative number of deaths (as of 29 April) as follows

$$p = \frac{\text{cumulative number of deaths}}{\text{cumulative number of reported cases}} = \frac{393}{13744}. \tag{10.21}$$

In Figure 10.10 we plot the cumulative number of $D(t)$ by using the same simulations as in Figures 10.8 and 10.9.

10.4.2 Model with age structure

To describe the confinement for the age-structured model (10.12)–(10.15) we will use for each age class $i = 1, \ldots, 10$ a different transmission rate having the following form

$$\begin{cases} \tau_i(t) = \tau_i, \, 0 \leq t \leq D_i, \\ \tau_i(t) = \tau_i \exp\left(-\mu_i \left(t - D_i\right)\right), \, D_i < t. \end{cases} \tag{10.22}$$

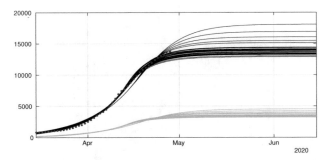

Fig. 10.8: *Cumulative number of cases. We plot the cumulative data (red dots) and the best fits of the model $CR(t)$ (black curve) and $CU(t)$ (green curve). We fix $f = 0.8$, $1/\eta = 7$ days and $1/\nu = 7$ and we apply the method described in Liu et al. [211]. The best fit is $d_1 = 2$ April, $d_2 = 5$ April, $D = 27$ April, $\mu = 0.6$, $\chi_1 = 179$, $\chi_2 = 0.085$, $\chi_3 = 1$ and $t_0 = 13$ January.*

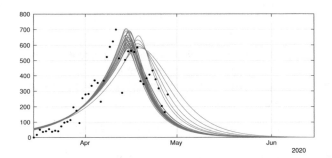

Fig. 10.9: *Daily number of cases. We plot the daily data (black dots) with $DR(t)$ (blue curve). We fix $f = 0.8$, $1/\eta = 7$ days and $1/\nu = 7$ and we apply the method described in Liu et al. [211]. The best fit is $d_1 = 2$ April, $d_2 = 5$ April, $N = 27$ April, $\mu = 0.6$, $\chi_1 = 179$, $\chi_2 = 0.085$, $\chi_3 = 1$ and $t_0 = 13$ January.*

The date D_i is the first day of public intervention for the age class i and μ_i is the intensity of the public intervention for each age class.

In Figure 10.11 we plot the cumulative number of reported cases as given by our model (10.12)–(10.15) (solid lines), compared with reported cases data (black dots). We used the method described in Section 10.6 to estimate the parameters τ_i from the data. In Figure 10.12 we plot the cumulative number of *unreported* cases (solid lines) as given by our model with the same parameter values, compared to the existing data of *reported* cases (black dots).

To understand the role of the transmission network between age groups in this epidemic, we plot in Figure 10.13 the transmission matrices computed at different times. The transmission matrix is the following

$$C(t) = \mathrm{diag}\,(\tau_1(t), \tau_2(t), \dots, \tau_{10}(t)) \times \phi, \qquad (10.23)$$

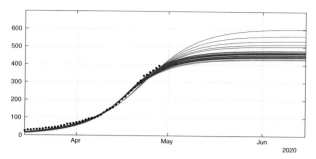

Fig. 10.10: *In this figure we plot the data for the cumulative number of deaths (black dots), and our best fits for $D(t)$ (red curves).*

where the matrix ϕ describes contacts and is given in (10.18), and the transmission rates are the ones fitted to the data as in Figure 10.11

$$\tau_i(t) = \tau_i^0(t) \exp(-\mu_i(t - D_i)_+).$$

During the early stages of the epidemic, the transmission seems to be evenly distributed among age classes, with a little bias towards younger age classes (Figure 10.13a). Younger age classes seem to react more quickly to social distancing policies than older classes, therefore their transmission rate drops rapidly (Figure 10.13b,c); one month after the start of social distancing measures, the transmission mostly occurs within elderly classes (60–100 years, Figure 10.13d).

10.5 Discussion

The recent COVID-19 pandemic has led many local governments to enforce drastic control measures to stop its progression. Those control measures were often taken in a state of emergency and without any real visibility concerning the later development of the epidemics, to prevent the collapse of the health systems under the pressure of severe cases. Mathematical models can help to clarify what the future of the pandemic could be, provided that the particularities of the pathogen under consideration are correctly identified. In the case of COVID-19, one of the features of the pathogen which makes it particularly dangerous is the existence of a high contingent of unidentified infectious individuals who spread the disease without notice. This makes non-intensive containment strategies such as quarantine and contact-tracing relatively inefficient but also renders predictions by mathematical models particularly challenging.

Early attempts to reconstruct the epidemics by using SIUR models were performed in Liu et al. [207, 208, 209, 210], who used them to fit the behavior of the epidemics in many countries, by including undetected cases into the mathematical model. Here we extend our modeling effort by adding the time series of deaths into the equation. In Section 10.4 we present an additional fit of the number of disease-induced deaths

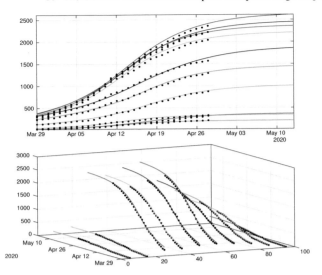

Fig. 10.11: *We plot a comparison between the model* (10.12)–(10.15) *and the age-structured data from Japan by age class. We took* $1/\nu = 1/\eta = 7$ *days for each age class. Our best fit is obtained for* f_i, *which depends linearly on the age class until it reaches 90%, with* $f_1 = 0.1$, $f_2 = 0.2$, $f_3 = 0.3$, $f_4 = 0.4$, $f_5 = 0.5$, $f_6 = 0.6$, $f_7 = 0.7$, $f_8 = 0.8$, $f_9 = 0.9$, *and* $f_{10} = 0.9$. *The values we used for the first day of public intervention are* $D_i = 13$ *April for the 0–20 years age class* $i = 1, 2$, $D_i = 11$ *April for the age class going from* $[20, 30[$ *to* $[60, 70[$, $i = 3, 4, 5, 6, 7$, *and* $D_i = 16$ *April for the remaining age classes. We fit the data from 30 March to 20 April to derive the value of* χ_1^i *and* χ_2^i *for each age class. For the intensity of confinement we use the values* $\mu_1 = \mu_2 = 0.4829$, $\mu_3 = \mu_4 = 0.2046$, $\mu_5 = \mu_6 = 0.1474$, $\mu_7 = 0.0744$, $\mu_8 = 0.1736$, $\mu_9 = \mu_{10} = 0.1358$. *By applying the method described in Section 10.6, we obtain* $\tau_1 = 0.1630$, $\tau_2 = 0.1224$, $\tau_3 = 0.3028$, $\tau_4 = 0.2250$, $\tau_5 = 0.1520$, $\tau_6 = 0.1754$, $\tau_7 = 0.1289$, $\tau_8 = 0.1091$, $\tau_9 = 0.1211$ *and* $\tau_{10} = 0.1642$. *The matrix* ϕ *is the one defined in* (10.18).

coming from symptomatic (reported) individuals (see Figure 10.10). To properly fit the data, we were forced to reduce the length of stay in the R-compartment to 6 days (on average), meaning that death induced by the disease should occur on average faster than recovery. A shorter period between infection and death (compared to remission) has also been observed, for instance, by Verity et al. [348].

The major improvement in this chapter is to combine our early SIUR model with chronological age. Early results using age-structured SIR models were obtained by Kucharski et al. [194] but no unreported individuals were considered and no comparison with age-structured data was performed. Indeed in this chapter, we provide a new method to fit the data and the model. The method extends our previous method for the SIUR model without age (see Section 10.6).

The data presented in Section 10.2 suggests that chronological age plays a very important role in the expression of the symptoms. The largest part of the reported

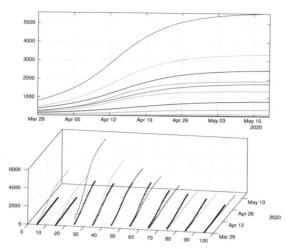

Fig. 10.12: *Cumulative number of unreported cases as given by the fit of the model (10.12)–(10.15) to Japanese data. The solid curves represent the solution of the model and the black dots correspond to the reported cases data. The parameters are the same as in Figure 10.11.*

patients is between 20 and 60 years old (see Figure 10.1), while the largest part of the deceased is between 60 and 90 years old (see Figure 10.3). This suggests that the symptoms associated with COVID-19 infection are more severe in elderly patients, which has been reported in the literature several times (see e.g., Lu et al. [219], Zhou et al. [390]). In particular, the probability of being asymptomatic (our parameter f) should depend on the age class.

Indeed, the best match for our model (see Figure 10.11) was obtained under the assumption that the proportion of symptomatic individuals among the infected increases with the age of the patient. This linear dependency of f as a function of age is consistent with the observations of Wu et al. [374] that the severity of the symptoms increases linearly with age. As a consequence, unreported cases are a majority for young age classes (for age classes less than 50 years) and become a minority for older age classes (more than 50 years), see Figure 10.12. Moreover, our model reveals the fact that the policies used by the government to reduce contacts between individuals have strongly heterogeneous effects depending on the age classes. Plotting the transmission matrix at different times (see Figure 10.13) shows that younger age classes react more quickly and more efficiently than older classes. This may be because the number of contacts in a typical day is higher among younger individuals. As a consequence, we predict that one month after the effective start of public measures, the new transmissions will almost exclusively occur in elderly classes. The observation that younger ages classes play a major role in the transmission of the disease has been highlighted several times in the literature, see e.g., Davies et al. [72], Cao et al. [48], Kucharski et al. [194] for the COVID-19 epidemic, but also Mossong et al. [259] in a more general context.

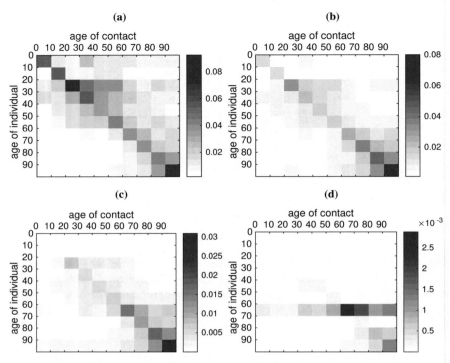

Fig. 10.13: *Rate of contact between age classes according to the fitted data. For each age class in the y-axis we plot the rate of contact between one individual of this age class and another individual of the age class indicated on the x-axis. (**a**) is the rate of contact before the start of public measures (11 April). (**b**) is the rate of contact at the date of effect of the public measures for the last age class (16 April). (**c**) is the rate of contact one week later (23 April). (**d**) is the rate of contact one month later (16 May). In this figure we use $\tau_1 = 0.1630$, $\tau_2 = 0.1224$, $\tau_3 = 0.3028$, $\tau_4 = 0.2250$, $\tau_5 = 0.1520$, $\tau_6 = 0.1754$, $\tau_7 = 0.1289$, $\tau_8 = 0.1091$, $\tau_9 = 0.1211$ and $\tau_{10} = 0.1642$, $\mu_1 = \mu_2 = 0.4829$, $\mu_3 = \mu_4 = 0.2046$, $\mu_5 = \mu_6 = 0.1474$, $\mu_7 = 0.0744$, $\mu_8 = 0.1736$, $\mu_9 = \mu_{10} = 0.1358$, and $D_1 = D_2 = 13$ April, $D_3 = D_4 = D_5 = D_6 = D_7 = 11$ April, $D_8 = D_9 = D_{10} = 16$ April.*

We develop a new model for an age-structured epidemic and provided a new and efficient method to identify the parameters of this model based on observed data. Our method differs significantly from the existing nonlinear least-squares and statistical inference methods and we believe that it produces high-quality results. Moreover, we only use the initial phase of the epidemic for the identification of the epidemiological parameters, which shows that the model itself is consistent with the observed phenomenon and argues against overfitting. Yet our study could be improved in several directions. We only use reported cases that were confirmed by PCR tests, and therefore the number of tests performed could introduce a bias in the observed data – and therefore our results. We are currently working on an integration of this number of tests in our model. We use a phenomenological model to describe the response of the population in terms of the number of contacts to the mitigation measures imposed by the government. This could probably be described more precisely by investigating the mitigation strategies in terms of a social network. Nevertheless, we believe that our study offers a precise and robust mathematical method that adds to the existing literature.

10.6 Method to Fit of Age Structured Model to Data

We first choose two days d_1 and d_2 between which each cumulative age group grows like an exponential. By fitting the cumulative age classes $[0, 10[$, $[10, 20[$, ... and $[90, 100[$ between d_1 and d_2, for each age class $j = 1, \ldots 10$ we can find χ_1^j and χ_2^j

$$CR_j^{data}(t) \simeq \chi_1^j e^{\chi_2^j t}.$$

We choose a starting time $t_0 \leq d_1$ and we fix

$$\chi_3^j = \chi_1^j e^{\chi_2^j t_0}, \forall j = 1, \ldots, n,$$

and we obtain

$$\begin{cases} CR_1(t) = \chi_1^1 e^{\chi_2^1 t} - \chi_3^1, \\ \vdots \\ CR_n(t) = \chi_1^n e^{\chi_2^n t} - \chi_3^n i \end{cases} \tag{10.24}$$

where

$$\chi_j^i \geq 0, \quad \forall i = 1, \ldots, n, \quad \forall j = 1, 2, 3.$$

We assume that

$$CR_1(t)' = v_1^1 I_1(t),$$
$$\vdots \tag{10.25}$$
$$CR_n(t)' = v_1^n I_n(t),$$

where

$$v_1^i = v f_i, \text{ and } v_2^i = v(1 - f_i), \forall i = 1, \ldots, n.$$

Therefore we obtain

$$I_j(t) = I_j^\star e^{\chi_2^j t} \tag{10.26}$$

where

$$I_j^\star := \frac{\chi_1^j \chi_2^j}{v_1^j}.$$

By assuming that the number of susceptible individuals remains constant we have

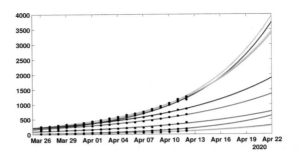

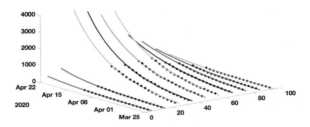

Fig. 10.14: *We plot an exponential fit for each age class using the data from Japan.*

$$\begin{cases} I_1'(t) = \tau_1 S_1 \left[\phi_{11} \dfrac{I_1(t) + U_1(t)}{N_1} + \cdots + \phi_{1n} \dfrac{I_n(t) + U_n(t)}{N_n} \right] - vI_1(t), \\ \qquad\qquad \vdots \\ I_n'(t) = \tau_n S_n \left[\phi_{n1} \dfrac{I_1(t) + U_1(t)}{N_1} + \cdots + \phi_{nn} \dfrac{I_n(t) + U_n(t)}{N_n} \right] - vI_n(t), \end{cases} \tag{10.27}$$

and

$$\begin{cases} U_1'(t) = v_2^1 I_1(t) - \eta U_1(t), \\ \qquad \vdots \\ U_n'(t) = v_2^n I_n(t) - \eta U_n(t). \end{cases} \tag{10.28}$$

If we assume that the $U_j(t)$ have the following form

$$U_j(t) = U_j^\star e^{\chi_2^j t}, \tag{10.29}$$

then by substituting in (10.28) we obtain

$$U_j^\star = \frac{v_2^j I_j^\star}{\eta + \chi_2^j}. \tag{10.30}$$

The cumulative number of unreported cases $CU_j(t)$ is computed as

$$CU_j(t)' = v_2^j I_j(t),$$

and we used the following initial condition:

$$CU_j(0) = CU_j^* = \int_{-\infty}^0 v_2^j I_j^* e^{\chi_2^j s} ds = \frac{v_2^j I_j^*}{\chi_2^j}.$$

We define the error between the data and the model as follows

$$
\begin{cases}
\varepsilon_1(t) = I_1'(t) - \tau_1 S_1 \left[\phi_{11} \dfrac{I_1(t) + U_1(t)}{N_1} + \cdots + \phi_{1n} \dfrac{I_n(t) + U_n(t)}{N_n} \right] + v I_1(t), \\
\qquad\qquad\qquad\qquad\qquad\vdots \\
\varepsilon_n(t) = I_n'(t) - \tau_n S_n \left[\phi_{n1} \dfrac{I_1(t) + U_1(t)}{N_1} + \cdots + \phi_{nn} \dfrac{I_n(t) + U_n(t)}{N_n} \right] + v I_n(t),
\end{cases}
\tag{10.31}
$$

or equivalently

$$
\begin{cases}
\varepsilon_1(t) = \left(\chi_2^1 + v\right) I_1^* e^{\chi_2^1 t} - \tau_1 S_1 \left[\phi_{11} \dfrac{I_1^\star + U_1^\star}{N_1} e^{\chi_2^1 t} + \cdots + \phi_{1n} \dfrac{I_n^\star + U_n^\star}{N_n} e^{\chi_2^n t} \right], \\
\qquad\qquad\qquad\qquad\qquad\vdots \\
\varepsilon_n(t) = \left(\chi_2^n + v\right) I_n^* e^{\chi_2^n t} - \tau_n S_n \left[\phi_{n1} \dfrac{I_1^\star + U_1^\star}{N_1} e^{\chi_2^1 t} + \cdots + \phi_{nn} \dfrac{I_n^\star + U_n^\star}{N_n} e^{\chi_2^n t} \right].
\end{cases}
\tag{10.32}
$$

Let the matrix ϕ be fixed. We look for the vector $\tau = (\tau_1, \ldots, \tau_n)$ which minimizes

$$\min_{\tau \in \mathbb{R}^n} \sum_{j=1,\ldots,n} \int_{d_1}^{d_2} \varepsilon_j(t)^2 dt.$$

Define for each $j = 1, \ldots, n$

$$K_j(t) := \left(\chi_2^j + v\right) I_j^* e^{\chi_2^j t}$$

and

$$H_j(t) := S_j \left[\phi_{j1} \dfrac{I_1^\star + U_1^\star}{N_1} e^{\chi_2^1 t} + \cdots + \phi_{jn} \dfrac{I_n^\star + U_n^\star}{N_n} e^{\chi_2^n t} \right],$$

so that

$$\varepsilon_j(t) = K_j(t) - \tau_j H_j(t).$$

Hence for each $j = 1, \ldots, n$

$$\int_{d_1}^{d_2} \varepsilon_j(t)^2 dt = \int_{d_1}^{d_2} K_j(t)^2 dt - 2\tau_j \int_{d_1}^{d_2} K_j(t) H_j(t) dt + \tau_j^2 \int_{d_1}^{d_2} H_j(t)^2 dt,$$

and by setting

$$0 = \frac{\partial}{\partial \tau_j} \int_{d_1}^{d_2} \varepsilon_j(t)^2 dt = -2 \int_{d_1}^{d_2} K_j(t) H_j(t) dt + 2\tau_j \int_{d_1}^{d_2} H_j(t)^2 dt$$

we deduce that

$$\tau_j = \frac{\int_{d_1}^{d_2} K_j(t) H_j(t) dt}{\int_{d_1}^{d_2} H_j(t)^2 dt}. \tag{10.33}$$

Remark 10.2 It does not seem possible to estimate the matrix of contact ϕ by using a similar optimization method. Indeed, if we look for a matrix $\phi = (\phi_{ij})$ which minimizes

$$\min_{\phi \in M_n(\mathbb{R})} \sum_{j=1,\dots,n} \int_{d_1}^{d_2} \varepsilon_j(t)^2 dt,$$

it turns out that

$$\sum_{j=1,\dots,n} \int_{d_1}^{d_2} \varepsilon_j(t)^2 dt = 0$$

whenever ϕ is diagonal. Therefore the optimum is reached for any diagonal matrix. Moreover, by using similar considerations, if several χ_j^2 are equal, we can find a multiplicity of optima (possibly with ϕ not diagonal). This means that trying to optimize by using the matrix ϕ does not yield significant and reliable information.

In Figure 10.15, we present an example of the application of our method to fit the Japanese data. We use the period going from 20 March to 15 April.

10.7 Construction of the Contact Matrix

The survey [281] presents reconstructed contact matrices for many countries including Japan for the 5-year age classes $[0, 5)$, $[5, 10)$, ..., $[75, 80)$ at various locations (work, school, home, and other locations) and a compilation of those contact matrices to account for all locations. The precise description of the compilation is presented in the paper. Note that this paper is a follow-up of Mossong et al. [259] where the survey procedure is described (including the data collection protocol) for several European countries participating in the POLYMOD study.

The data is publicly available online (Prem et al. [281], Supporting dataset, DOI: https://doi.org/10.1371/journal.pcbi.1005697.s002) and is presented in the form of a zipped collection of spreadsheets, containing the data for several countries in columns X1 X2 ... X16. The columns stand for the average number of contacts of one individual of the corresponding age class (0–5 years for X1, 5–10 years for X2, etc...), with an individual of the age class indicated by the row (the first row is 0–5 years, second is 5–10 years, etc...). Since the age span covered by the study stops at 80, we had to infer the number of contacts for people over the age of 80. We postulated that most people aged 80 or more are retired and that their behavior does not significantly differ from the behavior of people in the age class $[75, 80)$. Therefore we completed the missing columns by copying the last available information and shifting it to the bottom. We repeated the procedure for rows. We believe that the introduced bias is kept to a minimum since the numerical values are relatively low compared to the diagonal.

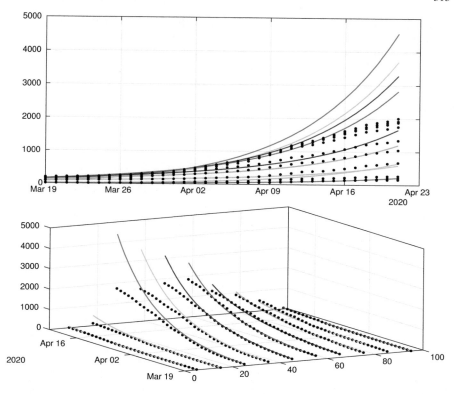

Fig. 10.15: *We plot a comparison between the model* (10.12)–(10.15) *(without public intervention) and the age-structured data from Japan. We set* $1/\nu = 1/\eta = 7$ *days,* f_i *which actually depends on the age class, with* $f_1 = 0.1$, $f_2 = 0.2$, $f_3 = 0.4$, $f_4 = 0.4$, $f_5 = 0.6$, $f_6 = 0.6$, $f_7 = 0.8$, $f_8 = 0.8$, $f_9 = 0.8$, *and* $f_{10} = 0.9$. *and we obtain* $\tau_1 = 0.1264$, $\tau_2 = 0.1655$, $\tau_3 = 0.3538$, $\tau_4 = 0.2966$, $\tau_5 = 0.1513$, $\tau_6 = 0.1684$, $\tau_7 = 0.1251$, $\tau_8 = 0.1168$, $\tau_9 = 0.1015$, $\tau_{10} = 0.1258$. *The matrix* ϕ *is the one defined in* (10.18).

Because we use 10-year age classes and the data is given in 5-year age classes, we had to combine adjacent columns to recover the average number of contacts. To combine columns, we used the weighted average

$$C_i' = \frac{N_{2(i-1)+1} C_{2(i-1)+1} + N_{2(i-1)+2} C_{2(i-1)+2}}{N_{2(i-1)+1} + N_{2(i-1)+2}},$$

where the column C_i' corresponds to the average number of contacts of an individual taken at random in the $[10(i-1), 10i)$ and C_i is the average number of contacts of an individual taken at random in the age class $[5(i-1), 5i)$. To combine two lines, we simply use the sum of the data

$$L_i' = L_{2(i-1)+1} + L_{2(i-1)+2}.$$

The matrix γ in (10.17) is the transpose of the array obtained by the former procedure applied to the "all locations" dataset. Then ϕ is obtained by scaling the rows of γ to 1, i.e.,

$$\phi_{ij} = \frac{\gamma_{ij}}{\sum_{k=1}^{10} \gamma_{ik}}.$$

Chapter 11
Clarifying Predictions for COVID-19 from Testing Data: The Example of New York State

This chapter is based on the article by Griette and Magal [125].

11.1 Introduction

The epidemic of novel coronavirus (COVID-19) infections began in China in December 2019 and rapidly spread worldwide in 2020. Since the early beginning of the epidemic, mathematicians and epidemiologists have developed models to analyze the data, characterize the spread of the virus and attempt to project the future evolution of the epidemic. Many of those models are based on the SIR or SEIR model which is classical in the context of epidemics. We refer to [334, 375] for the earliest articles devoted to such a question and to [7, 22, 33, 34, 35, 42, 86, 150, 174, 262, 338] for more models. In the course of the COVID-19 outbreak, it became clear to the scientific community that covert cases (asymptomatic or unreported infectious cases) play an important role. An early description of an asymptomatic transmission in Germany was reported by Rothe et al. [302]. It was also observed on the *Diamond Princess* cruise ship in Yokohama in Japan by Mizumoto et al. [257] that many of the passengers were tested positive for the virus, but never presented any symptoms. We also refer to Qiu [284] for more information about this problem. At the early stage of the COVID-19 outbreak, a new class of epidemic models was proposed in Liu et al. [207] to take into account the contamination of susceptible individuals by contact with unreported infectious. This class of models was presented earlier in Arino et al. [10]. In [207] a new method which uses the number of reported cases in SIR models was also proposed. This method and model were extended in several directions by the same group in [208, 209, 210] to include non-constant transmission rates and a period of exposure. More recently the method was extended and successfully applied to a Japanese age-structured dataset in [127]. The method was also extended to investigate the predictability of the outbreak in several countries, including China, South Korea, Italy, France, Germany, and the United Kingdom in [211]. The application of the Bayesian method was also considered in [67].

A. Ducrot et al., *Differential Equations and Population Dynamics I*, Lecture Notes on Mathematical Modelling in the Life Sciences, https://doi.org/10.1007/978-3-030-98136-5_11

In parallel with these modeling ideas, Bayesian methods have been widely used to identify the parameters in the models used for the COVID-19 pandemic (see e.g. Roques et al. [295, 296], where an estimate of the fatality ratio has been developed). A remarkable feature of those methods is to provide mechanisms to correct some of the known biases in the observation of cases, such as the daily number of tests. Here we embed the data for the daily number of tests into an epidemic model and compare the number of reported cases produced by the model and the data. Our goal is to understand the relationship between the data for the daily number of tests (which is an input of our model) and the data for the daily number of reported cases (which is an output of our model).

The plan of the chapter is the following. In Section 11.2, we present a model involving the daily number of tests. In Section 11.3, we apply the method presented in [207] to our new model. In Section 11.4, we present some numerical simulations and compare the model with the data. The last section is devoted to the discussion.

11.2 Epidemic with Testing Data

Let $n(t)$ be the number of tests per unit of time. Throughout this chapter, we use one day as the unit of time. Therefore $n(t)$ can be regarded as the daily number of tests at time t. The function $n(t)$ comes from a database for New York State.[1] Let $N(t)$ be the cumulative number of tests from the beginning of the epidemic. Then

$$N'(t) = n(t), \text{ for } t \geq t_1 \text{ and } N(t_1) = N_1.$$

Remark 11.1 Section 11.4 is devoted to numerical simulations. We use $n(t)$ as a piecewise constant function that varies day by day. Each day, $n(t)$ is equal to the number of tests that were performed that day. So $n(t)$ should be understood as the black curve in Figure 11.4.

The model consists of the following ordinary differential equations

$$\begin{cases} S'(t) = -\tau S(t)[I(t) + U(t) + D(t)], \\ E'(t) = \tau S(t)[I(t) + U(t)] + D(t)] - \alpha E(t), \\ I'(t) = \alpha E(t) - \nu I(t), \\ U'(t) = \nu (1 - f) I(t) + n(t) (1 - \sigma) g D(t) - \eta U(t), \\ D'(t) = \nu f I(t) - n(t) g D(t) - \eta D(t), \\ R'(t) = n(t) \sigma g D(t) - \eta R(t). \end{cases} \tag{11.1}$$

This system is supplemented by initial data (which are all non-negative)

$$S(t_1) = S_1, \ E(t_1) = E_1, \ I(t_1) = I_1, \ U(t_1) = U_1, \ D(t_1) = D_1 \text{ and } R(t_1) = R_1.$$

The time t_1 corresponds to the time where the tests started to be used constantly. Therefore the epidemic started before t_1.

[1] The COVID Tracking Project at *The Atlantic*. https://covidtracking.com/data/state/new-york#historical. Accessed June 23, 2021.

Here $t \geq t_1$ is the time in days. $S(t)$ is the number of individuals susceptible to infection. $E(t)$ is the number of exposed individuals (i.e. who are incubating the disease but not infectious). $I(t)$ is the number of individuals incubating the disease, but already infectious. $U(t)$ is the number of undetected infectious individuals (i.e. who are expressing mild or no symptoms), and the infectious that have been tested with a false negative result, are therefore not candidates for testing. $D(t)$ is the number of individuals who express severe symptoms and are candidates for testing. $R(t)$ is the number of individuals who have been tested positive for the disease. The flux diagram of our model is presented in Figure 11.1.

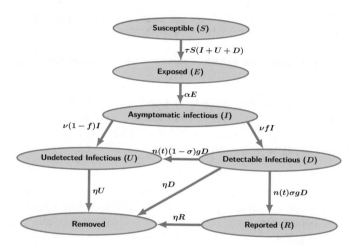

Fig. 11.1: *Flow chart of the epidemic model with tests* (11.1). *In this diagram* $n(t)$ *is the daily number of tests at time* t. *We consider a fraction* $(1 - \sigma)$ *of false negative tests and a fraction* σ *of true positive tests. The parameter g reflects the fact that the tests are devoted not only to the symptomatic patients but also to a large fraction of the population of New York state.*

Susceptible individuals $S(t)$ become infected by contact with an infectious individual $I(t)$, $U(t)$ or $D(t)$. When they get infected, susceptibles are first classified as exposed individuals $E(t)$, that is, they are incubating the disease but not yet infectious. The average length of this exposed period (or non-infectious incubation period) is $1/\alpha$ days.

After the exposure period, individuals become asymptomatic infectious $I(t)$. The average length of the asymptomatic infectious period is $1/\nu$ days. After this period, individuals either become mildly symptomatic individuals $U(t)$ or individuals with severe symptoms $D(t)$. The average length of this infectious period is $1/\eta$ days. Some of the U-individuals may show no symptoms at all.

In our model, the transmission can occur between an S-individual and an I-, U- or R-individual. Transmissions of SARS-CoV-2 are described in the model by the term $\tau S(t)[I(t) + U(t) + D(t)]$, where τ is the transmission rate. Here, even though transmission from an R-individual to an S-individual is possible in theory (e.g. if a tested patient infects their medical doctor), we consider that such a case is rare and we neglect it.

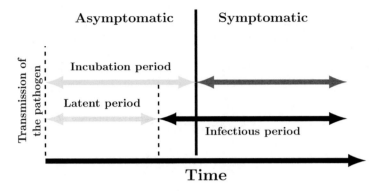

Fig. 11.2: *Key time periods of COVID-19 infection: the latent or exposed period before the onset of symptoms and transmissibility, the incubation period before symptoms appear, the symptomatic period, and the transmissibility period, which may overlap the asymptomatic period.*

The last part of the model is devoted to the testing. The parameter σ is the fraction of true positive tests and $(1 - \sigma)$ is the fraction of false-negative tests. The quantity σ has been estimated at $\sigma = 0.7$ in the case of nasal or pharyngeal swabs for SARS-CoV-2 [272].

Among the detectable infectious, we assume that only a fraction g are tested per unit of time. This fraction corresponds to individuals with symptoms suggesting a potential infection of SARS-CoV-2. The fraction g is the frequency of testable individuals in the population of New York State. We can rewrite g as

$$g = \frac{1}{\kappa P},$$

where P is the total number of individuals in the population of the state of New York and $0 \leq \kappa \leq 1$ is the fraction of the total population with mild or severe symptoms that may induce a test.

Individuals who were tested positive $R(t)$ are infectious on average during a period of $1/\eta$ days, but we assume that they become immediately isolated and do not contribute to the epidemic anymore. In this model, we focus on the testing of the D-individuals. The quantity $n(t) \sigma g D$ is a flux of successfully tested D-individuals which become R-individuals. The flux of tested D-individuals which are false negatives is $n(t) (1 - \sigma) g D$, which go from the class of D-individuals to the U-individuals. The parameters of the model and the initial conditions of the model are listed in Table 11.1.

Before describing our method we need to introduce a few useful identities. The cumulative number of reported cases is obtained by using the following equation

Symbol	Interpretation	Method
t_1	Date when the tests start to be used extensively	fixed
S_1	Number of susceptible at time t_1	fixed
E_1	Number of exposed at time t_1	fitted
I_1	Number of asymptomatic infectious at time t_1	fitted
U_1	Number of undetectable infectious at time t_1	fitted
D_1	Number of detectable infectious at time t_1	fitted
R_1	Number of reported (tested positive) cases at time t_1	fitted
τ	Transmission rate	fitted
$n(t)$	Number of tests per unit of time	fixed
$1/\alpha$	Average length of exposure	fixed
$1/\nu$	Average length of asymptomatic infectiousness	fixed
$1/\eta$	Average length of symptomatic infectiousness	fixed
f	Frequency of infectious with sever symptoms	fixed
σ	Fraction of true positive tests	fixed
g	Frequency of testable individuals	fixed

Table 11.1: *Parameters and initial conditions of the model.*

$$CR'(t) = n(t)\,\sigma\,g\,D(t). \tag{11.2}$$

The daily number of reported cases $DR'(t)$ is given by

$$DR(t)' = n(t)\,\sigma\,g\,D(t) - DR(t). \tag{11.3}$$

The cumulative number of detectable cases is given by

$$CD'(t) = \nu f I(t), \tag{11.4}$$

and the cumulative number of undetectable cases is given by

$$CU'(t) = \nu(1-f)I(t) + n(t)(1-\sigma)gD(t). \tag{11.5}$$

Symbol	Interpretation	Equation
t	Time (in days)	
$S(t)$	Number of susceptible at time t	(11.1)
$E(t)$	Number of exposed at time t	(11.1)
$I(t)$	Number of asymptomatic infectious at time t	(11.1)
$U(t)$	Number of undetectable infectious at time t	(11.1)
$D(t)$	Number of detectable infectious at time t	(11.1)
$R(t)$	Number of reported (tested positive) cases at time t	(11.1)
$CR(t)$	Cumulative number of reported (tested infectious) cases at time t	(11.2)
$DR(t)$	Daily number of reported (tested infectious) cases at time t	(11.3)
$CD(t)$	Cumulative number of detectable infectious at time t	(11.4)
$CU(t)$	Cumulative number of undetectable infectious at time t	(11.5)

Table 11.2: *Variables used in the model.*

11.3 Method to fit the cumulative number of reported cases

To deal with data, we need to understand how to set the parameters as well as some components of the initial conditions. To do so, we extend the method presented first in [207]. The main novelty here concerns the cumulative number of tests which is assumed to grow linearly at the beginning. This property is satisfied by the New York State data as we can see in Figure 11.3. The black curve in this figure is close to a line from March 15 to April 15. Figure 11.4 shows day-by-day fluctuations of the number of tests while in Figure 11.3 the day-by-day fluctuations are not visible and the cumulative data allow us to understand the growth tendency of the number of tests.

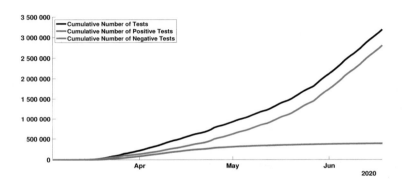

Fig. 11.3: *In this figure, we plot the cumulative number of tests for New York State. The black curve, orange curve, and blue curve correspond respectively to the number of tests, the number of positive tests, and the number of negative tests. We can see that at the early stages of the epidemic, the cumulative number of tests (black curve) grows linearly from mid-March to mid-April.*

Phenomenological models for the tests: We fit a line to the cumulative number of tests in a suitable interval of days $[t_1, t_2]$. This means that we can find a pair of numbers a and b such that

$$N(t) = a \times (t - t_1) + N_1, \text{ for } t_1 \leq t \leq t_2,$$

where a the daily number of tests and N_1 is the cumulative number of tests on day t_1.

By using the fact that $N(t)' = n(t)$ we deduce that

$$n(t) = a, \text{ for } t_1 \leq t \leq t_2. \tag{11.6}$$

Remark 11.2 In the simulations, we fit a line to the cumulative number of tests from mid-March to mid-April. Figure 11.3 shows that the linear growth assumption is reasonable for the New York State cumulative testing data.

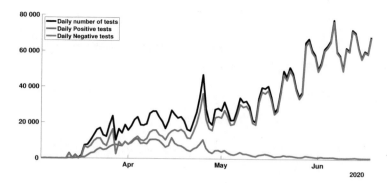

Fig. 11.4: *In this figure, we plot the daily number of tests for New York State. The black curve, orange curve, and blue curve correspond respectively to the number of tests, the number of positive tests, and the number of negative tests.*

Phenomenological models for the reported cases: At the early stage of the epidemic, we assume that all the infected components of the system grow exponentially while the number of susceptible remains unchanged during a relatively short period $t \in [t_1, t_2]$. Therefore, we assume that

$$E(t) = E_1 e^{\chi_2(t-t_1)}, I(t) = I_1 e^{\chi_2(t-t_1)}, D(t) = D_1 e^{\chi_2(t-t_1)} \text{ and } U(t) = U_1 e^{\chi_2(t-t_1)}.$$
$$(11.7)$$

We deduce that the cumulative number of reported cases satisfies

$$CR(t) = CR(t_1) + \int_{t_1}^{t} a\sigma g D(\theta) d\theta \qquad (11.8)$$

hence by replacing $D(t)$ by the exponential formula (11.7)

$$CR(t) = CR(t_1) + \frac{a\sigma g}{\chi_2} D_1 \left(e^{\chi_2(t-t_1)} - 1 \right) \qquad (11.9)$$

and it makes sense to assume that $CR(t) - CR(t_1)$ has the following form

$$CR(t) - CR(t_1) = \chi_1 e^{\chi_2(t-t_1)} - \chi_3. \qquad (11.10)$$

By identifying (11.9) and (11.10) we deduce that

$$\chi_1 = \chi_3 = \frac{a\sigma g}{\chi_2} D_1. \qquad (11.11)$$

Moreover, by using (11.6) and the fact that the number of susceptible $S(t)$ remains constant, equalling S_1 on the time interval $t \in [t_1, t_2]$, the E-equation, I-equation, U-equation and D-equation of the model (11.1) become

$$\begin{cases} E'(t) = \tau S_1 [I(t) + U(t) + D(t)] - \alpha E(t), \\ I'(t) = \alpha E(t) - \nu I(t), \\ U'(t) = \nu (1 - f) I(t) + a (1 - \sigma) g D(t) - \eta U(t), \\ D'(t) = \nu f I(t) - a g D(t) - \eta D(t). \end{cases}$$

By using (11.7) we obtain

$$\begin{cases} \chi_2 E_1 = \tau S_1 [I_1 + U_1 + D_1] - \alpha E_1, \\ \chi_2 I_1 = \alpha E_1 - \nu I_1, \\ \chi_2 U_1 = \nu (1 - f) I_1 + a (1 - \sigma) g D_1 - \eta U_1, \\ \chi_2 D_1 = \nu f I_1 - a g D_1 - \eta D_1. \end{cases}$$

Computing further, we get

$$\begin{cases} E_1 = \dfrac{\tau_1 S_1 (I_1 + U_1 + D_1)}{\chi_2 + \alpha} \\[2ex] I_1 = \dfrac{\alpha E_1}{\chi_2 + \nu} \\[2ex] U_1 = \dfrac{\nu I_1 + a (1 - \sigma) g D_1}{\chi_2 + \eta} \\[2ex] D_1 = \dfrac{\nu f I_1}{\chi_2 + a g + \eta}. \end{cases} \tag{11.12}$$

Finally by using (11.11)

$$D_1 = \frac{\chi_2 \chi_3}{\sigma a g} \tag{11.13}$$

and by using (11.12) we obtain

$$\begin{cases} I_1 = \dfrac{\chi_2 + a g + \eta}{\nu f} D_1 = \dfrac{\chi_2 + a g + \eta}{\nu} \times \dfrac{\chi_2 \chi_3}{f \sigma a g} \\[2ex] U_1 = \dfrac{\nu I_1 + (1 - \sigma) a g D_1}{\chi_2 + \eta} = \dfrac{(\chi_2 + \eta + [1 + f(1 - \sigma)] a g)}{\chi_2 + \eta} \times \dfrac{\chi_2 \chi_3}{f \sigma a g} \\[2ex] E_1 = \dfrac{(\chi_2 + \nu)}{\alpha} I_1 = \dfrac{(\chi_2 + \nu)}{\alpha} \times \dfrac{(\chi_2 + a g + \eta)}{\nu} \times \dfrac{\chi_2 \chi_3}{f \sigma a g} \\[2ex] \tau_1 = \dfrac{(\chi_2 + \alpha)}{S_1 (I_1 + U_1 + D_1)} E_1 \\[2ex] \quad = \dfrac{(\chi_2 + \alpha) (\chi_2 + \nu) (\chi_2 + \eta) (\chi_2 + a g + \eta)}{\alpha S_1 \left([\chi_2 + a g + \eta + \nu(f + 1)] (\chi_2 + \eta) + \nu [1 + f(1 - \sigma)] a g \right)}, \end{cases} \tag{11.14}$$

where I_1 is the number of incubating infectious individuals at time t_1, U_1 is the number of unreported infectious individuals at time t_1, E_1 is the number of incubating non-infectious individuals at time t_1 (see (11.7)), and finally τ_1 is the transmission rate at time t_1.

11.4 Numerical Simulations

We assume that the transmission coefficient takes the form

$$\tau(t) = \tau_0\big((1 - \gamma)\exp(-\mu(t - T_m)_+) + \gamma\big), \tag{11.15}$$

where $\tau_0 > 0$ is the initial transmission coefficient, $T_m > 0$ is the time at which the social distancing starts in the population, and $\mu > 0$ controls the speed at which this social distancing is taking place.

To take into account the effect of social distancing and public measures, we assume that the transmission coefficient $\tau(t)$ can be modulated by γ. Indeed by closing schools and non-essential shops and by imposing social distancing in New York State, the number of contacts per day is reduced. This effect was visible on the news during the first wave of the COVID-19 epidemic in New York City since the streets were almost empty on some occasions. The parameter $\gamma > 0$ is the percentage of the number of transmissions that remain after a transition period (depending on μ), compared to a normal situation. A similar non-constant transmission rate was considered by Chowell et al. [56].

In Figure 11.5 we consider a constant transmission rate $\tau(t) \equiv \tau_0$ which corresponds to $\gamma = 1$ in (11.15). To evaluate the distance between the model and the data, we compare the distance between the cumulative number of cases CR produced by the model and the data (see the orange dots and orange curve in Figure 11.5-(a)). In Figure 11.5-(c) we observe that the cumulative number of cases increases up to more than 14 million people, which indeed is not realistic. Nevertheless by choosing the parameter $g = 3.08 \times 10^{-7} = 1/\left(\frac{S_0}{6}\right)$ in Figure 11.5-(d) we can see that the orange dots and the blue curve match very well.

In the rest of this section, we focus on the model with confinement (or social distancing) measures. We assume that such social distancing measures have a strong impact on the transmission rate by assuming that $\gamma = 0.2 < 1$. This means that only 20% of the transmissions remain after a transition period.

In Figure 11.6-(c) we can observe that the cumulative number of cases increases up to 800 000 (blue curve) while the cumulative number of reported cases goes up to 350 000. In Figure 11.6-(d) we can see that the orange dots and the blue curve match very well again. In order to get this fit we fix the parameter $g = 10^{-5}$.

In Figure 11.7 (a) and (b), we aim at understanding the connection between the daily fluctuations of the number of reported cases (epidemic dynamic) and the daily number of tests (testing dynamics). The combination of the testing dynamics and the infection dynamics indeed gives a very complex curve parametrized by time. It seems that the only reasonable comparison that we can make is between the cumulative number of reported cases and the cumulative number of tests. In Figure 11.7 (c) and (d), the comparison of the model and the data gives a very decent fit. In Figure 11.7, all the curves are time-dependent parametrized curves. The abscissa is the number of tests (horizontal axis) and the ordinate is the number of reported cases (vertical axis). It corresponds (with our notations) to the parametric functions $t \to (n_{data}(t), DR(t))$ in figures (a) and (b) and their cumulative equivalent $t \to (N_{data}(t), CR(t))$ in figures (c) and (d). In figures (a) and (c) we use only the data,

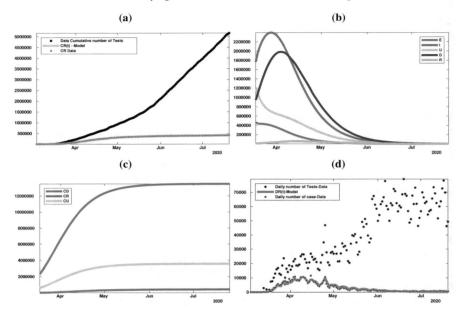

Fig. 11.5: *Best fit of the model without confinement (or social distancing) measures (i.e. $\gamma = 1$).* **Fitted parameters:** *The transmission rate $\tau(t) \equiv \tau_0$ is constant according to the formula (11.15) with $\gamma = 1$ and τ_0 is fixed to the value τ_1 computed by using (11.14).* **Parameter values:** $S_0 = 19453561$, $\alpha = 1$, $\nu = 1/6$, $\eta = 1/7$, $\sigma = 0.7$, $f = 0.8$ and $g = 6/S_0 = 3.08 \times 10^{-7}$. $t_1 = $ March 18, $t_2 = $ March 29, $a = 1.4874 \times 10^4$, $b = -2.1781 \times 10^5$, $\chi_1 = 2.8814 \times 10^4$, $\chi_2 = 0.1013$, $\chi_3 = 2.9969 \times 10^4$. *In figure (a) we plot the cumulative number of tests (black dots), the cumulative number of positive cases (red dots) for the state of New York and the cumulative number of cases $CD(t)$ (yellow curve) obtained by fitting the model to the data. In figures (b)–(c) we plot the number of cases obtained from the model. We observe that most of the cases are unreported. In figure (d) we plot the daily number of tests (black dots), the daily number of positive cases (red dots) for the state of New York and the daily number of cases $DD(t)$ obtained from the data.*

that is, we plot $t \rightarrow (n_{data}(t), DR_{data}(t))$ and $t \rightarrow (N_{data}(t), CR_{data}(t))$. In figures (b) and (d) we use only the model for the number of reported cases, that is, we plot $t \rightarrow (n_{data}(t), DR_{model}(t))$ and $t \rightarrow (N_{data}(t), CR_{model}(t))$.

In Figure 11.8, our goal is to investigate the effect of a change in the testing policy in New York State. We are particularly interested in estimating the effect of an increase in the number of tests on the epidemic. Indeed increasing the number of tests may be thought of as beneficial to reducing the number of cases. Here we challenge this idea by comparing an increase in the number of tests to the quantitative output of our model. In Figure 11.8, we replace the daily number of tests $n_{data}(t)$ (coming from the data for New York State) in the model by either $2 \times n_{data}(t)$, $5 \times n_{data}(t)$, $10 \times n_{data}(t)$ or $100 \times n_{data}(t)$.

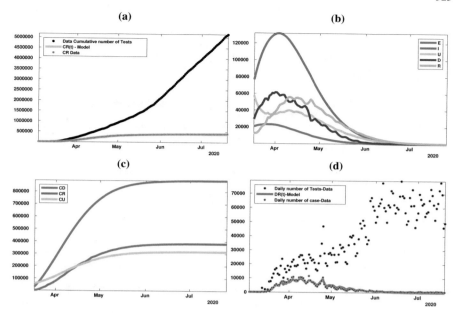

Fig. 11.6: *Best fit of the model with confinement (or social distancing) measures.* **Parameter values:** *Same as in Figure 11.5, except the transmission coefficient, which is not constant in time with* $\gamma = 0.2$, $T_m = 15$ *March (starting day of public measures),* $\mu = 0.0251$, $g = 10^{-5}$ *and* τ_0 *is fixed at the value* τ_1 *computed by using* (11.14). *In figure (a) we plot the cumulative number of tests (black dots), the cumulative number of positive cases (red dots) for the state of New York and the cumulative number of cases* $CD(t)$ *(yellow curve) obtained by fitting the model to the data. In figures (b)–(c) we plot the corresponding number of cases obtained from the model. With this set of parameters we observe that most of the cases are unreported. In figure (d) we plot the daily number of tests (black dots), the daily number of positive cases (red dots) for the state of New York and the daily number of cases* $DD(t)$ *obtained from the data.*

As expected, an increase in the number of tests helps to reduce the number of cases at first. However, after increasing the number of tests 10 times, there is no significant difference (in the number of reported) between 10 times and 100 times more tests. Therefore there must be an optimum between increasing the number of tests (which costs money and other limited resources) and efficiently slowing slow down the epidemic.

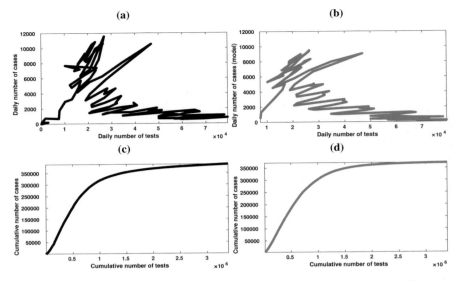

Fig. 11.7: *In this figure we plot the curves of the number of reported cases as a function of the number of tests parametrized by time. The top figures (a) and (b) correspond to the daily number of cases and the bottom figures (c) and (d) correspond to the cumulative number of cases. On the left-hand side, we plot the data (a) and (c) while on the right-hand side we plot the model (b) and (d).* **Parameter values:** *Same as in Figure 11.6. In figure (a) we plot the daily number of cases coming from the data as a function of the daily number of tests. In figure (b) we plot the daily number of cases given by the model as a function of the daily number of tests coming from the data. In figure (c) we plot the cumulative number of cases coming from the data as a function of the cumulative number of tests. In figure (d) we plot the cumulative number of cases coming from the model as a function of the cumulative number of tests from the data.*

11.5 Discussion

In this chapter, we proposed a new epidemic model involving the daily number of tests as an input of the model. The model itself extends our previous models presented in [127, 207, 208, 209, 210, 211]. We proposed a new method to use the data in such a context based on the fact that the cumulative number of tests grows linearly at the early stage of the epidemic. Figure 11.3 shows that this is a reasonable assumption for the New York State data from mid-March to mid-April.

Our numerical simulations show a very good concordance between the number of reported cases produced by the model and the data in two very different situations. Indeed, Figures 11.5 and 11.6 correspond respectively to an epidemic without and with public intervention to limit the number of transmissions. This is an important observation since this shows that testing data and reported cases are not sufficient to evaluate the real amplitude of the epidemic. To solve this problem, the only solution

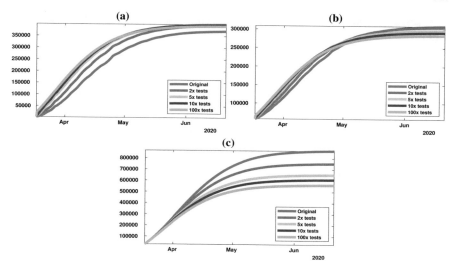

Fig. 11.8: *Cumulative number of cases for different testing strategies: Original (blue curve), doubled (red curve), multiplied by 5 (yellow curve), multiplied by 10 (purple line) and multiplied by 100 (green curve). The transmission coefficient depends on time, according to the formula (11.15) with $\gamma = 0.2$, and τ_0 is fitted by using (11.14). Parameter values: these are the same as in Figure 11.6. In figure (a) we plot the cumulated number of cases $CR(t)$ as a function of time. In figure (b) we plot the cumulative number of undetectable cases $CU(t)$ as a function of time. In figure (c) we plot the cumulative number of cases (including covert cases) $CD(t)$ as a function of time. Note that the total number of cases (including covert cases) is reduced by 35% when the number of tests is multiplied by 100.*

seems to include a different kind of data to the models. This could be done by studying statistically representative samples in the population. Otherwise, biases can always be suspected. Such a question is of particular interest to evaluate the fraction of the population that has been infected by the virus and their possible immunity.

In Figure 11.7, we compared the testing dynamic (day to day variation in the number of tests) and the reported cases dynamic (day to day variation in the number of reported). Indeed, the dynamics of daily cases are extremely complex, but we also obtain a relatively robust curve for the cumulative numbers. Our model gives a good fit for these cumulative cases.

In Figure 11.8, we compared multiple testing strategies. By increasing the number of tests 2, 5, 10, and 100 times, we can project the efficiency of an increase in the daily number of tests. We observe that it is efficient to increase this number up to 10 but the relative gain in the absolute number of infected individuals rapidly drops after that. In particular, our projections do not show a big difference between a 10-times increase in the number of tests and a 100-times increase. Therefore there is a balance to find between the number of tests and the efficiency in the evaluation of the number of cases, the optimal strategy being dependent on other factors like the monetary cost of the tests.

Chapter 12
SI Epidemic Model Applied to COVID-19 Data in Mainland China

This chapter was published as a paper by Demongeot, Griette and Magal [77].

12.1 Introduction

Estimating the average transmission rate is one of the most crucial challenges in the epidemiology of communicable diseases. This rate conditions the entry into the epidemic phase of the disease and its return to the extinction phase, if it has diminished sufficiently. It is the combination of three factors, one, the coefficient of virulence, linked to the infectious agent (in the case of infectious transmissible diseases), the other, the coefficient of susceptibility, linked to the host (all summarized as the probability of transmission), and also, the number of contacts per unit of time between individuals (see Magal and Ruan [235]). The coefficient of virulence may change over time due to mutation over the course of the disease history. The second and third coefficients may also vary, if mitigation measures have been taken. This was the case in China from the start of the pandemic (see Qiu, Chen and Shi [285]). Monitoring the decrease in the average transmission rate is an excellent way to monitor the effectiveness of these mitigation measures. Estimating the rate is therefore a central problem in the fight against epidemics.

The goal of this chapter is to understand how to compare the SI model to the reported epidemic data and therefore how the model can be used to predict the future evolution of epidemic spread and to test various possible scenarios of social mitigation measures. For $t \geq t_0$, the SI model is the following

$$\begin{cases} S'(t) = -\tau(t)S(t)I(t), \\ I'(t) = \tau(t)S(t)I(t) - \nu I(t), \end{cases} \tag{12.1}$$

where $S(t)$ is the number of susceptible and $I(t)$ the number of infectious at time t. This system is supplemented by initial data

$$S(t_0) = S_0 \geq 0, \ I(t_0) = I_0 \geq 0. \tag{12.2}$$

© The Author(s), under exclusive license to Springer Nature Switzerland AG 2022
A. Ducrot et al., *Differential Equations and Population Dynamics I*, Lecture Notes on
Mathematical Modelling in the Life Sciences, https://doi.org/10.1007/978-3-030-98136-5_12

In this model, the rate of transmission $\tau(t)$ combines the number of contacts per unit of time and the probability of transmission. The transmission of the pathogen from the infectious to the susceptible individuals is described by a mass action law $\tau(t) S(t) I(t)$ (which is also the flux of new infectious).

The quantity $1/\nu$ is the average duration of the infectious period and $\nu I(t)$ is the flux of recovering or dying individuals. At the end of the infectious period, we assume that a fraction $f \in (0, 1]$ of the infectious individuals is reported. Let $CR(t)$ be the cumulative number of reported cases. We assume that

$$CR(t) = CR_0 + \nu f\, CI(t), \text{ for } t \geq t_0, \tag{12.3}$$

where

$$CI(t) = \int_{t_0}^t I(\sigma)d\sigma. \tag{12.4}$$

Assumption 12.1 We assume that

- $S_0 > 0$ the number of susceptible individuals at time t_0 when we start to use the model;
- $\dfrac{1}{\nu} > 0$ the average duration of infectious period;
- $f > 0$ the fraction of reported individuals,

are known parameters.

Throughout this chapter, the parameter $S_0 = 1.4 \times 10^9$ will be the entire population of mainland China (since COVID-19 is a newly emerging disease). The actual number of susceptibles S_0 can be smaller since some individuals can be partially (or totally) immunized by previous infections or other factors. This is also true for Sars-CoV2, even if COVID-19 is a newly emerging disease. In fact, for COVID-19 the level of susceptibility may depend on blood group and genetic lineage. It is indeed suspected that the blood group O is associated with a lower susceptibility to SARS-CoV2 while a gene cluster inherited from Neanderthals has been identified as a risk factor for severe symptoms (see Zeberg et al. [382] and Guillon et al. [132]).

At the early beginning of the epidemic, the average duration of the infectious period $1/\nu$ is unknown, since the virus has never been investigated in the past. Therefore, at the early beginning of the COVID-19 epidemic, medical doctors and public health scientists used the previously estimated average duration of the infectious period to make some public health recommendations. Here we show that the average infectious period is impossible to estimate by using only the time series of reported cases, and must therefore be identified by other means. Actually, with the data of Sars-CoV2 in mainland China, we will fit the cumulative number of reported cases almost perfectly for any non-negative value $1/\nu < 3.3$ days. In the literature, several estimates have been obtained: 11 days in [390], 9.5 days in [381], 8 days in [220], and 3.5 days in [201]. The recent survey by Byrne et al. [46] focuses on this subject.

> **Result**
>
> In Section 12.3, our analysis shows that
>
> - It is hopeless to estimate the exact value of the duration of infectiousness by using SI models. Several values of the average duration of the infectious period give the exact same fit to the data.
> - We can estimate an upper bound for the duration of infectiousness by using SI models. In the case of Sars-CoV2 in mainland China, this upper bound is 3.3 days.

In [302], it is reported that transmission of COVID-19 infection may occur from an infectious individual who is not yet symptomatic. In [367] it is reported that COVID-19 infected individuals generally develop symptoms, including mild respiratory symptoms and fever, on average 5–6 days after the infection date (with 95% confidence, a range of 1–14 days). In [376] it is reported that the median time prior to symptom onset is 3 days, the shortest 1 day, and the longest 24 days. It is evident that these time periods play an important role in understanding COVID-19 transmission dynamics. Here the fraction of reported individuals f is unknown as well.

> **Result**
>
> In Section 12.3, our analysis shows that:
>
> - It is hopeless to estimate the fraction of reported by using the SI models. Several values for the fraction of reported give the exact same fit to the data.
> - We can estimate a lower bound for the fraction of unreported. We obtain $3.83 \times 10^{-5} < f \leq 1$. This lower bound is not significant. Therefore we cannot say anything about the fraction of unreported from this class of models.

As a consequence, the parameters $1/\nu$ and f have to be estimated by another method, for instance by a direct survey methodology that should be employed on an appropriate sample of the population in order to evaluate the two parameters.

The goal of this chapter is to focus on the estimation of the two remaining parameters. Namely, knowing the above-mentioned parameters, we plan to identify

- I_0, the initial number of infectious at time t_0;
- $\tau(t)$, the rate of transmission at time t.

This problem has already been considered in several articles. In the early 70s, London and Yorke [212, 378] already discussed the time-dependent rate of transmission in the context of measles, chickenpox, and mumps. More recently, in Wang and Ruan [359] the question of reconstructing the rate of transmission was considered for the 2002-2004 SARS outbreak in China. In Chowell et al. [56] a specific form was chosen for the rate of transmission and applied to the Ebola outbreak in Congo. Another approach was also proposed in Smirnova et al. [320].

In Section 12.2, we will explain how to apply the method introduced in Liu et al. [210] to fit the early cumulative data of Sars-CoV2 in China. This method provides a way to compute I_0 and $\tau_0 = \tau(t_0)$ at the early stage of the epidemic. In Section 12.3, we establish an identifiability result in the spirit of Hadeler [136].

In Section 12.4, we use the Bernoulli–Verhulst model as a phenomenological model to describe the data. As was observed in several articles, the data from mainland China (and other countries as well) can be fitted very well by using this model. As a consequence, we will obtain an explicit formula for $\tau(t)$ and I_0 expressed as a function of the parameters of the Bernoulli–Verhulst model and the remaining parameters of the SI model. This approach gives a very good description of this set of data. The disadvantage of this approach is that it requires an early evaluation of the final size CR_∞ (or at least it requires an estimate of this quantity).

Therefore, in order to be predictive, we will explore in the remaining sections of this chapter the possibility of constructing a day-by-day rate of transmission. Here we should refer to Bakhta et al. [23], where another novel forecasting method was proposed.

In Section 12.5, we will prove that the daily cumulative data can be approached perfectly by at most one sequence of day-by-day piecewise constant transmission rates. In Section 12.6, we propose numerical methods to compute such a (piecewise constant) rate of transmission. Section 12.7 is devoted to the discussion, and we will present some figures showing the daily basic reproduction number for the COVID-19 outbreak in mainland China.

12.2 Estimating $\tau(t_0)$ and I_0 at the Early Stage of the Epidemic

In this section, we apply the method presented in [207] to the SI model. At the early stage of the epidemic, we can assume that $S(t)$ is almost constant and equal to S_0. We can also assume that $\tau(t)$ remains constant equal to $\tau_0 = \tau(t_0)$. Therefore, by replacing these parameters into the I-equation of system (12.1) we obtain

$$I'(t) = (\tau_0 S_0 - \nu)I(t).$$

Therefore

$$I(t) = I_0 \exp\left(\chi_2 \left(t - t_0\right)\right),$$

where

$$\chi_2 = \tau_0 S_0 - \nu. \tag{12.5}$$

By using (12.3), we obtain

$$CR(t) = CR_0 + \nu f I_0 \frac{e^{\chi_2(t-t_0)} - 1}{\chi_2}. \tag{12.6}$$

We obtain a first phenomenological model for the cumulative number of reported cases (valid only at the early stage of the epidemic)

$$CR(t) = \chi_1 e^{\chi_2 t} - \chi_3. \tag{12.7}$$

In Figure 12.1, we compare the model to the COVID-19 data for mainland China. The data used are taken from various sources,[1, 2, 3] and reported in Section 12.8. In order to estimate the parameter χ_3, we minimize the distance between $CR_{Data}(t) + \chi_3$ and the best exponential fit $t \rightarrow \chi_1 e^{\chi_2 t}$ (i.e. we use the MATLAB function fit(t, data, 'exp1')).

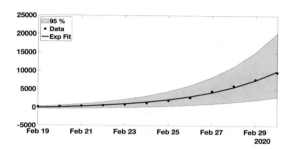

Fig. 12.1: *In this figure, we plot the best fit of the exponential model to the cumulative number of reported cases of COVID-19 in mainland China between February 19 and March 1. We obtain $\chi_1 = 3.7366$, $\chi_2 = 0.2650$ and $\chi_3 = 615.41$ with $t_0 = 19$ Feb. The parameter χ_3 is obtained by minimizing the error between the best exponential fit and the data.*

The estimated initial number of infected and transmission rate

By using (12.3) and (12.7) we obtain

$$I_0 = \frac{CR'(t_0)}{v\,f} = \frac{\chi_1 \chi_2 e^{\chi_2 t_0}}{v\,f}, \tag{12.8}$$

and by using (12.5)

$$\tau_0 = \frac{\chi_2 + v}{S_0}. \tag{12.9}$$

Remark 12.2 Fixing $f = 0.5$ and $v = 0.2$, we obtain

$$I_0 = 3.7366 \times 0.2650 \times \exp(0.2650 \times 19)/(0.2 \times 0.5) = 1521,$$

and

[1] Data sourced from Wikipedia, who used NHC daily reports : https://en.wikipedia.org/wiki/COVID-19_pandemic_in_mainland_China. Accessed June 23, 2021.

[2] The National Health Commission of the People's Republic of China : http://www.nhc.gov.cn/yjb/pzhgli/new_list.shtml. Accessed June 23, 2021.

[3] Chinese Center for Disease Control and Prevention : http://www.chinacdc.cn/jkzt/crb/zl/szkb_11803/jszl_11809/. Accessed June 23, 2021.

$$\tau_0 = \frac{0.2650 + 0.2}{1.4 \times 10^9} = 3.3214 \times 10^{-10}.$$

The influence of the errors made in the estimations (at the early stage of the epidemic) has been considered in the recent article by Roda et al. [291]. To understand this problem, let us first consider the case of the rate of transmission $\tau(t) = \tau_0$ in the model (12.1). In that case (12.1) becomes

$$\begin{cases} S'(t) = -\tau_0 S(t) I(t), \\ I'(t) = \tau_0 S(t) I(t) - \nu I(t). \end{cases} \tag{12.10}$$

By using the S-equation of model (12.10) we obtain

$$S(t) = S_0 \exp\left(-\tau_0 \int_{t_0}^{t} I(\sigma)\mathrm{d}\sigma\right) = S_0 \exp\left(-\tau_0 \mathrm{CI}(t)\right),$$

where $\mathrm{CI}(t)$ is the cumulated number of infectious individuals. Substituting $S(t)$ by this formula in the I-equation of (12.10) we obtain

$$I'(t) = S_0 \exp\left(-\tau_0 \mathrm{CI}(t)\right) \tau_0 \mathrm{CI}'(t) - \nu I(t).$$

Therefore, by integrating the above equation between t and t_0 we obtain

$$\mathrm{CI}'(t) = I_0 + S_0 \left[1 - \exp\left(-\tau_0 \mathrm{CI}(t)\right)\right] - \nu \mathrm{CI}(t). \tag{12.11}$$

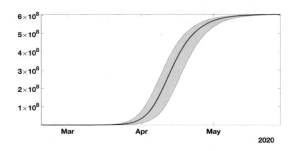

Fig. 12.2: *In this figure, the black curve corresponds to the cumulative number of reported cases* $\mathrm{CR}(t)$ *obtained from the model* (12.10) *with* $\mathrm{CR}'(t) = \nu f I(t)$ *by using the values* $I_0 = 1521$ *and* $\tau_0 = 3.32 \times 10^{-10}$ *obtained from our method and the early data from February 19 to March 1. The blue region corresponds to the 95% confidence interval when the rate of transmission* $\tau(t)$ *is constant and equal to the estimated value* $\tau_0 = 3.32 \times 10^{-10}$.

Remarkably, the equation (12.11) is monotone. We refer to Smith [326] for a comprehensive presentation on monotone systems. By applying a comparison principle to (12.11), we are in a position to confirm our intuition about epidemic SI models. Notice that the monotone properties are only true for the cumulative number of infectious (this is false for the number of infectious).

Theorem 12.3 *Let $t > t_0$ be fixed. The cumulative number of infectious* $\text{CI}(t)$ *is strictly increasing with respect to the following quantities*

(i) $I_0 > 0$, *the initial number of infectious individuals;*
(ii) $S_0 > 0$, *the initial number of susceptible individuals;*
(iii) $\tau > 0$, *the transmission rate;*
(iv) $1/v > 0$, *the average duration of the infectiousness period.*

Error in the estimated initial number of infected and transmission rate

Assume that the parameters χ_1 and χ_2 are estimated with a 95% confidence interval

$$\chi^-_{1,95\%} \leq \chi_1 \leq \chi^+_{1,95\%}$$

and

$$\chi^-_{2,95\%} \leq \chi_2 \leq \chi^+_{2,95\%}.$$

We obtain

$$I^-_{0,95\%} := \frac{\chi^-_{1,95\%}\,\chi^-_{2,95\%}\,e^{\chi^-_{2,95\%}\,t_0}}{v\,f} \leq I_0 \leq I^+_{0,95\%} := \frac{\chi^+_{1,95\%}\,\chi^+_{2,95\%}\,e^{\chi^+_{2,95\%}\,t_0}}{v\,f},$$

$$\tag{12.12}$$

and

$$\tau^-_{0,95\%} := \frac{\chi^-_{2,95\%} + v}{S_0} \leq \tau_0 \leq \tau^+_{0,95\%} := \frac{\chi^+_{2,95\%} + v}{S_0}. \tag{12.13}$$

Remark 12.4 By using the data for mainland China we obtain

$$\chi^-_{1,95\%} = 1.57, \ \chi^+_{1,95\%} = 5.89, \ \chi^-_{2,95\%} = 0.24, \ \chi^+_{2,95\%} = 0.28. \tag{12.14}$$

In Figure 12.2, we plot the upper and lower solutions $\text{CR}^+(t)$ (obtained by using $I_0 = I^+_{0,95\%}$ and $\tau_0 = \tau^+_{0,95\%}$) and $\text{CR}^-(t)$ (obtained by using $I_0 = I^-_{0,95\%}$ and $\tau_0 = \tau^-_{0,95\%}$) corresponding to the blue region and the black curve corresponds to the best estimated value $I_0 = 1521$ and $\tau_0 = 3.3214 \times 10^{-10}$.

Recall that the final size of the epidemic corresponds to the positive equilibrium of (12.11)

$$0 = I_0 + S_0 \left[1 - \exp\left(-\tau_0 \text{CI}_\infty\right)\right] - v\text{CI}_\infty. \tag{12.15}$$

In Figure 12.2 the changes in the parameters I_0 and τ_0 (in (12.12)–(12.13)) do not significantly affect the final size.

12.3 Theoretical Formula For $\tau(t)$

By using the S-equation of model (12.1) we obtain

$$S(t) = S_0 \exp\left(-\int_{t_0}^{t} \tau(\sigma) I(\sigma) d\sigma\right),$$

next by using the I-equation of model (12.1) we obtain

$$I'(t) = S_0 \exp\left(-\int_{t_0}^{t} \tau(\sigma) I(\sigma) d\sigma\right) \tau(t) I(t) - \nu I(t),$$

and by taking the integral between t and t_0 we obtain a Volterra integral equation for the cumulative number of infectious

$$\mathrm{CI}'(t) = I_0 + S_0 \left[1 - \exp\left(-\int_{t_0}^{t} \tau(\sigma) I(\sigma) d\sigma\right)\right] - \nu \mathrm{CI}(t), \tag{12.16}$$

which is equivalent to (by using (12.3))

$$\mathrm{CR}'(t) = \nu f \left(I_0 + S_0 \left[1 - \exp\left(-\frac{1}{\nu f}\int_{t_0}^{t} \tau(\sigma) \mathrm{CR}'(\sigma) d\sigma\right)\right]\right) + \nu \mathrm{CR}_0 - \nu \mathrm{CR}(t). \tag{12.17}$$

The following result permits us to obtain a perfect match between the SI model and the time-dependent rate of transmission $\tau(t)$.

Theorem 12.5 *Let $S_0, \nu, f, I_0 > 0$ and $\mathrm{CR}_0 \geq 0$ be given. Let $t \to I(t)$ be the second component of system (12.1). Let $\widehat{\mathrm{CR}} : [t_0, \infty) \to \mathbb{R}$ be a two times continuously differentiable function satisfying*

$$\widehat{\mathrm{CR}}(t_0) = \mathrm{CR}_0, \tag{12.18}$$

$$\widehat{\mathrm{CR}}'(t_0) = \nu f I_0, \tag{12.19}$$

$$\widehat{\mathrm{CR}}'(t) > 0, \forall t \geq t_0, \tag{12.20}$$

and

$$\nu f (I_0 + S_0) - \widehat{\mathrm{CR}}'(t) - \nu \left(\widehat{\mathrm{CR}}(t) - \mathrm{CR}_0\right) > 0, \forall t \geq t_0. \tag{12.21}$$

Then

$$\widehat{\mathrm{CR}}(t) = \mathrm{CR}_0 + \nu f \int_{t_0}^{t} I(s) \, ds, \forall t \geq t_0 \tag{12.22}$$

if and only if

$$\tau(t) = \frac{\nu f \left(\dfrac{\widehat{\mathrm{CR}}''(t)}{\widehat{\mathrm{CR}}'(t)} + \nu\right)}{\nu f (I_0 + S_0) - \widehat{\mathrm{CR}}'(t) - \nu \left(\widehat{\mathrm{CR}}(t) - \mathrm{CR}_0\right)}. \tag{12.23}$$

Proof Assume first (12.22) is satisfied. Then by using equation (12.16) we deduce that

$$S_0 \exp\left(-\int_{t_0}^{t} \tau(\sigma)I(\sigma)d\sigma\right) = I_0 + S_0 - I(t) - \nu\text{CI}(t).$$

Therefore

$$\int_{t_0}^{t} \tau(\sigma)I(\sigma)d\sigma = \ln\left[\frac{S_0}{I_0 + S_0 - I(t) - \nu\text{CI}(t)}\right]$$

$$= \ln(S_0) - \ln\left[I_0 + S_0 - I(t) - \nu\text{CI}(t)\right]$$

so by taking the derivative on both sides

$$\tau(t)I(t) = \frac{I'(t) + \nu I(t)}{I_0 + S_0 - I(t) - \nu\text{CI}(t)} \Leftrightarrow \tau(t) = \frac{\dfrac{I'(t)}{I(t)} + \nu}{I_0 + S_0 - I(t) - \nu\text{CI}(t)} \quad (12.24)$$

and by using the fact that $\text{CR}(t) - \text{CR}_0 = \nu f \text{CI}(t)$ we obtain (12.23).

Conversely, assume that $\tau(t)$ is given by (12.23). Then if we define $\widetilde{I}(t) = \widehat{\text{CR}}'(t)/\nu f$ and $\widetilde{\text{CI}}(t) = \left(\widehat{\text{CR}}(t) - \text{CR}_0\right)/\nu f$, by using (12.18) we deduce that

$$\widetilde{\text{CI}}(t) = \int_{t_0}^{t} \widetilde{I}(\sigma)d\sigma,$$

and by using (12.19)

$$\widetilde{I}(t_0) = I_0. \quad (12.25)$$

Moreover from (12.23) we deduce that $\widetilde{I}(t)$ satisfies (12.24). By using (12.25) we deduce that $t \to \widetilde{\text{CI}}(t)$ is a solution of (12.16). By uniqueness of the solution of (12.16), we deduce that $\widetilde{\text{CI}}(t) = \text{CI}(t), \forall t \geq t_0$ or equivalently $\text{CR}(t) = \text{CR}_0 + \nu f \int_{t_0}^{t} I(s)\,ds, \forall t \geq t_0$. The proof is complete. $\qquad\square$

The formula (12.23) was already obtained by Hadeler [136, see Corollary 2].

12.4 Explicit Formula For $\tau(t)$ and I_0

Many phenomenological models have been compared to the data during the first phase of the COVID-19 outbreak. We refer to the paper of Tsoularis and Wallace [342] for a nice survey on the generalized logistic equations. Let us consider here, for example, the Bernoulli–Verhulst equation

$$\text{CR}'(t) = \chi_2\,\text{CR}(t)\left(1 - \left(\frac{\text{CR}(t)}{\text{CR}_\infty}\right)^{\theta}\right), \forall t \geq t_0, \quad (12.26)$$

supplemented with the initial data

$$CR(t_0) = CR_0 \geq 0.$$

Let us recall the explicit formula for the solution of (12.26)

$$CR(t) = \frac{e^{\chi_2(t-t_0)} CR_0}{\left[1 + \frac{\chi_2 \theta}{CR_\infty^\theta} \int_{t_0}^t \left(e^{\chi_2(\sigma-t_0)} CR_0\right)^\theta d\sigma\right]^{1/\theta}} = \frac{e^{\chi_2(t-t_0)} CR_0}{\left[1 + \frac{CR_0^\theta}{CR_\infty^\theta} \left(e^{\chi_2 \theta(t-t_0)} - 1\right)\right]^{1/\theta}}.$$

(12.27)

Assumption 12.6 We assume that the cumulative numbers of reported cases $CR_{Data}(t_i)$ are known for a sequence of times $t_0 < t_1 < \cdots < t_{n+1}$.

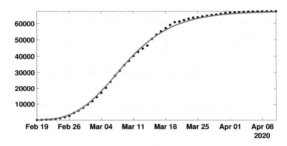

Fig. 12.3: *In this figure, we plot the best fit of the Bernoulli–Verhulst model to the cumulative number of reported cases of COVID-19 in China. We obtain $\chi_2 = 0.66$ and $\theta = 0.22$. The black dots correspond to data for the cumulative number of reported cases and the blue curve corresponds to the model.*

Estimated initial number of infected

By combining (12.3) and the Bernoulli–Verhulst equation (12.26) for $t \to CR(t)$, we deduce the initial number of infected

$$I_0 = \frac{CR'(t_0)}{v f} = \frac{\chi_2 CR_0 \left(1 - \left(\frac{CR_0}{CR_\infty}\right)^\theta\right)}{v f}.$$

(12.28)

Remark 12.7 We fix $f = 0.5$. From the COVID-19 data in mainland China and formula (12.28) (with $CR_0 = 198$), we obtain

$$I_0 = 1909 \text{ for } v = 0.1,$$

and

$$I_0 = 954 \text{ for } v = 0.2.$$

By using (12.26) we deduce that

$$\mathrm{CR}''(t) = \chi_2 \, \mathrm{CR}'(t) \left(1 - \left(\frac{\mathrm{CR}(t)}{\mathrm{CR}_\infty} \right)^\theta \right) - \frac{\chi_2 \theta}{\mathrm{CR}_\infty^\theta} \, \mathrm{CR}(t) \, (\mathrm{CR}(t))^{\theta-1} \, \mathrm{CR}'(t)$$

$$= \chi_2 \, \mathrm{CR}'(t) \left(1 - \left(\frac{\mathrm{CR}(t)}{\mathrm{CR}_\infty} \right)^\theta \right) - \frac{\chi_2 \theta}{\mathrm{CR}_\infty^\theta} \, (\mathrm{CR}(t))^\theta \, \mathrm{CR}'(t),$$

therefore

$$\mathrm{CR}''(t) = \chi_2 \, \mathrm{CR}'(t) \left(1 - (1+\theta) \left(\frac{\mathrm{CR}(t)}{\mathrm{CR}_\infty} \right)^\theta \right). \tag{12.29}$$

Estimated rate of transmission

By using the Bernoulli–Verhulst equation (12.26) and substituting (12.29) in (12.23), we obtain

$$\tau(t) = \frac{v \, f \left(\chi_2 \left(1 - (1+\theta) \left(\frac{\mathrm{CR}(t)}{\mathrm{CR}_\infty} \right)^\theta \right) + v \right)}{v \, f \, (I_0 + S_0) + v \mathrm{CR}_0 - \mathrm{CR}(t) \left(\chi_2 \left(1 - \left(\frac{\mathrm{CR}(t)}{\mathrm{CR}_\infty} \right)^\theta \right) + v \right)}. \tag{12.30}$$

This formula (12.30) combined with (12.27) gives an explicit formula for the rate of transmission.

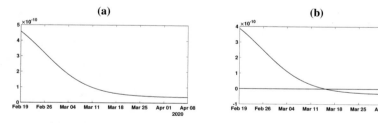

(a) **(b)**

Fig. 12.4: *In this figure, we plot the rate of transmission obtained from formula* (12.30) *with* $f = 0.5$, $\chi_2 \theta = 0.14 < v = 0.2$ *(in Figure (a)) and* $v = 0.1 < \chi_2 \theta = 0.14$ *(in Figure (b)),* $\chi_2 = 0.66$ *and* $\theta = 0.22$ *and* $\mathrm{CR}_\infty = 67102$, *which is the latest value obtained from the cumulative number of reported cases for China.*

Since $\mathrm{CR}(t) < \mathrm{CR}_\infty$, by considering the sign of the numerator and the denominator of (12.30), we obtain the following proposition.

Proposition 12.8 *The rate of transmission $\tau(t)$ given by* (12.30) *is non-negative for all $t \geq t_0$ if*

$$v \geq \chi_2 \, \theta, \tag{12.31}$$

and

$$f \, (I_0 + S_0) + v \mathrm{CR}_0 > \mathrm{CR}_\infty \, (\chi_2 + v) \,. \tag{12.32}$$

Compatibility of the model SI with the COVID-19 data for mainland China

The model SI is compatible with the data only when $\tau(t)$ stays positive for all $t \geq t_0$. From our estimation of the Chinese's COVID-19 data we obtain $\chi_2 \, \theta = 0.14$. Therefore from (12.31) we deduce that model is compatible with the data only when

$$1/v \leq 1/0.14 = 3.3 \text{ days.} \tag{12.33}$$

This means that the average duration of infectious period $1/v$ must be shorter than 3.3 days.

Similarly, the condition (12.32) implies

$$f \geq \frac{\mathrm{CR}_\infty \chi_2 + (\mathrm{CR}_\infty - \mathrm{CR}_0) \, v}{S_0 + I_0} \geq \frac{\mathrm{CR}_\infty \chi_2 + (\mathrm{CR}_\infty - \mathrm{CR}_0) \, \chi_2 \, \theta}{S_0 + I_0}$$

and since we have $CR_0 = 198$ and $\mathrm{CR}_\infty = 67102$, we obtain

$$f \geq \frac{67102 \times 0.66 + (67102 - 198) \times 0.14}{1.4 \times 10^9} \geq 3.83 \times 10^{-5}. \tag{12.34}$$

So according to this estimate, the fraction of unreported $0 < f \leq 1$ can be almost as small as we want.

Figure 12.4 illustrates Proposition 12.8. We observe that the formula for the rate of transmission (12.30) becomes negative whenever $v < \chi_2 \theta$.

In Figure 12.5 we plot the numerical simulation obtained from (12.1)–(12.3) when $t \to \tau(t)$ is replaced by the explicit formula (12.30). Surprisingly, we can perfectly reproduce the original Bernoulli–Verhulst model even when $\tau(t)$ becomes negative. This was not guaranteed at first, since the I-class of individuals loses some individuals which are recovering.

12.5 Computing Numerically a Day-By-Day Piecewise Constant Rate of Transmission

Assumption 12.9 We assume that the rate of transmission $\tau(t)$ is piecewise constant and for each $i = 0, \ldots, n$,

$$\tau(t) = \tau_i, \text{ whenever } t_i \leq t < t_{i+1}. \tag{12.35}$$

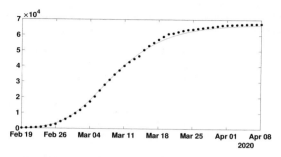

Fig. 12.5: *In this figure, we plot the number of reported cases by using model (12.1) and (12.3), and the rate of transmission is obtained in (12.30). The values of the parameters are $f = 0.5$, $v = 0.1$ or $v = 0.2$, $\chi_2 = 0.66$ and $\theta = 0.22$ and $CR_\infty = 67102$ is the latest value obtained from the cumulative number of reported cases for China. Furthermore, we use $S_0 = 1.4 \times 10^9$ for the total population of China and $I_0 = 954$, which is obtained from formula (12.28). The black dots correspond to data for the cumulative number of reported cases observed and the blue curve corresponds to the model.*

For $t \in [t_{i-1}, t_i]$, we deduce by using Assumption 12.9 that

$$\int_{t_0}^{t} \tau(\sigma) \, CR'(\sigma) d\sigma = \sum_{j=0}^{i-2} \int_{t_j}^{t_{j+1}} \tau_j \, CR'(\sigma) d\sigma + \int_{t_{i-1}}^{t} \tau_{i-1} \, CR'(\sigma) d\sigma.$$

Therefore by using (12.17), for $t \in [t_{i-1}, t_i]$, we obtain

$$CR'(t) = v f \left(I_0 + S_0 \left[1 - \Pi_{i-1} \exp\left(-\frac{\tau_{i-1}}{v f} [CR(t) - CR(t_{i-1})] \right) \right] \right)$$
$$+ v \, CR_0 - vCR(t), \tag{12.36}$$

where

$$\Pi_{i-1} = \exp\left(-\sum_{j=0}^{i-2} \frac{\tau_j}{v f} [CR(t_{j+1}) - CR(t_j)] \right). \tag{12.37}$$

By fixing $\tau_{i-1} = 0$ on the right-hand side of (12.36) we get

$$CR'(t) \geq v f \left(I_0 + S_0 \left[1 - \Pi_{i-1} \right] \right) + v \, CR_0 - vCR(t),$$

and when $\tau_{i-1} \to \infty$ we obtain

$$CR'(t) \leq v f \left(I_0 + S_0 \right) + v \, CR_0 - vCR(t).$$

By using the theory of monotone ordinary differential equations (see Smith [326]) we deduce that the map $\tau_i \to CR(t_i)$ is monotone increasing, and we get the following result.

Theorem 12.10 *Let assumptions 12.1, 12.6 and 12.9 be satisfied. Let I_0 be fixed. Then we can find a unique sequence $\tau_0, \tau_1, \ldots, \tau_n$ of non-negative numbers such that the solution $t \to CR(t)$ of (12.17) fits the data exactly at any time t_i, that is,*

$$CR(t_i) = CR_{Data}(t_i), \forall i = 1, \ldots, n + 1,$$

if and only if the following two conditions are satisfied for each $i = 0, 1, \ldots, n + 1$,

$$CR_{Data}(t_i) \geq e^{-\nu(t_i - t_{i_1})} CR_{Data}(t_{i-1})$$
$$+ \int_{t_{i-1}}^{t_i} \nu e^{-\nu(t_i - \sigma)} d\sigma \left(f \left(I_0 + S_0 \left[1 - \Pi_{i-1}^{Data} \right] \right) + CR_0 \right), \quad (12.38)$$

where

$$\Pi_{i-1}^{Data} = \exp \left(- \sum_{j=0}^{i-2} \frac{\tau_j}{\nu f} \left[CR_{Data}(t_{j+1}) - CR_{Data}(t_j) \right] \right), \quad (12.39)$$

and

$$CR_{Data}(t_i) \leq e^{-\nu(t_i - t_{i_1})} CR_{Data}(t_{i-1}) + \int_{t_{i-1}}^{t_i} \nu e^{-\nu(t_i - \sigma)} d\sigma \left(f \left(I_0 + S_0 \right) + CR_0 \right).$$
$$(12.40)$$

Remark 12.11 The above theorem means that the data are identifiable for this model SI if and only if the conditions (12.38) and (12.40) are satisfied. Moreover, in that case, we can find a unique sequence of transmission rates $\tau_i \geq 0$ which gives a perfect fit to the data.

12.6 Numerical Simulations

In this section, we propose a numerical method to fit the day-by-day rate of transmission. The goal is to take advantage of the monotone property of $CR(t)$ with respect to τ_i on the time interval $[t_i, t_{i+1}]$. Recently more sophisticated methods were proposed by Bakha et al. [23] by using several types of approximation methods for the rate of transmission.

We start with the simplest Algorithm 1 in order to show the difficulties in identifying the rate of transmission.

Algorithm 1

Step 1: *We fix $S_0 = 1.4 \times 10^9$, $\nu = 0.1$ or $\nu = 0.2$ and $f = 0.5$. We consider the system*

$$\begin{cases} S'(t) = -\tau S(t)I(t), \\ I'(t) = \tau S(t)I(t) - \nu I(t), \\ CR'(t) = \nu f I(t) \end{cases} \tag{12.41}$$

on the interval of time $t \in [t_0, t_1]$. This system is supplemented by initial values $S(t_0) = S_0$ and $I(t_0) = I_0$ is given by formula (12.8) (if we consider the data only at the early stage) or formula (12.28) (if we consider all the data) and $CR(t_0) = CR_{Data}(t_0)$ is obtained from the data.

Since the map $\tau \to CR(t_1)$ is monotone increasing, we can apply a bisection method to find the unique value τ_0 solving

$$CR(t_1) = CR_{Data}(t_1).$$

Then we proceed by induction.

Step i: *For each integer $i = 1, \ldots, n$ we consider the system*

$$\begin{cases} S'(t) = -\tau S(t)I(t), \\ I'(t) = \tau S(t)I(t) - \nu I(t), \\ CR'(t) = \nu f I(t) \end{cases} \tag{12.42}$$

on the interval of time $t \in [t_i, t_{i+1}]$. This system is supplemented by initial values $S(t_i)$ and $I(t_i)$ obtained from the previous iteration and with $CR(t_i) = CR_{Data}(t_i)$ obtained from the data.

Since the map $\tau \to CR(t_i)$ is monotone increasing, we can apply a bisection method to find the unique value τ_i solving

$$CR(t_i) = CR_{Data}(t_i).$$

In Figure 12.6, we plot an example of such a perfect fit, which is the same for $\nu = 0.1$ and $\nu = 0.2$. In Figure 12.7 we plot the rate of transmission obtained numerically for $\nu = 0.2$ in (a) and $\nu = 0.1$ in (b). This is an example of a negative rate of transmission. Figure 12.7 should be compared to Figure 12.4, which gives a similar result. In Figures 12.8–12.10 we use Algorithm 1 and we plot the rate of transmission obtained by using the reported cases of COVID-19 in China where the parameters are fixed as $f = 0.5$ and $\nu = 0.2$. In Figures 12.8–12.10, we observe an oscillating rate of transmission alternating back and forth from positive to negative. These oscillations are due to the amplification of the error in the numerical method itself. In Figure 12.8, we run the same simulation as in Figure 12.9 but during a shorter period. In Figure 12.8, we can see that the slope of $CR(t)$ at the $t = t_i$ between two days (the black dots) is amplified from one day to the next.

In Figure 12.10, we first smooth the original cumulative data by using the MAT-LAB function $CR_{Data}=$smoothdata(CR_{Data}, 'gaussian',50) to regularize the data and we apply Algorithm 1. Unfortunately, smoothing the data does not help to solve the instability problem in Figure 12.10.

We need to introduce a correction when choosing the next initial value $I(t_i)$. In Algorithm 1 the errors are due to the following relationship

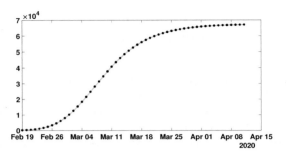

Fig. 12.6: *In this figure, we plot the perfect fit of the cumulative number of reported cases of COVID-19 in China. We fix the parameters $f = 0.5$ and $v = 0.2$ or $v = 0.1$ and we apply our algorithm 1 to obtain the perfect fit. The black dots correspond to data for the cumulative number of reported cases and the blue curve corresponds to the model.*

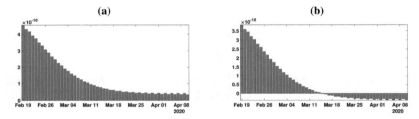

Fig. 12.7: *In this figure, we plot the rate of transmission obtained for the reported cases of COVID-19 in China with the parameters $f = 0.5$ and $v = 0.2$ in figure (a) and $v = 0.1$ in figure (b). This rate of transmission corresponds to the perfect fit obtained in Figure 12.6.*

$$CR'(t) = v f I(t)$$

not being respected at the points $t = t_i$, which should be reflected by the algorithm.

In Figure 12.11, we smooth the data first by using the MATLAB function CR_{Data}=smoothdata(CR_{Data},'gaussian',50), and we apply Algorithm 2 by approximating equation (12.46) by

$$I_i = [CR_{Data}(t_i) - CR_{Data}(t_{i-1})]/(v \times f). \tag{12.43}$$

In Figure 12.11 we no longer observe the oscillations of the rate of transmission.

Algorithm 2

We fix $S_0 = 1.4 \times 10^9$, $v = 0.1$ or $v = 0.2$ and $f = 0.5$. Then we fit the data by using the method described in Section 12.2 to estimate the parameters χ_1, χ_2 and χ_3 from

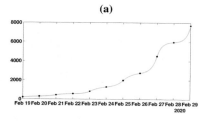
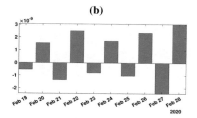

Fig. 12.8: *In figure (a), we plot the cumulative number of reported cases obtained from the data (black dots) and the model (blue curve). In figure (b), we plot the daily rate of transmission obtained by using Algorithm 1. We see that we can fit the data perfectly, but the method is very unstable. We obtain a rate of transmission that oscillates from positive to negative values back and forth.*

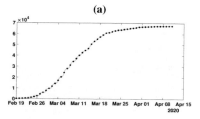
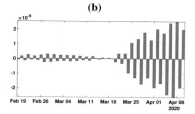

Fig. 12.9: *In figure (a), we plot the cumulative number of reported cases obtained from the data (black dots) and the model (blue curve). In figure (b), we plot the daily rate of transmission obtained by using Algorithm 1. We see that we can fit the data perfectly, but the method is very unstable. We obtain a rate of transmission that oscillates from positive to negative values back and forth.*

day 1 to 10. Then we use

$$S_0 = 1.40005 \times 10^9,$$
$$I_0 = \chi_2 \chi_1 \left[\exp(\chi_2 (t_0 - 1)) \right] / (f \, v), \qquad (12.44)$$
$$CR_0 = \chi_1 \exp(\chi_2 t_0) - \chi_3.$$

For each integer $i = 0, \ldots, n$, we consider the system

$$\begin{cases} S'(t) = -\tau S(t) I(t), \\ I'(t) = \tau S(t) I(t) - v I(t), \\ CR'(t) = v f I(t) \end{cases} \qquad (12.45)$$

for $t \in [t_i, t_{i+1}]$. Then since the map $\tau \to CR(t_{i+1})$ is monotone increasing, we can apply a bisection method to find the unique τ_i solving

$$CR(t_{i+1}) = CR_{\text{Data}}(t_{i+1}).$$

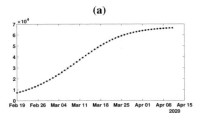
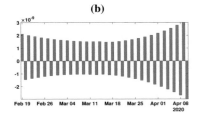

Fig. 12.10: *We apply Algorithm 1 to the regularized data. In figure (a), we plot the regularized cumulative number of reported cases obtained from the data (black dots) and the model (blue curve). In figure (b), we plot the daily rate of transmission obtained by using Algorithm 1. We see that we can fit the data perfectly, but the method is very unstable. We obtain a rate of transmission that oscillates from positive to negative values back and forth.*

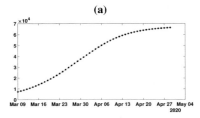
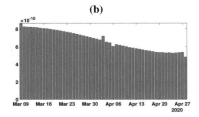

Fig. 12.11: *In this figure, we plot the rate of transmission obtained by using the reported cases of COVID-19 in China with the parameters $f = 0.5$ and $v = 0.2$. We first regularize the data by applying the MATLAB function $CR_{Data}=smoothdata(CR_{Data}, 'gaussian',50)$. Then we apply Algorithm 2 to the regularized data. In figure (a), we plot the regularized cumulative number of reported cases obtained after smoothing (black dots) and the model (blue curve). In figure (b), we plot the daily rate of transmission obtained by using Algorithm 2. We see that we can fit the data perfectly and this time the rate of transmission is becoming reasonable.*

The key idea of this new algorithm is the following correction on the I-component of the system. We start a new step by using the value $S(t_i)$ obtained from the previous iteration together with

$$I_i = CR'_{Data}(t_i)/(v\,f) \qquad (12.46)$$

and

$$CR_i = CR_{Data}(t_i). \qquad (12.47)$$

In Figure 12.12 we plot several types of regularized cumulative data in figure (a) and several types of regularized daily data in figure (b). Among the different regularization methods, an important one is the Bernoulli–Verhulst best fit approximation. In Figure 12.13 we plot the rate of transmission $t \rightarrow \tau(t)$ obtained by using Algorithm 2. We can see that the original data gives a negative transmission rate while at the other extreme the Bernoulli–Verhulst regularization seems to give the most regularized transmission rate. In Figure 12.13-(a) we observe that we now

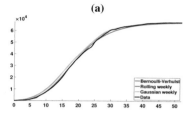
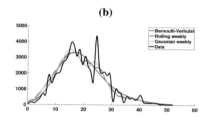

Fig. 12.12: *In this figure, we plot the cumulative number of reported cases (left) and the daily number of reported cases (right). The black curves are obtained by applying the cubic spline Matlab function spline(Days,DATA) to the cumulative data. The left-hand side is obtained by using the cubic spline function and the right-hand side is obtained by using the derivative of the cubic spline interpolation. The blue curves are obtained by applying the cubic spline function to the day-by-day values of the cumulative number of cases obtained from the best fit of the Bernoulli–Verhulst model. The orange curves are obtained by computing the rolling weekly daily number of cases (we use the Matlab function smoothdata(DAILY,'movmean',7)) and then by applying the cubic spline function the corresponding cumulative number of cases. The yellow curves are obtained by Gaussian the rolling weekly to the daily number of cases (we use the Matlab function smoothdata(DAILY,'gaussian',7)) and then by applying the cubic spline function to the corresponding cumulative number of cases.*

recover almost perfectly the theoretical transmission rate obtained in Section 12.4. In Figure 12.13-(b) the rolling weekly average regularization and in Figure 12.13-(c) the Gaussian weekly average regularization still vary a lot and in both cases, the transmission rate becomes negative after some time. In Figure 12.13-(c) the original data gives a transmission rate that is negative from the beginning. We conclude that it is crucial to find a "good" regularization of the daily number of cases. So far the best regularization method is obtained by using the best fit of the Bernoulli–Verhulst model.

Remark 12.12 For each simulation Figure 12.13-(b) and Figure 12.13-(c), it is possible to obtain a transmission $t \to \tau(t)$ that is non-negative for all time t by increasing the parameter v sufficiently. Nevertheless, we do not present these simulations here because the corresponding values of v to obtain a non-negative $\tau(t)$ are unrealistic.

In Figure 12.14 (a), (b), (c) and (d) (respectively) we plot the daily basic reproduction number corresponding to the Figure 12.13 (a), (b), (c) and (d) (respectively). The red line corresponds to $R_0 = 1$. We see some complex behavior for the Figure 12.14 (b) and (c) and the figure (d) is again unrealistic.

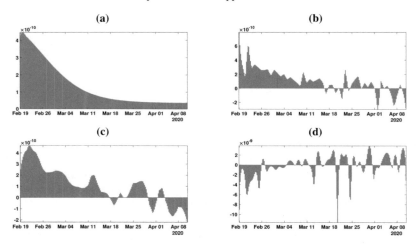

Fig. 12.13: *In this figure we plot the transmission rates $t \rightarrow \tau(t)$ obtained by using Algorithm 2 with the parameters $f = 0.5$ and $v = 0.2$. In figure (a) we use the cumulative data obtained by using the Bernoulli–Verhulst regularization. In figure (b) we use the cumulative data obtained by using the rolling weekly average regularization. In figure (c) we use the cumulative data obtained by using the Gaussian weekly average regularization. In figure (d) we use the original cumulative data.*

12.7 Discussion

Estimating the parameters of an epidemiological model is always difficult and generally requires strong assumptions about their value and their consistency and constancy over time. Despite this, it is often shown that many sets of parameter values are compatible with a good fit of the observed data. The new approach developed in this chapter consists first of all in postulating a phenomenological model of growth of infectious, based on the very classical model of Verhulst, proposed in demography in 1838 [347]. Then, obtaining explicit formulas for important parameter values such as the transmission rate or the initial number of infected (or for lower and/or upper limits of these values) gives an estimate allowing an almost perfect reconstruction of the observed dynamics.

The use of phenomenological models can also be regarded as a way of smoothing the data. Indeed, the errors concerning the observations of newly infected cases are numerous:

- the census is rarely regular and many countries report late cases that occurred during the weekend and at varying times over-add data from specific counts, such as those from homes for the elderly;
- the number of cases observed is still underestimated and the calculation of cases not reported as new cases of infected is always a difficult problem [207];
- the raw data are sometimes reduced for medical reasons of poor diagnosis or lack of detection tools, or for reasons of domestic policy of states.

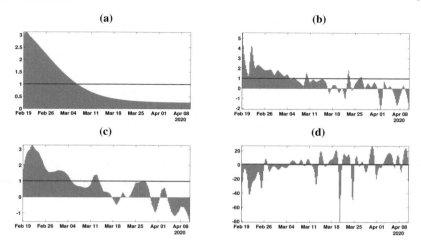

Fig. 12.14: *In this figure we plot the daily basic reproduction number $t \to R_0(t) = \tau(t)S(t)/\nu$ obtained by using Algorithm 2 with the parameters $f = 0.5$ and $\nu = 0.2$. In figure (a) we use the cumulative data obtained by using the Bernoulli–Verhulst regularization. In figure (b) we use the cumulative data obtained by using the rolling weekly average regularization. In figure (c) we use the cumulative data obtained by using the Gaussian weekly average regularization. In figure (d) we use the original cumulative data.*

For all these causes of error, it is important to choose the appropriate smoothing method (moving average, spline, Gaussian kernel, auto-regression, generalized linear model, etc.). In this article, several methods were used and the one which allowed the model to perfectly match the smoothed data was retained.

In this chapter, we developed several methods to understand how to reconstruct the rate of transmission from the data. In Section 12.2, we reconsidered the method presented in [207] based on an exponential fit of the early data. The approach gives a first estimation of I_0 and τ_0. In Section 12.3, we prove a result to connect the time-dependent cumulative reported data and the transmission rate. In Section 12.4, we compare the data to the Bernoulli–Verhulst model and we use this model as a phenomenological model. The Bernoulli–Verhulst model fits the data for mainland China very well. Next by replacing the data with the solution of the Bernoulli–Verhulst model, we obtain an explicit formula for the transmission rate. So we derive some conditions on the parameters for the applicability of the SI model to the data for mainland China. In Section 12.5, we discretized the rate of transmission and we observed that given some daily cumulative data, we can get at most one perfect fit of the data. Therefore, in Section 12.6, we provide two algorithms to numerically compute the daily rates of transmission. Such numerical questions turn out to be delicate. This problem was previously considered by another French group, Bakhta, Boiveau, Maday and Mula [23]. Here we use some simple ideas to approach the derivative of the cumulative reported cases combined with some smoothing methods applied to the data.

To conclude this chapter we plot the daily basic reproduction number

$$R_0(t) = \frac{\tau(t)S(t)}{\nu}$$

as a function of the time t and the parameters f or ν. The above simple formula for R_0 is not the real basic reproductive number in the sense of the number of newly infected produced by a single infectious, but it gives the tendency of the growth or decay of the number of infectious. In Figure 12.14-(a), the daily basic reproduction number is almost independent of f, while in Figure 12.14-(b), $R_0(t)$ is dependent on ν mostly for small values of ν. The red curve on each surface in Figure 12.14 corresponds to the turning point (i.e. the time $t \geq t_0$ for which $R_0(t) = 1$). We also see that the turning point does not depend much on these parameters.

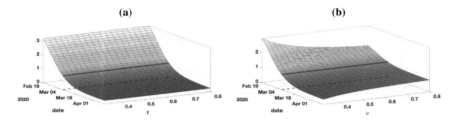

Fig. 12.15: *In this figure we plot the daily basic reproduction number $R_0(t) = \frac{\tau(t)S(t)}{\nu}$ and we vary the parameter f (left) and ν (right).*

Concerning contagious diseases, public health physicians are constantly facing four challenges. The first concerns the estimation of the average transmission rate. Until now, no explicit formula had been obtained in the case of the SIR model, according to the observed data of the epidemic, that is to say, the number of reported cases of infected patients. Here, from realistic simplifying assumptions, a formula is provided (formula (12.30)), making it theoretically possible to accurately reconstruct the curve of the observed cumulative cases. The second challenge concerns the estimation of the mean duration of the infectious period for infected patients. As for the transmission rate, the same realistic assumptions make it possible to obtain an upper limit for this duration (inequality (12.33)), which makes it possible to better guide the individual quarantine measures decided by the authorities in charge of public health. This upper bound also makes it possible to obtain a lower bound for the percentage of unreported infected patients (inequality (12.33)), which gives an idea of the quality of the census of cases of infected patients, which is the third challenge faced by epidemiologists, specialists of contagious diseases. The fourth challenge is the estimation of the average transmission rate for each day of the infectious period (dependent on the distribution of the transmission over the "ages" of infectivity), which will be the subject of further work and which poses formidable problems, in particular those related to the (biological or civil) age class of the patients concerned. Another interesting prospect is the extension of the methods developed in the present chapter to contagious non-infectious diseases (i.e., without a causal infectious agent), such as social contagious diseases, the best example being that of the pandemic linked to obesity [78, 79, 80], for which many concepts and modeling methods remain available.

12.8 Supplementary Tables

We use cumulative reported data from the National Health Commission of the People's Republic of China and the Chinese CDC for mainland China. Before February 11, the data was based on confirmed testing. From February 11 to February 15, the data included cases that were not tested for the virus but were clinically diagnosed based on medical imaging showing signs of pneumonia. There were 17,409 such cases from February 10 to February 15. The data from February 10 to February 15 specified both types of reported cases. From February 16, the data did not separate the two types of reporting but reported the sum of both types. We subtracted 17,409 cases from the cumulative reported cases after February 15 to obtain the cumulative reported cases based only on confirmed testing after February 15. The data is given in Table 2 with this adjustment.

January						
19	20	21	22	23	24	25
198	291	440	571	830	1287	1975
26	27	28	29	30	31	
2744	4515	5974	7711	9692	11791	
February						
1	2	3	4	5	6	7
14380	17205	20438	24324	28018	31161	34546
8	9	10	11	12	13	14
37198	40171	42638	44653	46472	48467	49970
15	16	17	18	19	20	21
51091	70548 − 17409	72436 − 17409	74185 − 17409	75002 − 17409	75891 − 17409	76288 − 17409
22	23	24	25	26	27	28
76936 − 17409	77150 − 17409	77658 − 17409	78064 − 17409	78497 − 17409	78824 − 17409	79251 − 17409
29						
79824 − 17409						
March						
1	2	3	4	5	6	7
79824 − 17409	79824 − 17409	79824 − 17409	80409 − 17409	80552 − 17409	80651 − 17409	80695 − 17409
8	9	10	11	12	13	14
80735 − 17409	80754 − 17409	80778 − 17409	80793 − 17409	80813 − 17409	80824 − 17409	80844 − 17409
15	16	17	18			
80860 − 17409	80881 − 17409	80894 − 17409	80928 − 17409			

Table 12.1: *Cumulative data describing confirmed cases in mainland China from January 20, 2020 to March 18, 2020. The data are taken from various sources.*

Chapter 13
A Robust Phenomenological Approach to Investigating COVID-19 Data for France

This chapter was published as a paper by Demongeot, Griette and Magal [122]. The method presented in this chapter has been extended and successfully applied to cumulative data on reported cases of COVID-19 for seven countries and the state of California in Griette, Demongeot and Magal [123].

13.1 Introduction

Modeling endemic and epidemic phases of infectious diseases such as smallpox, which by the 16th century had become a predominant cause of mortality in Europe until the vaccination by E. Jenner in 1796, and the present Covid-19 pandemic outbreak, has always been a means of describing and predicting disease. Daniel Bernoulli proposed in 1760 a differential model [28], taking into account the virulence of the infectious agent and the mortality of the host, which showed a logistic formula [28, p.13] of the same type as the logistic equation of Verhulst [347]. The succession of an epidemic phase followed by an endemic phase had been introduced by Bernoulli and, for example, appears clearly in Figures 9 and 10 in [90].

The aim of this chapter is to propose a new approach to compare epidemic models with data from reported cumulative cases. Here we propose a phenomenological model to fit the observed data of cumulative infectious cases of COVID-19 that describes the successive epidemic phases and endemic intermediate phases. This type of problem dates back to the 1970s with the work of London and Yorke [212]. More recently, Chowell et al. [56] have proposed a specific function to model the temporal transmission speeds $\tau(t)$. In the context of COVID-19, a two-phase model has been proposed by Liu et al. [209] to describe the South Korean data with an epidemic phase followed by an endemic phase.

In this chapter, we use a phenomenological model to fit the data (see Figure 13.1). The phenomenological model is used in the modeling process between the data and the epidemic models. The difficulty here is to propose a simple phenomenological model (with a limited number of parameters) that would give a meaningful result for the time-dependent transmission rates $\tau(t)$. Many models could potentially be used as phenomenological models to represent the data (e.g. cubic spline and others). The major difficulty here is to provide a model that gives a good description of the tendency for the data. It has been observed in our previous work that it is difficult to choose between the possible phenomenological models (see Figures 12–14 in [77]). The phenomenological model can also be viewed as a regularization of data that should not fluctuate too much to keep the essential information. An advantage in our phenomenological model is the limited number of parameters (five parameters during each epidemic phase and two parameters during each endemic phase). The last advantage of our approach is that once the phenomenological model has been chosen, we can compute an explicit formula for the transmission rate and derive some estimates for the other parameters.

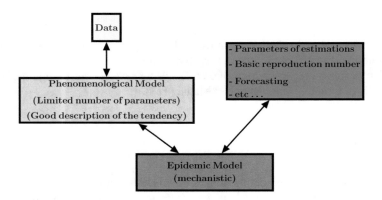

Fig. 13.1: *We can apply statistical methods to estimate the parameters of the proposed phenomenological model and derive their average values with some confidence intervals. The phenomenological model is used at the first step of the modeling process, providing regularized data to the epidemic model and allowing the identification of its parameters.*

13.2 Material and Methods

13.2.1 Phenomenological model

In this chapter, the phenomenological model is compared with the cumulative reported case data taken from WHO.[1] The phenomenological model deals with data series of new infectious cases decomposed into two types of successive phases, 1) endemic phases, followed by 2) epidemic phases.

---

[1] Data from WHO. Accessed: June 9, 2021. `https://covid19.who.int/WHO-COVID-19-global-data.csv`

Endemic phase: During the endemic phase, the dynamics of new cases appear to fluctuate around an average value independently of the number of cases. Therefore the average cumulative number of cases is given by

$$CR(t) = N_0 + (t - t_0) \times a, \text{ for } t \in [t_0, t_1], \tag{13.1}$$

where t_0 denotes the beginning of the endemic phase. a is the average value of $CR(t_0)$ and N_0 the average value of the daily number of new cases.

In other words, we assume that the average daily number of new cases is constant. Therefore the daily number of new cases is given by

$$CR'(t) = a. \tag{13.2}$$

Epidemic phase: In the epidemic phase, the new cases contribute to produce secondary cases. Therefore the daily number of new cases is no longer constant but varies with time as follows

$$CR(t) = N_{\text{base}} + N(t), \text{ for } t \in [t_0, t_1], \tag{13.3}$$

where

$$N(t) = \frac{e^{\chi(t-t_0)} N_0}{\left[1 + \dfrac{N_0^\theta}{N_\infty^\theta} \left(e^{\chi\theta(t-t_0)} - 1\right)\right]^{1/\theta}}. \tag{13.4}$$

In other words, the daily number of new cases follows the Bernoulli–Verhulst [28, 347] equation. Namely, by setting $N(t) = CR(t) - N_{\text{base}}$ we obtain

$$N'(t) = \chi N(t) \left[1 - \left(\frac{N(t)}{N_\infty}\right)^\theta\right] \tag{13.5}$$

with the initial value

$$N(t_0) = N_0. \tag{13.6}$$

In the model $N_{\text{base}} + N_0$ corresponds to the value $CR(t_0)$ of the cumulative number of cases at time $t = t_0$. The parameter $N_\infty + N_{\text{base}}$ is the maximal increase of the cumulative reported case after the time $t = t_0$. $\chi > 0$ is a Malthusian growth parameter, and θ regulates the speed at which the $CR(t)$ increases to $N_\infty + N_{\text{base}}$.

Regularized model

Because the formula for $\tau(t)$ involves derivatives of the phenomenological model regularizing $CR(t)$ (see equation (13.13)), we need to connect the phenomenological models of the different phases as smoothly as possible. We let $\widetilde{CR}(t)$ be the model obtained by placing phenomenological models side by side for different phases. Outside of the time window where phenomenological models are used, we consider the function $\widetilde{CR}(t)$ to be constant. We define the regularized model by using the convolution formula:

$$\text{CR}(t) = \int_{-\infty}^{+\infty} \widetilde{\text{CR}}(t-s) \times \frac{1}{\sigma\sqrt{2\pi}} e^{-\frac{s^2}{2\sigma^2}} \, ds = (\widetilde{\text{CR}} * \mathcal{G})(t), \qquad (13.7)$$

where $\mathcal{G}(t) := \frac{1}{\sigma\sqrt{2\pi}} e^{-\frac{t^2}{2\sigma^2}}$ is the Gaussian function with variance σ^2. The parameter σ controls the trade-off between smoothness and precision: increasing σ reduces the variations in $\text{CR}(t)$ and decreasing σ reduces the distance between $\text{CR}(t)$ and $\widetilde{\text{CR}}(t)$. In any case the resulting function $\text{CR}(t)$ is very smooth (as well as its derivatives) and close to the original model $\widetilde{\text{CR}}(t)$ when σ is not too large. In numerical applications, we take $\sigma = 2$ days.

Remark 13.1 Numerically, we can compute some derivatives of $t \to \text{CR}(t)$. Therefore it is convenient to take advantage of the convolution (13.7) and deduce that

$$\frac{d^n \text{CR}(t)}{dt^n} = \int_{-\infty}^{+\infty} \frac{d^n \mathcal{G}(t-s)}{dt^n} \times \widetilde{\text{CR}}(s) ds,$$

for $n = 1, 2, 3$.

Procedure to fit the phenomenological model to the data

To fit the model to the data, we used the regularized model (13.7) where the periods of the different phases are fixed as in Table 13.1. We use a standard curve-fitting algorithm to find the parameters of the regularized model. In numerical applications we used the Levenberg–Marquardt nonlinear least-squares algorithm provided by the MATLAB function `fit`. Our 95% confidence intervals are the ones provided as an output of this algorithm. The best-fit parameters and the corresponding confidence intervals are provided in Table 13.1.

13.2.2 SI Epidemic model

The SI epidemic model used in this work is the same as in [77] (see Chapter 12). It is summarized by the flux diagram in Figure 13.2.

The goal of this chapter is to understand how to compare the SI model to the reported epidemic data, and therefore the model can be used to predict the future evolution of epidemic spread and to test various possible scenarios of social mitigation measures. For $t \geq t_0$, the SI model is the following

$$\begin{cases} S'(t) = -\tau(t)S(t)I(t), \\ I'(t) = \tau(t)S(t)I(t) - \nu I(t), \end{cases} \qquad (13.8)$$

where $S(t)$ is the number of susceptible and $I(t)$ the number of infectious at time t. This system is supplemented by initial data

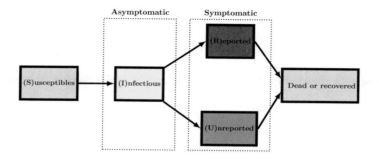

Fig. 13.2: *Schematic view showing the different compartments and transition arrows in the epidemic model.*

$$S(t_0) = S_0 \geq 0, \; I(t_0) = I_0 \geq 0. \qquad (13.9)$$

In this model, the rate of transmission $\tau(t)$ combines the number of contacts per unit of time and the probability of transmission. The transmission of the pathogen from the infectious to the susceptible individuals is described by a mass action law $\tau(t) S(t) I(t)$ (which is also the flux of new infectious).

The quantity $1/\nu$ is the average duration of the infectious period, and $\nu I(t)$ is the flux of recovering or dying individuals. At the end of the infectious period, we assume that a fraction $f \in (0, 1]$ of the infectious individuals are reported. Let $CR(t)$ be the cumulative number of reported cases. We assume that

$$CR(t) = CR_0 + \nu f \, CI(t), \text{ for } t \geq t_0, \qquad (13.10)$$

where

$$CI(t) = \int_{t_0}^{t} I(\sigma)\mathrm{d}\sigma. \qquad (13.11)$$

Assumption 13.2 (Given parameters) We assume that

- the number of susceptible individuals when we start to use the model, $S_0 = 67$ million;
- the average duration of infectious period, $\dfrac{1}{\nu} = 3$ days;
- the fraction of reported individuals, $f = 0.9$,

are known parameters.

Parameters estimated in the simulations: As described in [77] (see Chapter 12) the number of infectious at time t_0 is

$$I_0 = \frac{CR'(t_0)}{\nu f}. \qquad (13.12)$$

The rate of transmission $\tau(t)$ at time t is given by

$$\tau(t) = \frac{v f \left(\dfrac{CR''(t)}{CR'(t)} + v \right)}{v f \left(I_0 + S_0 \right) - CR'(t) - v \left(CR(t) - CR_0 \right)}.$$ (13.13)

Parameters estimated in the endemic phase: The initial number of infectious is given by

$$I_0 = \frac{a}{v f},$$

and the transmission rate is given by the explicit formula

$$\tau(t) = \frac{v^2 f}{v f \left(I_0 + S_0 \right) - a - v(t - t_0) \times a}, \forall t \in [t_0, t_1].$$

Parameters estimated in the epidemic phase: The initial number of infectious is given by

$$I_0 = \frac{\chi N_0 \left[1 - \left(\dfrac{N_0}{N_\infty} \right)^\theta \right]}{v f},$$

and the transmission rate is given by the explicit formula

$$\tau(t) = \frac{v f \left(\dfrac{N''(t)}{N'(t)} + v \right)}{v f \left(I_0 + S_0 \right) - N'(t) - v \left(N(t) - N_0 \right)},$$

and since (recall (13.5))

$$N'(t) = \chi N(t) \left[1 - \left(\frac{N(t)}{N_\infty} \right)^\theta \right]$$

and

$$N''(t) = \chi N'(t) \left[1 - (1 + \theta) \left(\frac{N(t)}{N_\infty} \right)^\theta \right],$$ (13.14)

we obtain an explicit formula

$$\tau(t) = \frac{v f \left(\chi \left[1 - (1 + \theta) \left(\dfrac{N(t)}{N_\infty} \right)^\theta \right] + v \right)}{v f \left(I_0 + S_0 \right) - \chi N(t) \left[1 - \left(\dfrac{N(t)}{N_\infty} \right)^\theta \right] - v \left(N(t) - N_0 \right)},$$ (13.15)

where $N(t)$ is given by (13.4):

$$N(t) = \frac{e^{\chi(t-t_0)} N_0}{\left[1 + \frac{N_0^\theta}{N_\infty^\theta} \left(e^{\chi\theta(t-t_0)} - 1 \right) \right]^{1/\theta}} \cdot$$

Using the Bernoulli–Verhulst model to represent the data, the daily number of new cases is nothing but the derivative $N'(t)$ (whenever the unit of time is one day). The daily number of new cases reaches its maximum at the turning point $t = t_p$, and by using (13.14), we obtain

$$N''(t_p) = 0 \Leftrightarrow N(t_p) = \left(\frac{1}{1+\theta} \right)^{1/\theta} N_\infty.$$

Therefore by using (13.5), the maximum of the daily number of cases equals

$$N'(t_p) = \chi N(t_p) \left[1 - \left(\frac{N(t_p)}{N_\infty} \right)^\theta \right].$$

By using the above formula, we obtain a new indicator for the amplitude of the epidemic.

Theorem 13.3 *The maximal daily number of cases in the course of the epidemic phase is given by*

$$\chi \times N_\infty \times \theta \times \left(\frac{1}{1+\theta} \right)^{\frac{1}{\theta}+1}. \tag{13.16}$$

13.2.3 Parameter bounds

The epidemic model (13.8) with time-dependent transmission rate is consistent only insofar as the transmission rate remains positive. This gives us a criterion to judge if a set of epidemic parameters has a chance of being consistent with the observed data: since we know the parameters N_0, N_∞, χ and θ from the phenomenological model, the formula (13.15) allows us to compute a criterion on v and f which decides whether a given set of parameter values is compatible with the observed data or not. That is, a set of parameter values is compatible if the transmission rate $\tau(t)$ in (13.15) remains positive for all $t \geq t_0$, and it is not compatible if the sign of $\tau(t)$ in (13.15) changes for some $t \geq t_0$. We refer to Proposition 12.8 for more results.

The value of the parameter v is compatible with the model (13.15) if and only if

$$0 \leq \frac{1}{v} \leq \frac{1}{\chi\theta}, \tag{13.17}$$

and the value of the parameter f is compatible with the model (13.15) if and only if

$$f \geq \frac{N_\infty - N_0}{I_0 + S_0}. \tag{13.18}$$

Therefore, we obtain information on the parameters v and f, even though they are not directly identifiable (two different values of v or f can produce exactly the same cumulative reported cases).

13.2.4 Computation of the basic reproduction number

In order to compute the reproduction number in Figure 13.5 we use Algorithm 2 in Chapter 12 and the day-by-day values of the phenomenological model.

13.3 Results

13.3.1 Phenomenological model compared to the French data

In Figure 13.3, we present the best fit of our phenomenological model for the cumulative reported case data of the COVID-19 epidemic in France. The yellow regions correspond to the endemic phases, and the blue regions correspond to the epidemic phases. Here we consider the two epidemic waves for France, and the chosen period, as well as the parameters values for each period, are listed in Table 13.1. In Table 13.1 we also give 95% confidence intervals for the fitted parameters values.

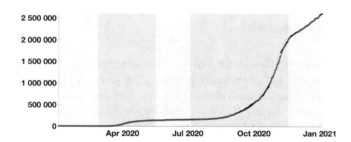

Fig. 13.3: *The red curve corresponds to the phenomenological model and the black dots correspond to the cumulative number of reported cases in France.*

Figure 13.4 shows the corresponding daily number of new reported case data (black dots) and the first derivative of our phenomenological model (red curve).

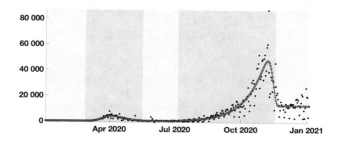

Fig. 13.4: *The red curve corresponds to the first derivative of the phenomenological model and the black dots correspond to daily number of new reported cases in France.*

Period	Parameters value	Method	95% Confidence interval
Period 1: Endemic phase Jan 03 - Feb 27	$N_0 = -4.368$ $a = 1.099 \times 10^{-1}$	computed fitted	$a \in [-8.582 \times 10^1, 8.604 \times 10^1]$
Period 2: Epidemic phase Feb 27 - May 17	$N_{base} = 0$ $N_0 = 1.675$ $N_\infty = 1.445 \times 10^5$ $\chi = 1.263$ $\theta = 6.315 \times 10^{-2}$	fixed fitted fitted fitted fitted	$N_0 \in [-3.807 \times 10^1, 4.142 \times 10^1]$ $N_\infty \in [1.367 \times 10^5, 1.523 \times 10^5]$ $\chi \in [-1.171 \times 10^1, 1.424 \times 10^1]$ $\theta \in [-6.086 \times 10^{-1}, 7.349 \times 10^{-1}]$
Period 3: Endemic phase May 17 - Jul 05	$N_0 = 1.405 \times 10^5$ $a = 3.11 \times 10^2$	computed computed	
Period 4: Epidemic phase Jul 05 - Nov 18	$N_{base} = 1.403 \times 10^5$ $N_0 = 1.517 \times 10^4$ $N_\infty = 1.953 \times 10^6$ $\chi = 3.671 \times 10^{-2}$ $\theta = 7.679$	fitted fitted fitted fitted fitted	$N_{base} \in [1.367 \times 10^5, 1.439 \times 10^5]$ $N_0 \in [1.427 \times 10^4, 1.607 \times 10^4]$ $N_\infty \in [1.92 \times 10^6, 1.986 \times 10^6]$ $\chi \in [3.62 \times 10^{-2}, 3.722 \times 10^{-2}]$ $\theta \in [6.256, 9.102]$
Period 5: Endemic phase Nov 18 - Jan 04	$N_0 = 4.45 \times 10^{-84}$ $a = 1.099 \times 10^{-1}$	computed fitted	$a \in [1.222 \times 10^4, 1.265 \times 10^4]$

Table 13.1: *Fitted parameters and computed parameters for the whole epidemic going from January 03 2020 to January 04 2021.*

13.3.2 SI epidemic model compared to the French data

Some parameters of the model are known, for instance $S_0 = 67$ million for France (although this is questionable). Some parameters of the epidemic model cannot be precisely evaluated [77].

> **Result**
>
> By using (13.17) we obtain the following conditions for the average duration of the infectious period
>
> - $0 < \dfrac{1}{\nu} \leq 1/(\chi\theta) = 12.5$ days during the first epidemic wave;
> - $0 < \dfrac{1}{\nu} \leq 1/(\chi\theta) = 3.5$ days during the second epidemic wave.
>
> We obtain no constraint for the fraction $f \in (0, 1]$ of reported new cases (between 0 and 1 for France).
>
> Moreover by using the formula (13.16) we deduce that the maximal daily number of cases is
>
> - 4110 during the first epidemic wave;
> - 47875 during the second epidemic wave.

Importantly, by combining the phenomenological model from Section 13.3.1 and the epidemiological model from Section 13.2.2, we can reconstruct the time-dependent transmission rate given by (13.13) and the corresponding time-dependent basic reproduction number $\mathcal{R}_0(t) = \tau(t)S(t)/\nu$ (sometimes called the "effective basic reproductive ratio"). The obtained basic reproduction number is presented in Figure 13.5. We observe that $\mathcal{R}_0(t)$ is decreasing during each epidemic wave, except at the very end where it becomes increasing. This is not necessarily surprising since the lockdown becomes less strictly respected towards the end. During the endemic phases, $\mathcal{R}_0(t)$ becomes effectively equal to one, except again near the end. The variations observed close to the transition between two phases may be partially due to the smoothing method, which has an impact on the size of the "bumps". However, they remain very limited in number and size.

13.4 Discussion

In this chapter, we use a phenomenological model to reduce the number of parameters necessary for summarizing observed data without loss of pertinent information. The process of reduction consists of three stages: qualitative or quantitative detection of the boundaries between the different phases of the dynamics (here endemic and epidemic phases), choice of a reduction model (among different possible approaches: logistic, regression polynomials, splines, autoregressive time series, etc.) and smoothing of the derivatives at the boundary points corresponding to the breaks in the model.

In Figure 13.3, we have a very good agreement between the data and the phenomenological model for both the original curve and its derivative. The relative error in Figure 13.3 is of order 10^{-2}, which means that the error is at most of the order of

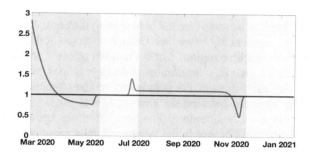

Fig. 13.5: *In this figure we plot the time-dependent basic reproduction number* $\mathcal{R}_0(t) := \tau(t)S(t)/\nu$. *We fix the average length of the asymptotic infectious period to 3 days. Notice that, in contrast to Figure 13.3 and 13.4, we do not plot the first endemic phase because the basic reproduction number is meaningless before the first wave.*

100 000 individuals. In Figure 13.4 the red curve also gives a good tendency of the black dots corresponding to raw data.

In Figure 13.5, the phenomenological models are necessary to derive a significant basic reproduction number. Otherwise, the resulting $\mathcal{R}_0(t)$ is not interpretable and even not computable after some time. Similar results were obtained in Figures 12–14 in [77]. The method to compute $\mathcal{R}_0$ can also be applied directly to the original data. We did not show the result here because the noise in the data is amplified by the method, and the results are not usable. This shows that it is important to use the phenomenological model to provide a good regularization of the data.

In Figure 13.5, the major difficulty is to know how to make the transition from an epidemic phase to an endemic phase and vice versa. This is a non-trivial problem that is solved by our regularization approach (using a convolution with a Gaussian). As we can see in Figure 13.5, the number of oscillations is very limited between two phases.

Without regularization, there is a sharp corner at the transition between two phases which leads to infinite values in $\tau(t)$. The choice of the convolution with a Gaussian kernel for the regularization method is the result of an experimental process. We tried several different regularization methods, including a smooth explicit interpolation function and Hermite polynomials. Eventually, the convolution with a Gaussian kernel gives the best results.

To minimize the variations of the curve of $\mathcal{R}_0(t)$, the choice of the transition dates between two phases is critical. In Figure 13.5 we choose the transition dates so that the derivatives of the phenomenological model do not oscillate too much. Other choices lead to higher variations or increase the number of oscillations. Finally, the qualitative shape of the curve presented in Figure 13.5 is very robust to changes in the epidemic parameters, even though the quantitative values of $\mathcal{R}_0(t)$ are different for other values of the parameters ν and f.

In Figure 13.5, we observe that the quantitative value of $\mathcal{R}_0(t)$ during the first part of the second epidemic wave (second blue region) is almost constant and equals 1.11. This value is significantly lower than the one observed at the beginning of the first epidemic wave (first blue region). Yet the number of cases produced during the second wave is much higher than the number of cases produced during the first wave.

We observe that the values of the parameters of the phenomenological model are quantitatively different between the first wave and the second wave. Several phenomena can explain this difference. The population was better prepared for the second wave. The huge difference in the number of daily reported cases during the second phase can be partially attributed to the huge increase in the number of tests in France during this period. But this is only a partial explanation for the explosion of cases during the second wave. We also observe that the average duration of the infectious period varies between the first epidemic wave (12.5 days) and the second epidemic wave (3.5 days). This may indicate a possible adaptation of the virus SARS CoV-2 circulating in France during the two periods, or the effect of the mitigation measures, with better respect of the social distancing and compulsory mask-wearing.

The huge difference between the initial values of $\mathcal{R}_0(t)$ in the first and the second waves is an apparent paradox which shows that $\mathcal{R}_0(t)$ has a limited explanatory value regarding the severity of the epidemic: even if the quantitative value of $\mathcal{R}_0(t)$ is higher at the start of the first wave, the number of cases produced during an equivalent period in the second wave is much higher. This paradox can be partially resolved by observing that $\mathcal{R}_0(t)$ behaves like an exponential rate and the number of secondary cases produced in the whole population is therefore very sensitive to the number of active cases at time t. In other words, $\mathcal{R}_0(t)$ is blind to the epidemic state of the population and cannot be used as a reliable indicator of the severity of the epidemic. Other indicators have to be found for that purpose; we propose, for instance, the maximal value of the daily number of new cases, which can be forecasted by our method (see equation (13.16)), although other indicators can be imagined.

In Figure 13.6 we present an exploratory scenario assuming that during the endemic period preceding the second epidemic wave (May 17 – Jul 05) the daily number of cases is divided by 10. The resulting cumulative number of cases obtained is five times lower than the original one. We summarize this observation in the following statement.

Result

- The level of the daily number of cases during an endemic phase preceding an epidemic phase strongly influences the severity of this epidemic wave.

- In other words, maintaining social distancing between epidemic waves is essential.

In Figure 13.4, there are two orders of magnitude in the daily number of cases in between $CR'(t_1) \approx 1$ (with $t_1 = $ Feb 27) at the early beginning of the first epidemic wave and $CR'(t_2) = 422$ (with $t_2 = $ July 05) at the early beginning of the second

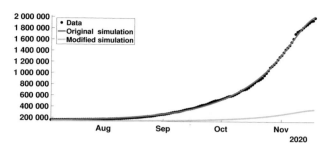

Fig. 13.6: *Cumulative number of cases for the second epidemic wave obtained by using the SI model* (13.8) *with* $\tau(t)$ *given by* (13.13), *the parameters from Table 13.1. We start the simulation at time* $t_0 = $ *July 05 with the initial value* $I_0 = \frac{CR'(t_2)}{vf}$ *for the red curve and with* $I_0 = \frac{1}{10}\frac{CR'(t_2)}{vf}$ *for the yellow curve. The remaining parameters used are* $v = 1/3$, $f = 0.9$, $S_0 = 66841266$. *We observe that the number is five times lower than then the original number of cases.*

epidemic wave. That confirms our result. After the second wave, the average daily number of cases $CR'(t)$ in France is stationary and approximately equal to 12440. Therefore, if the above observation remains true and if a third epidemic wave occurs, the third epidemic wave is expected to be more severe than the first and second epidemic waves.

Chapter 14
What Can We Learn From COVID-19 Data By Using Epidemic Models With Unidentified Infectious Cases?

This chapter is based on the paper by Griette, Demongeot and Magal [123].

14.1 Introduction

Since the first cases occurred in early December 2019, the COVID-19 crisis has been accompanied by unprecedented data release. The first cluster of cases was reported on December 31, 2019, by WHO (World Health Organization) [369]. Chinese authorities confirmed on January 7 that this cluster was caused by a novel coronavirus [368]. The disease then rapidly spread throughout the world; a case was identified in the U.S.A. as early as January 19, 2020, for instance [159]. According to the WHO database [370], the first cases in Japan date back to January 14, in Italy to January 29 (even though the cluster of cases was announced on January 21, 2020 [9]), in France to January 24, 2020, etc. The spread of the epidemic across countries was monitored, and the data was made publicly available at the international level by recognized scientific institutions such as WHO [370] and the Johns Hopkins University [92], who collected data provided by national health agencies. To the best of our knowledge, this is the first time in history that such detailed epidemiological data have been made publicly available on a global scale; this opens up new questions and new challenges for the scientific community.

Modeling efforts in order to analyze and predict the dynamics of the epidemics were initiated from the start [194, 207, 354]. Forecasting the propagation of the epidemic is, in particular, a key challenge in infectious disease epidemiology. It has quickly become clear to medical doctors and epidemiologists that covert cases (asymptomatic or unreported infectious cases) play an important role in the spread of the COVID-19. An early description of an asymptomatic transmission in Germany was reported by Rothe et al. [301]. It was also observed on the *Diamond Princess* cruise ship in Yokohama in Japan [257] that many of the passengers were tested positive for the virus but never presented any symptoms. On the French aircraft carrier *Charles de Gaulle*, clinical and biological data for all 1739 crew members were collected on arrival at Toulon harbor and during quarantine: 1121

A. Ducrot et al., *Differential Equations and Population Dynamics I*, Lecture Notes on Mathematical Modelling in the Life Sciences, https://doi.org/10.1007/978-3-030-98136-5_14

crew members (64%) were tested positive for COVID-19 using RT-PCR, and among these, 24% were asymptomatic [45]. The importance of covert cases in the silent propagation of the epidemic was highlighted by Qiu [284]. Models accounting for asymptomatic transmission, which agree with reported cases data, have been used from the start of the epidemic [207, 208, 209, 210]. The implementation of such models depends, however, on the *a priori* knowledge of some characteristic parameters of the host-pathogen interaction, among which is the ascertainment rate. Nishiura and collaborators [267] estimated this ascertainment rate as 9.2% on a 7.5-day detection window, based on testing data of repatriated Japanese nationals from Wuhan. This was corrected later to 44% for non-severe cases [270]. An early review of SARS-CoV-2 facts can be found in the work of Bar-On et al. [24].

To describe the spread of COVID-19 mathematically, Liu et al. [207] first took into account the infection of susceptible individuals by contacts with unreported infectious individuals. A new method using the number of reported cases in SIR models was also proposed in the same work. This method and the model were extended in several directions by the same group [208, 209, 210, 211] to include non-constant transmission rates and a period of exposure. More recently, the method was extended and successfully applied to a Japanese age-structured dataset by Griette, Magal and Seydi [127]. The method was also extended to investigate the predictability of the outbreak in several countries, including China, South Korea, Italy, France, Germany, and the United Kingdom by Liu, Magal and Webb [211].

Phenomenological models were extensively used in the literature even before the SARS-CoV-2 pandemic to describe reported cases data, see e.g., [162, 391] for the 2003 SARS outbreak, and also [163, 361], to cite a few. In the case of the SARS-CoV-2 epidemic, articles related to phenomenological models are particularly numerous, see e.g., [15, 49, 63, 106, 252, 271, 294, 318, 358, 394]. More precisely, Castro et al. [49] investigate the possibility of predicting the turning point of an epidemic wave. Many studies use phenomenological models to issue short-term predictions on the epidemic [252, 294, 318, 358]. But these models can also be used to reconstruct the evolution of the epidemic *a posteriori* [15, 63, 394].

In previous works [207, 208, 209, 210], we have replaced the data with the phenomenological model, and we use this continuous description as the output of the epidemic model. This allows us to understand how to express part of the initial distribution and some parameters (e.g., the transmission rate) from the data and the given parameters of the model. By using this approach, we obtain an explicit formula for the time-dependent transmission rate expressed by using some given parameters of the model and some parameters of the phenomenological model. In [77], we used a Bernoulli–Verhulst phenomenological model to describe a single epidemic wave and compute a time-dependent transmission rate.

There are many potential phenomenological models to represent a single epidemic wave [15, 63, 361]. However, except in the case of the logistic equation, there is usually no explicit formula for the solution. The explicit formula in the case considered here enables us to develop a comprehensive statistical analysis. Phenomenological models also serve to regularize the data, which is a complex question. Indeed the idea is to get rid of the stochastic oscillations (due for example to the way the data are collected, or the stochastic nature of the contact between individuals). Some phenomenological models also redistribute the reported cases to dampen the fluctuations in the data. Let us stress here the fact that some oscillations in cases data may not be random and might correspond to complex transmission dynamics (delayed infection, peak in contact numbers during the day, etc.) This highlights one of the drawbacks of phenomenological models: while they allow a precise description of epidemic waves, they might also hide some valuable information on how the disease is transmitted in the population.

A key parameter in understanding the dynamics of the COVID-19 epidemic is the transmission rate, defined as the fraction of all possible contacts between susceptible and infected individuals that effectively result in a new infection per unit of time. Estimating the average transmission rate is one of the most crucial challenges in the epidemiology of communicable diseases. In practice, many factors can influence the actual transmission rate, (i) the coefficient of susceptibility; (ii) the coefficient of virulence; (iii) the number of contacts per unit of time [235]; (iv) the environmental conductivity [76].

Epidemic models with time-dependent transmission rates have been considered in several articles in the literature. The classical approach is to fix a function of time that depends on some parameters and to fix these parameters by using the best fit to the data. In Chowell et al. [55] a specific form was chosen for the rate of transmission and applied to the Ebola outbreak in Congo. Huo et al [165] used a predefined transmission rate which is a Legendre polynomial depending on a tunable number of parameters. Let us also mention that the kinetic model idea has been used to understand this problem in the paper by Dimarco et al. [91]. Here we are going the other way around. We reconstruct the transmission rate from the data by using the model without choosing a predefined function for the transmission rate. Such an approach was used in the early 70s by London and Yorke [212, 378], who used a discrete-time model and discussed the time-dependent rate of transmission in the context of measles, chickenpox, and mumps. More recently, several authors [23, 77, 122] used both an explicit formula and algorithms to reconstruct the transmission rate. These studies allow us to understand that the regularization of the data is a complex problem and is crucial in order to rebuild a meaningful time-dependent transmission rate.

In this chapter, we apply a new method to compute the transmission rate from cumulative reported cases data. While the use of a predefined transmission rate $\tau(t)$ as a function of time can lead to very good fits of the data, here we are looking for a more intrinsic relationship between the data and the transmission rate. Therefore we propose a different approach and use a two-step procedure. Firstly, we use a phenomenological model to describe the data and extract the general trend of the epidemiological dynamics while removing the insignificant noise. Secondly, we derive an explicit relationship between the phenomenological model and the transmission rate. In other words, we compute the transmission rate directly from the data. As a result, we can reconstruct an estimation of the state of the population at each time, including covert cases. Our method also provides new indicators for the epidemiological dynamics that are related to the reproductive number.

14.2 Methods

14.2.1 COVID-19 data and phenomenological model

We regularized the time series of cumulative reported cases by fitting standard curves to the data to reconstruct the time-dependent transmission rate. We first identified the epidemic waves for each of the eight geographic areas. A Bernoulli–Verhulst curve was then fitted to each epidemic wave using the Levenberg–Marquardt algorithm [118]. We reported the detailed output of the algorithm in the supplementary material, including confidence bounds on the parameters. The model was completed by filling the time windows between two waves with straight lines. Finally, we applied a Gaussian filter with a standard deviation of 7 days to the curve to obtain a smooth model.

14.2.1.1 Data sources

We used reported cases data for 8 different geographic areas, namely California, France, India, Israel, Japan, Peru, Spain, and the UK. Apart from California State, for which we used data from the COVID tracking project,[1] the reported cases data were taken from the WHO database [370].

14.2.1.2 Phenomenological model used for multiple epidemic waves

To represent the data, we used a phenomenological model to fit the curve of cumulative rate cases. Such an idea is not new since it was already proposed by Bernoulli [28] in 1760 in the context of the smallpox epidemic. Here we used the so-called Bernoulli–Verhulst [347] model to describe the epidemic phase. Bernoulli [28] investigated an epidemic phase followed by an endemic phase. This appears clearly in Figures 9 and 10 of the paper by Dietz and Heesterbeek [90] who revisited the original article of Bernoulli. We also refer to Blower [29] for another article revisiting the original work of Bernoulli. Several works comparing cumulative reported cases data and the Bernoulli–Verhulst model appear in the literature (see [163, 361, 391]). The Bernoulli–Verhulst model is sometimes called Richard's model, although Richard's work came much later in 1959.

The phenomenological model deals with data series of new infectious cases decomposed into two successive phases: 1) endemic phases followed by 2) epidemic phases.

Endemic phase: During the endemic phase, the dynamics of new cases appears to fluctuate around an average value independently of the number of cases. Therefore the average cumulative number of cases is given by

---

[1] The COVID Tracking Project at *The Atlantic*. Accessed June 30, 2021. https://covidtracking.com/.

$$CR(t) = N_0 + (t - t_0) \times a, \text{ for } t \in [t_0, t_1], \tag{14.1}$$

where t_0 denotes the beginning of the endemic phase, and a is the average value of the daily number of new cases.

We assume that the average daily number of new cases is constant. Therefore the daily number of new cases is given by

$$CR'(t) = a. \tag{14.2}$$

Epidemic phase: In the epidemic phase, the new cases are contributing to produce secondary cases. Therefore the daily number of new cases is no longer constant, but varies with time as follows

$$CR(t) = N_{\text{base}} + \frac{e^{\chi(t-t_0)} N_0}{\left[1 + \dfrac{N_0^\theta}{N_\infty^\theta} \left(e^{\chi\theta(t-t_0)} - 1 \right) \right]^{1/\theta}}, \text{ for } t \in [t_0, t_1]. \tag{14.3}$$

In other words, the daily number of new cases follows the Bernoulli–Verhulst equation [28, 347]. Namely, by setting

$$N(t) = CR(t) - N_{\text{base}}, \tag{14.4}$$

we obtain

$$N'(t) = \chi N(t) \left[1 - \left(\frac{N(t)}{N_\infty} \right)^\theta \right], \tag{14.5}$$

completed with the initial value

$$N(t_0) = N_0.$$

In the model, $N_{\text{base}} + N_0$ corresponds to the value $CR(t_0)$ of the cumulative number of cases at time $t = t_0$. The parameter $N_\infty + N_{\text{base}}$ is the maximal value of the cumulative reported cases after the time $t = t_0$. $\chi > 0$ is a Malthusian growth parameter, and θ regulates the speed at which $CR(t)$ increases to $N_\infty + N_{\text{base}}$.

Regularize the junction between the epidemic phases: Because the formula for $\tau(t)$ involves derivatives of the phenomenological model regularizing $CR(t)$ (see Eqs (14.12)–(14.15)), we need to connect the phenomenological models of the different phases as smoothly as possible. Let $t_0, \ldots, t_n$ denote the $n + 1$ breaking points of the model, that is, the times at which there is a transition between one phase and the next one. We let $\widetilde{CR}(t)$ be the global model obtained by placing the phenomenological models of the different phases side by side.

More precisely, $\widetilde{CR}(t)$ is defined by Eq (14.3) during an epidemic phase $[t_i, t_{i+1}]$, or during the initial phase $(-\infty, t_0]$ or the last phase $[t_n, +\infty)$. During an endemic phase, $\widetilde{CR}(t)$ is defined by Eq (14.1). The parameters are chosen so that the resulting global model $\widetilde{CR}$ is continuous. We define the regularized model by using the convolution formula:

$$CR(t) = \int_{-\infty}^{+\infty} \mathcal{G}(t - s) \times \widetilde{CR}(s)ds = (\mathcal{G} * \widetilde{CR})(t), \qquad (14.6)$$

where

$$\mathcal{G}(t) := \frac{1}{\sigma\sqrt{2\pi}} e^{-\frac{t^2}{2\sigma^2}}$$

is the Gaussian function with mean 0 and variance σ^2. The parameter σ controls the trade-off between smoothness and precision: increasing σ reduces the variations in $CR(t)$ and reducing σ reduces the distance between $CR(t)$ and $\widetilde{CR}(t)$. In any case the resulting function $CR(t)$ is very smooth (as well as its derivatives) and close to the original model $\widetilde{CR}(t)$ when σ is not too large. In the results section (Section 14.3), we fix $\sigma = 7$ days.

Numerically, we will need to compute some $t \to CR(t)$ derivatives. Therefore it is convenient to take advantage of the convolution Eq (14.6) and deduce that

$$\frac{d^n CR(t)}{dt^n} = \int_{-\infty}^{+\infty} \frac{d^n \mathcal{G}(t - s)}{dt^n} \times \widetilde{CR}(s)ds, \qquad (14.7)$$

for $n = 1, 2, 3$.

14.2.2 Epidemic model

To reconstruct the transmission rate, we used the underlying mathematical model described by the flowchart presented in Figure 14.1.

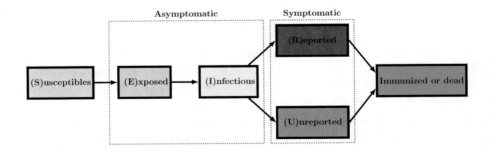

Fig. 14.1: *Flowchart for the model.*

The model itself includes five parameters whose values were taken from the literature: the average length of the noninfectious incubation period (1 day, (E)xposed); the average length of the infectious incubation period (3 days, (I)nfectious); the average length of the symptomatic period (7 days, (R)eported or (U)nreported); the ascertainment rate (0.8). Additional parameters appear in the initial condition and could not be computed from the initial number of unreported individuals. The transmission rate was computed from the regularized data and the assumed parameters according to a methodology adapted from Demongeot et al. [77].

Many epidemiological models are based on the SIR or SEIR model, which is classical in epidemic modeling. We refer to [334, 374] for the earliest articles devoted to such a question and to [7, 22, 33, 34, 36, 42, 86, 150, 174, 262, 338] for more models. In this chapter, we will compare the following SEIUR model to the cumulative reported cases data

$$
\begin{cases}
S'(t) = -\tau(t) \left[I(t) + \kappa U(t) \right] S(t), \\
E'(t) = \tau(t) \left[I(t) + \kappa U(t) \right] S(t) - \alpha E(t), \\
I'(t) = \alpha E(t) - v I(t), \\
U'(t) = v (1 - f) I(t) - \eta U(t), \\
R'(t) = v f I(t) - \eta R(t),
\end{cases}
\tag{14.8}
$$

where at time t, $S(t)$ is the number of susceptible, $E(t)$ the number of exposed (not yet capable of transmitting the pathogen), $I(t)$ the number of asymptomatic infectious, $R(t)$ the number of reported symptomatic infectious and $U(t)$ the number of unreported symptomatic infectious. This system is supplemented by initial data

$$
S(t_0) = S_0, \ E(t_0) = E_0, \ I(t_0) = I_0, \ U(t_0) = U_0, \text{ and } R(t_0) = R_0.
\tag{14.9}
$$

In this model, $\tau(t)$ is the rate of transmission, $1/\alpha$ is the average duration of the exposure period, $1/v$ is the average duration of the asymptomatic infectious period, and for simplicity, we subdivide the class of symptomatic patients into the fraction $0 \le f \le 1$ of patients showing some severe symptoms, and the fraction $1 - f$ of patients showing some mild symptoms assumed to be not detected. The quantity $1/\eta$ is the average duration of the symptomatic infectious period. In the model, we assume that the average time of infection is the same for Reported and Unreported infectious individuals. We refer to [173, 182] for more information about this topic. Finally, we assume that reported symptomatic individuals do not contribute significantly to the transmission of the virus.

The cumulative number of reported cases $CR(t)$ is connected to the epidemic model by the following relationship

$$
CR(t) = CR_0 + v f \, CI(t), \text{ for } t \ge t_0,
\tag{14.10}
$$

where

$$
CI(t) = \int_{t_0}^{t} I(\sigma) d\sigma.
\tag{14.11}
$$

Given and estimated parameters

We assume that the following parameters of the model are known

$$S_0, U_0, R_0, f, \kappa, \alpha, \nu, \eta.$$

The goal of our method is to focus on the estimation of the three remaining parameters. Namely, knowing the parameters mentioned above, we plan to identify

$$E_0, I_0, \tau(t).$$

Computation of the rate of transmission

The transmission rate is fully determined by the parameters $\kappa, \alpha, \nu, \eta, f, S_0, E_0, I_0, U_0$, and the data that are represented by the function $t \rightarrow CR(t)$, by using the three following equations

$$\tau(t) = \frac{1}{I(t) + \kappa U(t)} \times \frac{CE''(t) + \alpha CE'(t)}{E_0 + S_0 - CE'(t) - \alpha CE(t)}, \tag{14.12}$$

where

$$I(t) = \frac{CR'(t)}{\nu f}, \tag{14.13}$$

$$CE(t) = \frac{1}{\alpha \nu f} \left[CR'(t) - \nu f I_0 + \nu \left(CR(t) - CR_0 \right) \right], \tag{14.14}$$

$$U(t) = e^{-\eta(t-t_0)} U_0 + \int_{t_0}^{t} e^{-\eta(t-s)} \frac{(1-f)}{f} CR'(s) ds. \tag{14.15}$$

14.2.2.1 Instantaneous reproduction number computed for COVID-19 data

We have only a single epidemic phase in the standard SI epidemic model because the epidemic exhausts the susceptible population. Here, the changes of regimes (epidemic phase versus endemic phase) are partly due to the decay in the number of susceptible. But these changes are also influenced by the changes in the transmission rate. These changes in the transmission rate are due to the limitation of contacts between individuals or to changes in climate (in summer) or other factors influencing transmissions.

In this section, we will observe that the main factors for the changes in the epidemic regimes are the changes in the transmission rate. To investigate this for the COVID-19 data, we use our method to compute the transmission rate, and we consider the *instantaneous reproduction number*

$$R_e(t) = \frac{\tau(t) S(t)}{\eta \nu} (\eta + \nu(1 - f)) \tag{14.16}$$

and the *quasi-instantaneous reproduction number*

$$R_e^0(t) = \frac{\tau(t)S_0}{\eta v}(\eta + v(1 - f)), \tag{14.17}$$

in which the transmission varies, but the size of the susceptible population remains constant equal to S_0. We refer to Section A8 of the supplementary material for detailed computations to obtain Eq (14.16).

The comparison between $R_e(t)$ and $R_e^0(t)$ permits us to understand the contribution of the decay of the susceptible population in the variations of $R_e(t)$. Another interesting aspect is that $R_e^0(t)$ is proportional to the transmission rate $\tau(t)$. Therefore plotting $R_e^0(t)$ permits us to visualize the variation of $t \to \tau(t)$ only.

14.2.2.2 Computation of the initial value of the epidemic model

Based on Eq (14.4), we can recover the initial number of asymptomatic infectious $I_0 = I(t_0)$ and the initial number of exposed $E_0 = E(t_0)$ for an epidemic phase starting at time t_0. Indeed by definition, we have $CR'(t) = v f I(t)$ and therefore

$$I_0 = \frac{CR'(t_0)}{v f} = \frac{\chi N_0 \left(1 - \left(\frac{N_0}{N_\infty}\right)^\theta\right)}{v f}.$$

Estimated initial number of infected

The initial number of asymptomatic infectious is given by

$$I_0 = \frac{CR'(t_0)}{v f}. \tag{14.18}$$

In the special case of the Bernoulli–Verhulst model we obtain

$$I_0 = \frac{\chi}{v f} N_0 \left(1 - \left(\frac{N_0}{N_\infty}\right)^\theta\right). \tag{14.19}$$

By differentiating Eq (14.5) we deduce that

$$N''(t) = \chi N'(t) \left(1 - \left(\frac{N(t)}{N_\infty}\right)^\theta\right) - \frac{\chi \theta}{N_\infty^\theta} N(t) \, (N(t))^{\theta-1} \, N'(t)$$

$$= \chi N'(t) \left(1 - \left(\frac{N(t)}{N_\infty}\right)^\theta\right) - \frac{\chi \theta}{N_\infty^\theta} \, (N(t))^\theta \, N'(t),$$

therefore

$$\text{CR}''(t) = N''(t) = \chi^2 N(t) \left(1 - \left(\frac{N(t)}{N_\infty}\right)^\theta\right) \left(1 - (1+\theta)\left(\frac{N(t)}{N_\infty}\right)^\theta\right).$$

By using the third equation in Eq (14.8) we obtain

$$E_0 = \frac{I'(t_0) + \nu I(t_0)}{\alpha} = \frac{\text{CR}''(t_0) + \nu\text{CR}'(t_0)}{\alpha} = \frac{N''(t_0) + \nu N'(t_0)}{\alpha}.$$

Estimated initial number of exposed

The initial number of exposed is given by

$$E_0 = \frac{\text{CR}''(t_0) + \nu\text{CR}'(t_0)}{\alpha}. \tag{14.20}$$

In the special case of the Bernoulli–Verhulst model, we obtain

$$E_0 = \frac{\chi}{\alpha \, \nu \, f} N_0 \left(1 - \left(\frac{N_0}{N_\infty}\right)^\theta\right) \left(\chi + \nu - \chi\,(1+\theta)\left(\frac{N_0}{N_\infty}\right)^\theta\right). \tag{14.21}$$

14.2.2.3 Theoretical formula for $\tau(t)$

We first remark that the S-equation of model (14.8) can be written as

$$\frac{d}{dt}\ln(S(t)) = \frac{S'(t)}{S(t)} = -\tau(t)\big[I(t) + \kappa U(t)\big],$$

therefore by integrating between t_0 and t we get

$$S(t) = S_0 \exp\left(-\int_{t_0}^t \tau(\sigma)\,[I(\sigma) + \kappa U(\sigma)]\,d\sigma\right).$$

Next we plug the above formula for $S(t)$ into the E-equation of model (14.8) and obtain

$$E'(t) = S_0 \exp\left(-\int_{t_0}^t \tau(\sigma)\,[I(\sigma) + \kappa U(\sigma)]\,d\sigma\right)\tau(t)\,[I(t) + \kappa U(t)] - \alpha\,E(t)$$

$$= -S_0 \frac{d}{dt}\left(-\int_{t_0}^t \tau(\sigma)\,[I(\sigma) + \kappa U(\sigma)]\,d\sigma\right)\exp\left(-\int_{t_0}^t \tau(\sigma)\,[I(\sigma) + \kappa U(\sigma)]\,d\sigma\right)$$

$$- \alpha\,E(t),$$

and by integrating this equation between t_0 and t we obtain

$$E(t) = E_0 + S_0\left[1 - \exp\left(-\int_{t_0}^t \tau(\sigma)\,[I(\sigma) + \kappa U(\sigma)]\,d\sigma\right)\right] - \alpha\int_{t_0}^t E(\sigma)\,d\sigma. \tag{14.22}$$

Define the cumulative numbers of exposed, infectious and unreported individuals by

$$\text{CE}(t) := \int_{t_0}^t E(\sigma)\mathrm{d}\sigma, \ \text{CI}(t) := \int_{t_0}^t I(\sigma)\mathrm{d}\sigma, \ \text{and } \text{CU}(t) := \int_{t_0}^t U(\sigma)\mathrm{d}\sigma,$$

and note that $\text{CE}'(t) = E(t)$. We can rewrite Eq (14.22) as

$$S_0 \exp\left(-\int_{t_0}^t \tau(\sigma)\,[I(\sigma) + \kappa U(\sigma)]\,\mathrm{d}\sigma\right) = E_0 + S_0 - \text{CE}'(t) - \alpha\,\text{CE}(t).$$

By taking the logarithm of both sides we obtain

$$\int_{t_0}^t \tau(\sigma)\,[I(\sigma) + \kappa U(\sigma)]\,\mathrm{d}\sigma = \ln(S_0) - \ln\left(E_0 + S_0 - \text{CE}'(t) - \alpha\,\text{CE}(t)\right),$$

and by differentiating with respect to t:

$$\tau(t) = \frac{1}{I(t) + \kappa U(t)} \times \frac{\text{CE}''(t) + \alpha \text{CE}'(t)}{E_0 + S_0 - \text{CE}'(t) - \alpha\,\text{CE}(t)}. \tag{14.23}$$

Therefore we have an explicit formula giving $\tau(t)$ as a function of $I(t)$, $U(t)$ and $\text{CE}(t)$ and its derivatives. Next we explain how to identify those three remaining unknowns as a function of $\text{CR}(t)$ and its derivatives. We first recall that, from Eq (14.10), we have

$$\text{CR}(t) = \text{CR}(t_0) + \nu f\,\text{CI}(t).$$

The I-equation of model (14.8) can be rewritten as

$$\alpha E(t) = I'(t) + \nu I(t),$$

and by integrating this equation between t_0 and t we obtain

$$\alpha\,\text{CE}(t) = \text{CI}'(t) - I_0 + \nu\,\text{CI}(t) = \frac{1}{\nu f}\left(\text{CR}'(t) + \nu\text{CR}(t) - \nu\text{CR}(t_0)\right). \tag{14.24}$$

Finally, by applying the variation of constants formula to the U-equation of system (14.8) we obtain

$$U(t) = e^{-\eta(t-t_0)}U_0 + \int_{t_0}^t e^{-\eta(t-s)}\nu\,(1-f)\,I(s)\mathrm{d}s$$

$$= e^{-\eta(t-t_0)}U_0 + \int_{t_0}^t e^{-\eta(t-s)}\frac{1-f}{f}\text{CR}'(s)\mathrm{d}s. \tag{14.25}$$

From these computations we deduce that $\tau(t)$ can be computed thanks to Eq (14.23) from $\text{CR}(t)$, α, ν, η, κ, f and U_0. The following theorem is a precise statement of this result.

Theorem 14.1 *Let $S_0 > 0$, $E_0 > 0$, $I_0 > 0$, $U_0 > 0$, $\text{CR}_0 \geq 0$, α, ν, η and $f > 0$ be given. Let $t \mapsto \tau(t) \geq 0$ be a given continuous function and $t \to I(t)$ be the second component of system (14.8). Let $\widehat{\text{CR}} : [t_0, \infty) \to \mathbb{R}$ be a twice continuously* *differentiable function. Then*

$$\widehat{CR}(t) = CR_0 + v f \int_{t_0}^{t} I(s)\,ds, \forall t \geq t_0, \qquad (14.26)$$

if and only if $\widehat{CR}$ *satisfies*

$$\widehat{CR}(t_0) = CR_0, \qquad (14.27)$$

$$\widehat{CR}'(t_0) = v f I_0, \qquad (14.28)$$

$$\widehat{CR}''(t_0) + v\widehat{CR}'(t_0) = \alpha v f E_0, \qquad (14.29)$$

$$\widehat{CR}'(t) > 0, \forall t \geq t_0, \qquad (14.30)$$

$$v f (E_0 + S_0) - \left[\widehat{CR}''(t) + v\widehat{CR}'(t)\right] - \alpha \left[\widehat{CR}'(t) - v f I_0 + v\widehat{CR}(t)\right] > 0, \forall t \geq t_0, \qquad (14.31)$$

and $\tau(t)$ *is given by*

$$\tau(t) = \frac{1}{\widehat{I}(t) + \kappa\widehat{U}(t)} \times \frac{\widehat{CE}''(t) + \alpha\widehat{CE}'(t)}{E_0 + S_0 - \widehat{CE}'(t) - \alpha\widehat{CE}(t)}, \qquad (14.32)$$

where

$$\widehat{I}(t) := \frac{\widehat{CR}'(t)}{v f}, \qquad (14.33)$$

$$\widehat{CI}(t) := \frac{1}{v f}\left[\widehat{CR}(t) - \widehat{CR}(t_0)\right], \qquad (14.34)$$

$$\widehat{CE}(t) := \frac{1}{\alpha}\left[\widehat{CI}'(t) - I_0 + v\widehat{CI}(t)\right] = \frac{1}{\alpha v f}\left[\widehat{CR}'(t) - v f I_0 + v\left(\widehat{CR}(t) - CR_0\right)\right], \qquad (14.35)$$

$$\widehat{U}(t) := e^{-\eta(t-t_0)}U_0 + \int_{t_0}^{t} e^{-\eta(t-s)}\frac{(1-f)}{f}\widehat{CR}'(s)ds. \qquad (14.36)$$

Proof Assume first that $\widehat{CR}(t)$ satisfies Eq (14.26). Then by using the first equation of system (14.8) we deduce that

$$S_0 \exp\left(-\int_{t_0}^{t}\tau(\sigma)\left[I(\sigma) + \kappa U(\sigma)\right]d\sigma\right) = E_0 + S_0 - E(t) - \alpha CE(t). \qquad (14.37)$$

Therefore

$$\int_{t_0}^{t}\tau(\sigma)\left[I(\sigma) + \kappa U(\sigma)\right]d\sigma = \ln\left[\frac{S_0}{E_0 + S_0 - E(t) - \alpha CE(t)}\right]$$

$$= \ln(S_0) - \ln\left[E_0 + S_0 - E(t) - \alpha CE(t)\right],$$

and by taking the derivative of both sides we obtain

$$\tau(t)\left[I(t) + \kappa U(t)\right] = \frac{E'(t) + \alpha E(t)}{E_0 + S_0 - E(t) - \alpha CE(t)},$$

which is equivalent to

$$\tau(t) = \frac{E(t)}{I(t) + \kappa U(t)} \times \frac{\dfrac{E'(t)}{E(t)} + \alpha}{E_0 + S_0 - E(t) - \alpha \mathrm{CE}(t)}.$$

By using the fact that $E(t) = \mathrm{CE}'(t)$ and $I = \mathrm{CR}'(t)/(vf)$, we deduce Eq (14.32). By differentiating Eq (14.26), we get Eqs (14.28) and (14.30). Equation (14.29) is a consequence of the E-component of Eq (14.8). We get Eq (14.31) by combining Eqs (14.37) and (14.35) (since $\widehat{\mathrm{CE}}(t) = \mathrm{CE}(t)$).

Conversely, assume that $\tau(t)$ is given by Eq (14.31) and all the Eqs (14.27)–(14.36) hold. We define $\widehat{I}(t) = \widehat{\mathrm{CR}}'(t)/vf$ and $\widehat{\mathrm{CI}}(t) = \left(\widehat{\mathrm{CR}}(t) - \mathrm{CR}_0\right)/vf$. Then, by using Eq (14.27), we deduce that

$$\widehat{\mathrm{CI}}(t) = \int_{t_0}^{t} \widehat{I}(\sigma)\mathrm{d}\sigma, \tag{14.38}$$

and by using Eq (14.28), we deduce

$$\widehat{I}(t_0) = I_0. \tag{14.39}$$

Moreover, from Eq (14.31) and $\widehat{I}(t) = \widehat{\mathrm{CR}}'(t)/vf$ we deduce that

$$\tau(t) = \frac{1}{\widehat{I}(t) + \kappa \widehat{U}(t)} \times \frac{\widehat{\mathrm{CE}}''(t) + \alpha \widehat{\mathrm{CE}}'(t)}{E_0 + S_0 - \widehat{\mathrm{CE}}'(t) - \alpha \widehat{\mathrm{CE}}(t)}. \tag{14.40}$$

Multiplying Eq (14.40) by $\widehat{I}(t) + \kappa \widehat{U}(t)$ and integrating, we obtain

$$\int_{t_0}^{t} \tau(\sigma) \left[\widehat{I}(\sigma) + \kappa \widehat{U}(\sigma)\right] \mathrm{d}\sigma = \ln\left(E_0 + S_0 - \widehat{\mathrm{CE}}'(t_0) - \alpha \widehat{\mathrm{CE}}(t_0)\right) \\ - \ln\left(E_0 + S_0 - \widehat{\mathrm{CE}}'(t) - \alpha \widehat{\mathrm{CE}}(t)\right), \tag{14.41}$$

where the right-hand side is well defined thanks to Eq (14.31). By combining Eqs (14.27), (14.28) and (14.35) we obtain

$$\widehat{\mathrm{CE}}(t_0) = 0, \tag{14.42}$$

and by taking the derivative in Eq (14.35) we obtain

$$\widehat{\mathrm{CE}}'(t_0) = \frac{1}{\alpha v f}\left[\widehat{\mathrm{CR}}''(t) + v\widehat{\mathrm{CR}}'(t)\right]$$

therefore by using Eq (14.29) we deduce that

$$\widehat{\mathrm{CE}}'(t_0) = E_0. \tag{14.43}$$

In particular, $E_0 + S_0 - \widehat{\mathrm{CE}}'(t_0) - \alpha \widehat{\mathrm{CE}}(t_0) = S_0$ and, by taking the exponential of Eq (14.41), we obtain

$$S_0 e^{-\int_{t_0}^{t} \tau(\sigma)\left[\widehat{I}(\sigma)+\kappa\widehat{U}(\sigma)\right]d\sigma} = E_0 + S_0 - \widehat{CE}'(t) - \alpha\widehat{CE}(t),$$

which, differentiating both sides, yields

$$-S_0 e^{-\int_{t_0}^{t} \tau(\sigma)\left[\widehat{I}(\sigma)+\kappa\widehat{U}(\sigma)\right]d\sigma}\tau(t)\left[\widehat{I}(t)+\kappa\widehat{U}(t)\right] = -\widehat{CE}''(t) - \alpha\widehat{CE}'(t)$$

$$= -\widehat{E}'(t) - \alpha\widehat{E}(t),$$

and therefore

$$\widehat{E}'(t) = \tau(t)\widehat{S}(t)\left[\widehat{I}(t)+\kappa\widehat{U}(t)\right] - \alpha\widehat{E}(t), \tag{14.44}$$

where $\widehat{E}(t) := \widehat{CE}'(t)$ and $\widehat{S}(t) := S_0 e^{-\int_{t_0}^{t} \tau(\sigma)\left[\widehat{I}(\sigma)+\kappa\widehat{U}(\sigma)\right]d\sigma}$. Differentiating the definition of $\widehat{S}(t)$, we get

$$\widehat{S}'(t) = -\left[\widehat{I}(t)+\kappa\widehat{U}(t)\right]\widehat{S}(t). \tag{14.45}$$

Next the derivative of Eq (14.35) can be rewritten as

$$\widehat{I}'(t) = \frac{1}{\nu f}\widehat{CR}''(t) = \alpha\widehat{CE}'(t) - \nu\frac{1}{\nu f}\widehat{CR}'(t) = \alpha\widehat{E}(t) - \nu\widehat{I}(t). \tag{14.46}$$

Finally, differentiating Eq (14.36) yields

$$\widehat{U}'(t) = \nu(1-f)\widehat{I}(t) - \eta\widehat{U}(t). \tag{14.47}$$

By combining Eqs (14.44)–(14.47) we see that $\left(\widehat{S}(t), \widehat{E}(t), \widehat{I}(t), \widehat{U}(t)\right)$ satisfies Eq (14.8) with the initial condition $\left(\widehat{S}(t_0), \widehat{E}(t_0), \widehat{I}(t_0), \widehat{U}(t_0)\right) = (S_0, E_0, I_0, U_0)$. By the uniqueness of the solutions of Eq (14.8) for a given initial condition, we conclude that $\left(\widehat{S}(t), \widehat{E}(t), \widehat{I}(t), \widehat{U}(t)\right) = \left(S(t), E(t), I(t), U(t)\right)$. In particular, CR$(t)$ satisfies Eq (14.26). The proof is complete.   □

Remark 14.2 The condition Eq (14.31) is equivalent to

$$E_0 + S_0 - \widehat{CE}'(t) - \alpha\widehat{CE}(t) > 0, \forall t \geq t_0.$$

Remark 14.3 The present computations have previously been done, in a different context, by Hadeler [136].

14.2.3 Computing the explicit formula for $\tau(t)$ during an epidemic phase

In this section, we assume that the curve of cumulative reported cases is given by the Bernoulli–Verhulst formula

$$N(t) := \mathrm{CR}(t) - N_{\mathrm{base}} = \frac{e^{\chi(t-t_0)} N_0}{\left[1 + \dfrac{N_0^\theta}{N_\infty^\theta}\left(e^{\chi\theta(t-t_0)} - 1\right)\right]^{1/\theta}}, \quad \text{for } t \in [t_0, t_1],$$

and we recall that

$$N'(t) = \chi N(t)\left(1 - \left(\frac{N(t)}{N_\infty}\right)^\theta\right).$$

Then we can compute an explicit formula for the components of the system (14.8). By definition we have

$$I(t) = \frac{\mathrm{CR}'(t)}{vf} = \frac{\chi}{vf} N(t)\left(1 - \left(\frac{N(t)}{N_\infty}\right)^\theta\right), \tag{14.48}$$

which gives

$$I'(t) = \frac{\mathrm{CR}''(t)}{vf} = \frac{\chi^2}{vf} N(t)\left(1 - \left(\frac{N(t)}{N_\infty}\right)^\theta\right)\left(1 - (1+\theta)\left(\frac{N(t)}{N_\infty}\right)^\theta\right),$$

so that by using the I-component in the system (14.8) we get

$$E(t) = \frac{1}{\alpha}\left(I'(t) + vI(t)\right) = \frac{1}{\alpha vf}\left(\mathrm{CR}''(t) + v\mathrm{CR}'(t)\right).$$

By integration, we get

$$\begin{aligned}
\mathrm{CE}(t) &= \frac{1}{\alpha vf}\left[\left(\mathrm{CR}'(t) - \mathrm{CR}_0'\right) + v\left[\mathrm{CR}(t) - \mathrm{CR}(t_0)\right]\right], \\
&= \frac{1}{\alpha vf}\left[\chi N(t)\left(1 - \left(\frac{N(t)}{N_\infty}\right)^\theta\right) - vf I_0 + v\left[N(t) - N_0\right]\right], \\
&= \frac{1}{\alpha vf}\left[N(t)\left(\chi + v - \chi\left(\frac{N(t)}{N_\infty}\right)^\theta\right) - vf I_0 - vN_0\right],
\end{aligned}$$

and since

$$vf I_0 = \mathrm{CR}'(t_0) = N'(t_0) = \chi N_0\left(1 - \left(\frac{N_0}{N_\infty}\right)^\theta\right),$$

we obtain

$$\mathrm{CE}(t) = \frac{1}{\alpha vf}\left[N(t)\left(\chi + v - \chi\left(\frac{N(t)}{N_\infty}\right)^\theta\right) - N_0\left(\chi + v - \chi\left(\frac{N_0}{N_\infty}\right)^\theta\right)\right].$$

Note also that we have explicit formulas for $E(t) = \mathrm{CE}'(t)$ and $E'(t) = \mathrm{CE}''(t)$,

$$E(t) = CE'(t) = \frac{\chi}{\alpha v f} \left[N(t) \left(1 - \left(\frac{N(t)}{N_\infty} \right)^\theta \right) \left(\chi + v - \chi(1+\theta) \left(\frac{N(t)}{N_\infty} \right)^\theta \right) \right]$$
$$\tag{14.49}$$

and

$$E'(t) = CE''(t) = \frac{\chi^2}{\alpha v f} N(t) \left(1 - \left(\frac{N(t)}{N_\infty} \right)^\theta \right)$$
$$\times \left[\chi + v - (\chi(2+\theta) + v)(1+\theta) \left(\frac{N(t)}{N_\infty} \right)^\theta + \chi(1+\theta)(1+2\theta) \left(\frac{N(t)}{N_\infty} \right)^{2\theta} \right].$$

Next, recall the U-equation of Eq (14.8), that is,

$$U'(t) = v(1-f)I(t) - \eta U(t),$$

therefore by the variation of constant formula we have

$$U(t) = e^{-\eta(t-t_0)} U(t_0) + \int_{t_0}^t e^{-\eta(t-s)} (1-f) v I(s) ds$$
$$= e^{-\eta(t-t_0)} U_0 + \int_{t_0}^t e^{-\eta(t-s)} \frac{1-f}{f} CR'(s) ds. \tag{14.50}$$

Explicit formula for the transmission rate during an epidemic phase

The transmission rate $\tau(t)$ can be computed as

$$\tau(t) = \frac{\chi N(t) \left(1 - \left(\frac{N(t)}{N_\infty} \right)^\theta \right)}{I(t) + \kappa U(t)} \times \frac{\left[A \left(\frac{N(t)}{N_\infty} \right)^{2\theta} - B \left(\frac{N(t)}{N_\infty} \right)^\theta + C \right]}{E_0 + S_0 - E(t) - \alpha CE(t)}, \tag{14.51}$$

where

$$N(t) = \frac{e^{\chi(t-t_0)} N_0}{\left[1 + \frac{N_0^\theta}{N_\infty^\theta} \left(e^{\chi\theta(t-t_0)} - 1 \right) \right]^{1/\theta}}, \quad \text{for } t \geq t_0, \tag{14.52}$$

and

$$A := \chi^2(1+\theta)(1+2\theta), \tag{14.53}$$
$$B := \chi(1+\theta)\left[\chi(2+\theta) + v + \alpha \right], \tag{14.54}$$
$$C := (\alpha + \chi)(\chi + v), \tag{14.55}$$

and $I(t)$ is given by Eq (14.48), $E(t)$ by Eq (14.49) and $U(t)$ by Eq (14.50).

14.2.3.1 Compatibility conditions for the positivity of the transmission rate

Recall from Eq (14.51):

$$\tau(t) = \frac{\chi N(t)\left(1 - \left(\frac{N(t)}{N_\infty}\right)^\theta\right)}{I(t) + \kappa U(t)} \times \frac{\left[A\left(\frac{N(t)}{N_\infty}\right)^{2\theta} - B\left(\frac{N(t)}{N_\infty}\right)^\theta + C\right]}{E_0 + S_0 - E(t) - \alpha CE(t)}.$$

Here we require that the numerator and the denominator of the last fraction stay positive for all times.

Positivity of the numerator: The model is compatible with the data if the transmission rate $\tau(t)$ stays positive for all times $t \in \mathbb{R}$. The numerator

$$p(N) := AN^2 - BN + C$$

is a second-order polynomial with $N \in (0, 1)$. Let $\Delta := B^2 - 4AC$ be the discriminant of $p(N)$. Since $p'(0) = -B < 0$ and

$$p'(N) = 0 \Leftrightarrow N = \frac{B}{2A}$$

we have two cases: 1) $\frac{B}{2A} \geq 1$; or 2) $0 < \frac{B}{2A} < 1$.

Case 1: If $\frac{B}{2A} \geq 1$, $p(N)$ is non-negative for all $N \in [0, 1]$ if and only if

$$p(1) > 0 \Leftrightarrow A + C - B > 0. \tag{14.56}$$

Substituting A, B, C by their expressions, we get

$$
\begin{aligned}
A + C - B &= \chi^2(1+\theta)(1+2\theta) + (\alpha+\chi)(\chi+\nu) - \chi(1+\theta)(\chi(2+\theta)+\alpha+\nu) \\
&= \chi^2 + 2\chi^2\theta + \chi^2\theta + 2\chi^2\theta^2 + \alpha\chi + \alpha\nu + \chi^2 + \chi\nu \\
&\quad - 2\chi^2 - \chi\theta - 2\chi^2\theta - \chi^2\theta^2 - \alpha\chi - \nu\chi - \alpha\chi\theta - \nu\chi\theta \\
&= \chi^2\theta^2 + \alpha\nu - \alpha\chi\theta - \nu\chi\theta \\
&= (\alpha - \chi\theta)(\nu - \chi\theta).
\end{aligned}
$$

Case 2: If $\frac{B}{2A} < 1$, $p(N)$ is non-negative for all $N \in [0, 1]$ if and only if

$$p\left(\frac{B}{2A}\right)(1) > 0 \Leftrightarrow \Delta < 0 \Leftrightarrow B^2 - 4AC < 0. \tag{14.57}$$

Lemma 14.4 $\Delta < 0 \Rightarrow A + C - B > 0$.

Proof We have

$$\Delta < 0 \Rightarrow B^2 - 4AC \leq (B - 2A)^2 \Leftrightarrow B^2 - 4AC \leq B^2 - 4AB + 4A^2$$

and after simplifying the result follows.   □

Positivity of the denominator: Next we turn to the denominator in the expression of τ, i.e., we want to ensure

$$E_0 + S_0 - E(t) - \alpha CE(t) > 0 \text{ for all } t \in \mathbb{R}. \tag{14.58}$$

We let $Y := \dfrac{N(t)}{N_\infty}$ and observe that $E(t) + \alpha CE(t)$ can be written as

$$
\begin{aligned}
E(t) + \alpha CE(t) &= \frac{1}{\alpha v f}\big[\chi N_\infty Y(1 - Y^\theta)(\chi + v - \chi(1 + \theta)Y^\theta) \\
&\quad + \alpha N_\infty Y(\chi + v - \chi Y^\theta) - \alpha N_\infty Y_0(\chi + v - Y_0^\theta)\big] \\
&= \frac{N_\infty}{\alpha v f} Y\big[(\chi + \alpha)(\chi + v) - \chi(\alpha + v + \chi(2 + \theta))Y^\theta + \chi^2(1 + \theta)Y^{2\theta}\big] \\
&\quad - \frac{N_0}{v f}\left(\chi + v - Y_0^\theta\right),
\end{aligned}
$$

since we know that $A > 0$. Therefore Eq (14.58) becomes

$$
\begin{aligned}
Y\big[(\chi + \alpha)(\chi + v) &- \chi(\chi + v + \chi(1 + \theta) + \alpha)Y^\theta + \chi^2(1 + \theta)Y^{2\theta}\big] \\
&\leq \frac{\alpha v f}{N_\infty}\left[E_0 + S_0 + \frac{N_0}{v f}\left(\chi + v - \left(\frac{N_0}{N_\infty}\right)^\theta\right)\right].
\end{aligned}
$$

We let

$$g(Y) := Y\big[(\chi + \alpha)(\chi + v) - \chi(\alpha + v + \chi(2 + \theta))Y^\theta + \chi^2(1 + \theta)Y^{2\theta}\big]$$

and notice that

$$g'(Y) = (\chi + \alpha)(\chi + v) - \chi(1 + \theta)(\alpha + v + \chi(2 + \theta))Y^\theta + \chi^2(1 + 2\theta)(1 + \theta)Y^{2\theta}$$

is exactly $p(N) := AN^2 - BN + C$.

Therefore, assuming that $A + C - B > 0$, the derivative $g'(Y)$ is positive and g is strictly increasing. So we only have to check the final value $g(1)$. We get

$$
\begin{aligned}
\frac{\alpha v f}{N_\infty}\left(S_0 + E_0 + \frac{N_0}{v f}\left(\chi + v - \left(\frac{N_0}{N_\infty}\right)^\theta\right)\right) \\
\geq (\chi + \alpha)(\chi + v) - \chi(\alpha + v - \chi(2 + \theta)) + \chi^2(1 + \theta) \\
= \chi^2 + \alpha v + \alpha\chi + v\chi + \chi^2 + \chi^2\theta - \alpha\chi - v\chi - 2\chi^2 - \chi^2\theta \\
= \alpha v.
\end{aligned}
$$

Compatibility for the positivity

The SEIUR model is compatible with the data only when $\tau(t)$ stays positive for all $t \geq t_0$. Therefore the following two conditions should be met:

$$(\nu - \chi\theta)(\alpha - \chi\theta) \geq 0 \tag{14.59}$$

and

$$f + \frac{1}{\nu}\frac{N_0}{S_0 + E_0}\left(\chi + \nu - \left(\frac{N_0}{N_\infty}\right)^\theta\right) \geq \frac{N_\infty}{S_0 + E_0}. \tag{14.60}$$

14.2.3.2 Computing the explicit formula for $\tau(t)$ during an endemic phase

Recall that during an endemic phase, the cumulative number of cases is assumed to be a line. Therefore,

$$CR(t) = A(t - t_0) + B$$

and

$$CR'(t) = A \text{ and } CR''(t) = 0.$$

Therefore

$$I(t) = \frac{CR'(t)}{\nu f} = \frac{A}{\nu f} \tag{14.61}$$

and

$$E(t) = \frac{I'(t) + \nu I(t)}{\alpha} = \frac{A}{\alpha f}. \tag{14.62}$$

Hence

$$CE(t) = \frac{A}{\alpha f}(t - t_0). \tag{14.63}$$

Moreover

$$U(t) = e^{-\eta(t - t_0)}U_0 + \int_{t_0}^{t} e^{-\eta(t-s)}\nu(1 - f)I(s)ds,$$

and we obtain

$$U(t) = e^{-\eta(t - t_0)}U_0 + \frac{(1 - f)A}{\eta f}\left(1 - e^{-\eta(t - t_0)}\right). \tag{14.64}$$

By combining Eqs (14.12) and (14.61)–(14.64) we obtain the following explicit formula.

Explicit formula for the transmission rate during an endemic phase

The transmission rate $\tau(t)$ can be computed as

$$\tau(t) = \frac{1}{\frac{A}{vf} + \kappa \left(e^{-\eta(t-t_0)} U_0 + \frac{1-f}{\eta f} A \left(1 - e^{-\eta(t-t_0)} \right) \right)} \times \frac{A}{fS_0 - A(t-t_0)},$$

(14.65)

with the compatibility condition

$$t_0 \leq t < \frac{fS_0}{A} + t_0.$$

Remark 14.5 The above transmission rate corresponds to a constant number of daily infected A. Therefore it is impossible to maintain such a constant flux of new infected whenever the number of susceptible individuals is finite. The time $t = \dfrac{fS_0}{A} + t_0$ corresponds to the maximal time starting from t_0 during which we can maintain such a regime.

14.3 Results

14.3.1 Phenomenological model applied to COVID-19 data

Our method to regularize the data was applied to the eight geographic areas. The resulting curves are presented in Figure 14.2. The blue background color regions correspond to epidemic phases, and the yellow background color regions to endemic phases. We added a plot of the daily number of cases (black dots) and the derivative of the regularized model for comparison, even though the daily number of cases is not used in the fitting procedure. In general, the figures show an extremely good agreement between the time series of reported cases (top row, black dots) and the regularized model (top row, blue curve). The match between the daily number of cases (bottom row, black dots) and the derivative of the regularized model (bottom row, blue curve) is also excellent, even though it is not a part of the optimization process. Of course, we lose some of the information like the extremal values ("peaks") of the daily number of cases. This is because we focus on an averaged value of the number of cases. More information could be retrieved by studying statistically the variation around the phenomenological model. However, we leave such a study for future work. The relative error between the regularized curve and the data may be relatively high at the beginning of the epidemic because of the stochastic nature of the infection process and the small number of infected individuals but quickly drops below 1% (see the supplementary material for more details).

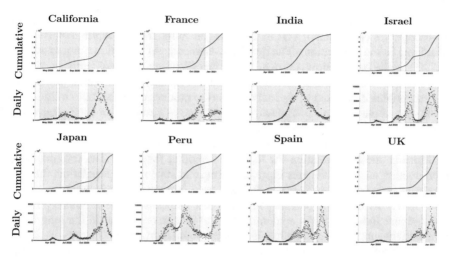

Fig. 14.2: *In the top rows, we plot the cumulative number of reported cases (black dots) and the best fit of the phenomenological model (blue curve). In the bottom rows, we plot the daily number of reported cases (black dots) and the first derivative of the phenomenological model (blue curve).*

14.3.2 Bounds for the value of non-identifiable parameters

Even if some parameters of the mathematical model are not identifiable, we were able to gain some information on possible values for those parameters. Indeed, a mathematical model with a negative transmission rate $\tau(t)$ cannot be consistent with the real phenomenon. Therefore, parameter values which produce such negative transmission rates cannot be compatible with the data. Using this argument, we found that the average incubation period cannot exceed eight days. The actual value of the upper bound is highly variable across countries and epidemic waves. We report the values of the upper bound in the supplementary material.

14.3.3 Instantaneous reproduction number computed for COVID-19 data

Our analysis allows us to compute the instantaneous transmission rate $\tau(t)$. We use this transmission rate to compute two different indicators of the epidemiological dynamics for each geographic area, the instantaneous reproduction number and the quasi-instantaneous reproduction number. Both coincide with the basic reproduction number R_0 on the first day of the epidemic. The instantaneous reproduction number at time t, $R_e(t)$, is the basic reproduction number corresponding to an epidemic starting at time t with a constant transmission rate equal to $\tau(t)$ and with an initial population of susceptibles composed of $S(t)$ individuals (the number of susceptible individuals remaining in the population). The quasi-instantaneous reproduction number at time t, $R_e^0(t)$, is the basic reproduction number corresponding to an epidemic starting at time t with a constant transmission rate equal to $\tau(t)$ and with an initial population of susceptibles composed of S_0 individuals (the number of susceptible individuals at the start of the epidemic). The two indicators are represented for each geographic area in the top row of Figure 14.3 (black curve: instantaneous reproduction number; green curve: quasi-instantaneous reproduction number).

There is one interpretation for $R_e(t)$ and another for $R_e^0(t)$. The instantaneous reproduction number indicates if, given the current state of the population, the epidemic tends to persist or die out in the long term (note that our model assumes that recovered individuals are perfectly immunized). The quasi-instantaneous reproduction number indicates if the epidemic tends to persist or die out in the long term, provided the number of susceptible is the total population. In other words, we forget about the immunity already obtained by recovered individuals. Also, it is directly proportional to the transmission rate and therefore allows monitoring of its changes. Note that the value of $R_e^0(t)$ changed drastically between epidemic phases, revealing that $\tau(t)$ is far from constant. In any case, the difference between the two values starts to be visible in the figures one year after the start of the epidemic.

We also computed the reproduction number by using the method described in Cori et al. [66], which we denote by $R_e^c(t)$. The precise implementation is described in the supplementary material. It is plotted in the bottom row of Figure 14.3 (green curve), along with the instantaneous reproduction number $R_e(t)$ (green curve).

Remark 14.6 In the bottom of Figure 14.3, we compare the instantaneous reproduction numbers obtained by our method in black and the classical method of Cori et al. [66] in green. We observe that the two approaches are not the same at the beginning. This is because the method of Cori et al. [66] does not take into account the initial values I_0 and E_0 while we do. Indeed the method of Cori et al. [66] assumes that I_0 and E_0 are close to 0 at the beginning when it is viewed as a Volterra equation reformulation of the Bernoulli–Kermack–McKendrick model with the age of infection. Our method, on the other hand, does not require such an assumption since it provides a way to compute the initial states I_0 and E_0.

Remark 14.7 It is essential to "regularize" the data to obtain a comprehensive outcome from SIR epidemic models. In general, the rate of transmission in the SIR model (applying identification methods) is not very noisy, and is meaningless. For example, at the beginning of the first epidemic wave, the transmission rate should be decreasing since people tend to have less and less contact during epidemic growth. Standard regularization methods (like, for example, the rolling weekly average method) have been tested for COVID-19 data in Demongeot, Griette and Magal [77]. The outcome in terms of transmission rate is very noisy and even shows negative transmission (which is impossible). Regularizing the data is not an easy task, and the method used is very important in order to obtain a meaningful outcome for the models. Here, we tried several approaches to link an epidemic phase to the next endemic phase. So far, this regularization procedure is the best one we have tested.

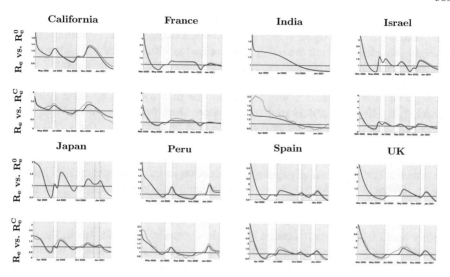

Fig. 14.3: *In the top rows, we plot the instantaneous reproduction number $R_e(t)$ (in black) and the quasi instantaneous reproduction number $R_e^0(t)$ (in green). In the bottom rows, we plot the instantaneous reproduction number $R_e(t)$ (in black) and the one obtained by the standard method [66, 309] $R_e^c(t)$ (in green).*

14.4 Discussion

In this chapter, we presented a new phenomenological model to describe cumulative reported cases data. This model allows us to handle multiple epidemic waves and fits the data for the eight geographic areas considered very well. The use of Bernoulli–Verhulst curves to fit an epidemic wave is not necessary. We expect that a number of different phenomenological models could be employed for the same purpose; however, our method has the advantage of involving a limited number of parameters. Moreover, the Bernoulli–Verhulst model leads to an explicit algebraic formula for the compatibility conditions of non-identifiable parameters. It is far from obvious that the same computations can be carried out with other models. Our method also provides a very smooth curve with controlled upper bound for the first (four) derivatives, and we use the regularity obtained to compute the transmission rate. We refer to Demongeot, Griette and Magal [77] for several examples of problems that may occur when using other methods to regularize the data (rolling weekly average, etc.).

The first goal of the chapter is to understand how to connect successive epidemic waves. As far as we know, this is new compared to the existing literature. A succession of epidemic waves separated by a short period of time with random transmissions is regularly observed in the COVID-19 epidemic data. But several consecutive epidemic phases may happen without endemic transition. An illustration of this situation is provided by the case of Japan, where the parameters of the Bernoulli–Verhulst model changed three times during the last epidemic phases (without endemic interruption). Therefore we subdivide this last epidemic wave into three epidemic phases.

Another advantage of our method is the connection with an epidemiological model. Our study provides a way to explain the data by using a single epidemic model with a time-dependent transmission rate. More precisely, we find that there exists precisely one model that matches the best fit to the data. The fact that the transmission rate corresponding to the data is not constant is, therefore, meaningful. This means that the depletion of susceptible hosts due to natural epidemiological dynamics is not sufficient to explain the reduction in the epidemic spread. Indeed, due to the social changes involving the distancing between individuals, the transmission rate should vary to take into account the changes in the number of contacts per unit of time. The variations in the observed dynamics of the number of cases mainly result from the modification of people's behavior. In other words, the social changes in the population have a stronger impact on the propagation of the disease than the pure epidemiological dynamics. By computing the transmission rate and the associated reproduction numbers, we propose a new method to quantify those social changes. Other factors may also influence the dynamics of the COVID-19 outbreak (temperature, humidity, etc.) and should be taken into account. However, the correlation between the dates of the waves and the mitigation measures imposed by local governments suggests that the former phenomenon plays a more significant role in the epidemiological dynamics.

Precisely because it involves an epidemiological model, our method provides an alternative, robust way to compute indicators for the future behavior of the epidemic: the instantaneous and quasi-instantaneous reproductive numbers $R_e(t)$ and $R_e^0(t)$. It is natural to compare them to an alternative in the literature, sometimes called "effective reproductive number". The method of Cori et al. [66] is a popular framework to estimate its value. Compared with this standard method, our indicators perform better near the beginning of the epidemic and close to the last data point and are less variable in time. That we require an *a priori* definition of epidemic waves can be considered as both an advantage and a drawback. It is a drawback because the computed value of the indicator may slightly depend on the choice of the dates of the epidemic waves. On the other hand, this flexibility also allows testing different scenarios for the future evolution of the epidemic. Thanks to the explicit formula for $R_e(t)$ expressed as a function of the parameters, we can also explore the dependency on the parameters (see supplementary material Section A6).

It appears from our results that the instantaneous reproduction number in almost every geographic area considered is less than 3.5. Therefore, an efficient policy to eliminate the COVID-19 would be to vaccinate a fraction of $75 - 80\%$ of the population. Once this threshold is reached, the situation should go back to normal in all the geographic areas considered in this study. This proportion can even be reduced at the expense of partially maintaining the social distancing and the other anti-COVID measures for a sufficiently long period of time.

With a few modifications, our method could also include several other features. It is likely, for instance, that the vaccination of a large part of the population has an impact on the epidemiological dynamics, and this impact is not taken into account for the time being. Different distributions of serial intervals could be taken into account by replacing the mathematical model of ordinary differential equations with integral equations. What we have shown is that the coupling of a phenomenological model to describe the data, with an epidemiological model to take into account the nature of the underlying phenomenon, should provide us with a new, untapped source of information on the epidemic.

Supplementary Material

A1 Table of estimated parameters for the phenomenological model

California

Period	Parameters value	Method	95% Confidence interval
Period 1: Epidemic phase Mar 26, 2020 - Jun 11, 2020	$N_0 = 7.34 \times 10^3$	fitted	$N_0 \in [4.16 \times 10^3, 1.05 \times 10^4]$
	$N_{base} = 1.14 \times 10^{-5}$	fitted	$N_{base} \in [-4.33 \times 10^3, 4.33 \times 10^3]$
	$N_\infty = 3.24 \times 10^5$	fitted	$N_\infty \in [2.52 \times 10^5, 3.96 \times 10^5]$
	$\chi = 4.14 \times 10^4$	fitted	$\chi \in [7.74 \times 10^2, 8.20 \times 10^4]$
	$\theta = 4.62 \times 10^{-7}$	fitted	$\theta \in [2.39 \times 10^{-8}, 9.00 \times 10^{-7}]$
Period 2: Endemic phase Jun 11, 2020 - Jun 23, 2020	$a = 3.81 \times 10^3$	computed	
	$N_0 = 1.36 \times 10^5$	computed	
Period 3: Epidemic phase Jun 23, 2020 - Sep 20, 2020	$N_0 = 1.57 \times 10^5$	fitted	$N_0 \in [5.96 \times 10^4, 2.55 \times 10^5]$
	$N_{base} = 2.45 \times 10^4$	fitted	$N_{base} \in [-7.58 \times 10^4, 1.25 \times 10^5]$
	$N_\infty = 8.22 \times 10^5$	fitted	$N_\infty \in [7.36 \times 10^5, 9.08 \times 10^5]$
	$\chi = 5.54 \times 10^{-2}$	fitted	$\chi \in [5.32 \times 10^{-3}, 1.05 \times 10^{-1}]$
	$\theta = 7.18 \times 10^{-1}$	fitted	$\theta \in [-3.59 \times 10^{-2}, 1.47]$
Period 4: Endemic phase Sep 20, 2020 - Nov 01, 2020	$a = 3.66 \times 10^3$	computed	
	$N_0 = 7.76 \times 10^5$	computed	
Period 5: Epidemic phase Nov 01, 2020 - Feb 25, 2021	$N_0 = 6.27 \times 10^4$	fitted	$N_0 \in [4.95 \times 10^4, 7.59 \times 10^4]$
	$N_{base} = 8.67 \times 10^5$	fitted	$N_{base} \in [8.45 \times 10^5, 8.88 \times 10^5]$
	$N_\infty = 2.66 \times 10^6$	fitted	$N_\infty \in [2.64 \times 10^6, 2.67 \times 10^6]$
	$\chi = 6.36 \times 10^{-2}$	fitted	$\chi \in [5.73 \times 10^{-2}, 6.98 \times 10^{-2}]$
	$\theta = 1.02$	fitted	$\theta \in [8.79 \times 10^{-1}, 1.16]$

Table A1: *In this table we list the parameters of the phenomenological model which gives the best fit to the cumulative number of cases data in California from January 03 2020 to February 25 2021.*

France

Period	Parameters value	Method	95% Confidence interval
Period 1: Epidemic phase Feb 27, 2020 - May 17, 2020	$N_0 = 3.61 \times 10^{-4}$	fitted	$N_0 \in [-3.77, 3.77]$
	$N_{base} = 0.00$	fixed	
	$N_\infty = 1.43 \times 10^5$	fitted	$N_\infty \in [-1.58 \times 10^4, 3.01 \times 10^5]$
	$\chi = 1.17 \times 10^2$	fitted	$\chi \in [-1.09 \times 10^7, 1.09 \times 10^7]$
	$\theta = 7.29 \times 10^{-4}$	fitted	$\theta \in [-6.84 \times 10^1, 6.84 \times 10^1]$
Period 2: Endemic phase May 17, 2020 - Jul 05, 2020	$a = 3.14 \times 10^2$	computed	
	$N_0 = 1.39 \times 10^5$	computed	
Period 3: Epidemic phase Jul 05, 2020 - Nov 26, 2020	$N_0 = 1.50 \times 10^4$	fitted	$N_0 \in [1.36 \times 10^4, 1.65 \times 10^4]$
	$N_{base} = 1.40 \times 10^5$	fitted	$N_{base} \in [1.33 \times 10^5, 1.46 \times 10^5]$
	$N_\infty = 1.99 \times 10^6$	fitted	$N_\infty \in [1.97 \times 10^6, 2.01 \times 10^6]$
	$\chi = 3.68 \times 10^{-2}$	fitted	$\chi \in [3.60 \times 10^{-2}, 3.76 \times 10^{-2}]$
	$\theta = 6.55$	fitted	$\theta \in [5.52, 7.58]$
Period 4: Endemic phase Nov 26, 2020 - Dec 20, 2020	$a = 1.28 \times 10^4$	computed	
	$N_0 = 2.11 \times 10^6$	computed	
Period 5: Epidemic phase Dec 20, 2020 - Feb 25, 2021	$N_0 = 2.73 \times 10^5$	fitted	$N_0 \in [-2.43 \times 10^3, 5.48 \times 10^5]$
	$N_{base} = 2.15 \times 10^6$	fitted	$N_{base} \in [1.86 \times 10^6, 2.43 \times 10^6]$
	$N_\infty = 2.13 \times 10^6$	fitted	$N_\infty \in [1.88 \times 10^6, 2.39 \times 10^6]$
	$\chi = 5.88 \times 10^{-2}$	fitted	$\chi \in [-6.11 \times 10^{-2}, 1.79 \times 10^{-1}]$
	$\theta = 5.47 \times 10^{-1}$	fitted	$\theta \in [-9.19 \times 10^{-1}, 2.01]$

Table A2: *In this table we list the parameters of the phenomenological model which gives the best fit to the cumulative number of cases data in France from January 03 2020 to February 25 2021.*

India

Period	Parameters value	Method	95% Confidence interval
Period 1: Epidemic phase Feb 01, 2020 - Feb 25, 2021	$N_0 = 5.83 \times 10^2$	fitted	$N_0 \in [3.45 \times 10^2, 8.20 \times 10^2]$
	$N_{base} = 1.97 \times 10^4$	fitted	$N_{base} \in [5.36 \times 10^3, 3.39 \times 10^4]$
	$N_\infty = 1.10 \times 10^7$	fitted	$N_\infty \in [1.10 \times 10^7, 1.11 \times 10^7]$
	$\chi = 4.89 \times 10^{-2}$	fitted	$\chi \in [4.59 \times 10^{-2}, 5.20 \times 10^{-2}]$
	$\theta = 5.12 \times 10^{-1}$	fitted	$\theta \in [4.71 \times 10^{-1}, 5.54 \times 10^{-1}]$

Table A3: *In this table we list the parameters of the phenomenological model which gives the best fit to the cumulative number of cases data in India from January 03 2020 to February 25 2021.*

Israel

Period	Parameters value	Method	95% Confidence interval
Period 1: Epidemic phase Feb 27, 2020 - Jun 01, 2020	$N_0 = 1.08 \times 10^{-2}$	fitted	$N_0 \in [-3.85 \times 10^{-2}, 6.02 \times 10^{-2}]$
	$N_{base} = 4.27 \times 10^1$	fitted	$N_{base} \in [-3.36 \times 10^1, 1.19 \times 10^2]$
	$N_\infty = 1.71 \times 10^4$	fitted	$N_\infty \in [1.70 \times 10^4, 1.72 \times 10^4]$
	$\chi = 9.18 \times 10^{-1}$	fitted	$\chi \in [1.71 \times 10^{-1}, 1.67]$
	$\theta = 1.05 \times 10^{-1}$	fitted	$\theta \in [1.55 \times 10^{-2}, 1.94 \times 10^{-1}]$
Period 2: Endemic phase Jun 01, 2020 - Jun 25, 2020	$a = 2.04 \times 10^2$	computed	
	$N_0 = 1.70 \times 10^4$	computed	
Period 3: Epidemic phase Jun 25, 2020 - Aug 08, 2020	$N_0 = 2.48 \times 10^3$	fitted	$N_0 \in [3.43 \times 10^2, 4.61 \times 10^3]$
	$N_{base} = 1.95 \times 10^4$	fitted	$N_{base} \in [1.70 \times 10^4, 2.20 \times 10^4]$
	$N_\infty = 8.66 \times 10^4$	fitted	$N_\infty \in [7.78 \times 10^4, 9.55 \times 10^4]$
	$\chi = 2.93 \times 10^{-1}$	fitted	$\chi \in [-2.61 \times 10^{-1}, 8.48 \times 10^{-1}]$
	$\theta = 2.04 \times 10^{-1}$	fitted	$\theta \in [-2.43 \times 10^{-1}, 6.50 \times 10^{-1}]$
Period 4: Endemic phase Aug 08, 2020 - Sep 03, 2020	$a = 1.54 \times 10^3$	computed	
	$N_0 = 7.97 \times 10^4$	computed	
Period 5: Epidemic phase Sep 03, 2020 - Oct 20, 2020	$N_0 = 4.59 \times 10^4$	fitted	$N_0 \in [2.88 \times 10^4, 6.31 \times 10^4]$
	$N_{base} = 7.38 \times 10^4$	fitted	$N_{base} \in [5.53 \times 10^4, 9.23 \times 10^4]$
	$N_\infty = 2.35 \times 10^5$	fitted	$N_\infty \in [2.19 \times 10^5, 2.52 \times 10^5]$
	$\chi = 5.05 \times 10^{-2}$	fitted	$\chi \in [3.77 \times 10^{-2}, 6.34 \times 10^{-2}]$
	$\theta = 3.45$	fitted	$\theta \in [1.96, 4.93]$
Period 6: Endemic phase Oct 20, 2020 - Nov 14, 2020	$a = 8.90 \times 10^2$	computed	
	$N_0 = 3.04 \times 10^5$	computed	
Period 7: Epidemic phase Nov 14, 2020 - Feb 25, 2021	$N_0 = 3.16 \times 10^3$	fitted	$N_0 \in [2.16 \times 10^3, 4.17 \times 10^3]$
	$N_{base} = 3.23 \times 10^5$	fitted	$N_{base} \in [3.21 \times 10^5, 3.25 \times 10^5]$
	$N_\infty = 4.87 \times 10^5$	fitted	$N_\infty \in [4.79 \times 10^5, 4.95 \times 10^5]$
	$\chi = 8.28 \times 10^{-2}$	fitted	$\chi \in [7.22 \times 10^{-2}, 9.34 \times 10^{-2}]$
	$\theta = 7.06 \times 10^{-1}$	fitted	$\theta \in [5.69 \times 10^{-1}, 8.43 \times 10^{-1}]$

Table A4: *In this table we list the parameters of the phenomenological model which gives the best fit to the cumulative number of cases data in Israel from January 03 2020 to February 25 2021.*

Japan

Period	Parameters value	Method	95% Confidence interval
Period 1: Epidemic phase Feb 20, 2020 - May 27, 2020	$N_0 = 5.83$	fitted	$N_0 \in [1.91, 9.74]$
	$N_{base} = 3.25 \times 10^2$	fitted	$N_{base} \in [2.55 \times 10^2, 3.95 \times 10^2]$
	$N_\infty = 1.63 \times 10^4$	fitted	$N_\infty \in [1.62 \times 10^4, 1.64 \times 10^4]$
	$\chi = 1.48 \times 10^{-1}$	fitted	$\chi \in [1.30 \times 10^{-1}, 1.65 \times 10^{-1}]$
	$\theta = 8.29 \times 10^{-1}$	fitted	$\theta \in [6.88 \times 10^{-1}, 9.70 \times 10^{-1}]$
Period 2: Endemic phase May 27, 2020 - Jun 13, 2020	$a = 7.07 \times 10^1$	computed	
	$N_0 = 1.65 \times 10^4$	computed	
Period 3: Epidemic phase Jun 13, 2020 - Sep 10, 2020	$N_0 = 1.49 \times 10^2$	fitted	$N_0 \in [8.52 \times 10^1, 2.13 \times 10^2]$
	$N_{base} = 1.75 \times 10^4$	fitted	$N_{base} \in [1.73 \times 10^4, 1.78 \times 10^4]$
	$N_\infty = 6.02 \times 10^4$	fitted	$N_\infty \in [5.93 \times 10^4, 6.10 \times 10^4]$
	$\chi = 1.19 \times 10^{-1}$	fitted	$\chi \in [1.03 \times 10^{-1}, 1.35 \times 10^{-1}]$
	$\theta = 6.28 \times 10^{-1}$	fitted	$\theta \in [5.04 \times 10^{-1}, 7.52 \times 10^{-1}]$
Period 4: Endemic phase Sep 10, 2020 - Oct 18, 2020	$a = 5.36 \times 10^2$	computed	
	$N_0 = 7.27 \times 10^4$	computed	
Period 5: Epidemic phase Oct 18, 2020 - Dec 05, 2020	$N_0 = 6.33 \times 10^3$	fitted	$N_0 \in [4.64 \times 10^3, 8.01 \times 10^3]$
	$N_{base} = 8.68 \times 10^4$	fitted	$N_{base} \in [8.48 \times 10^4, 8.88 \times 10^4]$
	$N_\infty = 9.10 \times 10^4$	fitted	$N_\infty \in [7.75 \times 10^4, 1.05 \times 10^5]$
	$\chi = 5.60 \times 10^{-2}$	fitted	$\chi \in [4.74 \times 10^{-2}, 6.46 \times 10^{-2}]$
	$\theta = 2.58$	fitted	$\theta \in [1.00, 4.16]$
Period 6: Epidemic phase Dec 05, 2020 - Dec 30, 2020	$N_0 = 1.23 \times 10^5$	fitted	$N_0 \in [-2.43 \times 10^5, 4.90 \times 10^5]$
	$N_{base} = 3.43 \times 10^4$	fitted	$N_{base} \in [-3.33 \times 10^5, 4.01 \times 10^5]$
	$N_\infty = 3.49 \times 10^5$	fitted	$N_\infty \in [-2.92 \times 10^7, 2.99 \times 10^7]$
	$\chi = 1.78 \times 10^{-2}$	fitted	$\chi \in [-3.59 \times 10^{-2}, 7.15 \times 10^{-2}]$
	$\theta = 7.84$	fitted	$\theta \in [-1.28 \times 10^3, 1.30 \times 10^3]$
Period 7: Epidemic phase Dec 30, 2020 - Feb 25, 2021	$N_0 = 2.00 \times 10^4$	fitted	$N_0 \in [1.59 \times 10^3, 3.84 \times 10^4]$
	$N_{base} = 2.05 \times 10^5$	fitted	$N_{base} \in [1.85 \times 10^5, 2.25 \times 10^5]$
	$N_\infty = 2.29 \times 10^5$	fitted	$N_\infty \in [2.11 \times 10^5, 2.47 \times 10^5]$
	$\chi = 7.98 \times 10^{-1}$	fitted	$\chi \in [-2.54, 4.13]$
	$\theta = 9.61 \times 10^{-2}$	fitted	$\theta \in [-3.15 \times 10^{-1}, 5.07 \times 10^{-1}]$

Table A5: *In this table we list the parameters of the phenomenological model which gives the best fit to the cumulative number of cases data in Japan from January 03 2020 to February 25 2021.*

Peru

Period	Parameters value	Method	95% Confidence interval
Period 1: Epidemic phase Mar 20, 2020 - Jul 01, 2020	$N_0 = 8.36 \times 10^2$	fitted	$N_0 \in [2.63 \times 10^2, 1.41 \times 10^3]$
	$N_{base} = 3.00 \times 10^{-5}$	fitted	$N_{base} \in [-1.74 \times 10^3, 1.74 \times 10^3]$
	$N_\infty = 3.61 \times 10^5$	fitted	$N_\infty \in [3.44 \times 10^5, 3.79 \times 10^5]$
	$\chi = 1.08 \times 10^{-1}$	fitted	$\chi \in [7.59 \times 10^{-2}, 1.41 \times 10^{-1}]$
	$\theta = 4.20 \times 10^{-1}$	fitted	$\theta \in [2.41 \times 10^{-1}, 5.98 \times 10^{-1}]$
Period 2: Endemic phase Jul 01, 2020 - Jul 30, 2020	$a = 3.67 \times 10^3$	computed	
	$N_0 = 2.83 \times 10^5$	computed	
Period 3: Epidemic phase Jul 30, 2020 - Nov 10, 2020	$N_0 = 1.86 \times 10^5$	fitted	$N_0 \in [-2.61 \times 10^4, 3.98 \times 10^5]$
	$N_{base} = 2.03 \times 10^5$	fitted	$N_{base} \in [-1.11 \times 10^4, 4.18 \times 10^5]$
	$N_\infty = 7.69 \times 10^5$	fitted	$N_\infty \in [5.65 \times 10^5, 9.72 \times 10^5]$
	$\chi = 4.84 \times 10^{-1}$	fitted	$\chi \in [-6.23, 7.20]$
	$\theta = 5.95 \times 10^{-2}$	fitted	$\theta \in [-7.74 \times 10^{-1}, 8.93 \times 10^{-1}]$
Period 4: Endemic phase Nov 10, 2020 - Jan 11, 2021	$a = 1.80 \times 10^3$	computed	
	$N_0 = 9.16 \times 10^5$	computed	
Period 5: Epidemic phase Jan 11, 2021 - Feb 25, 2021	$N_0 = 3.23 \times 10^5$	fitted	
	$N_{base} = 7.04 \times 10^5$	fitted	
	$N_\infty = 7.00 \times 10^6$	fitted	
	$\chi = 1.36 \times 10^{-2}$	fitted	
	$\theta = 3.67 \times 10^1$	fitted	

Table A6: *In this table we list the parameters of the phenomenological model which gives the best fit to the cumulative number of cases data in Peru from January 03 2020 to February 25 2021.*

Spain

Period	Parameters value	Method	95% Confidence interval
Period 1: Epidemic phase Feb 15, 2020 - May 10, 2020	$N_0 = 5.19 \times 10^{-4}$	fitted	$N_0 \in [-5.00 \times 10^{-3}, 6.04 \times 10^{-3}]$
	$N_{base} = 5.77 \times 10^2$	fitted	$N_{base} \in [-4.50 \times 10^2, 1.60 \times 10^3]$
	$N_\infty = 2.32 \times 10^5$	fitted	$N_\infty \in [2.30 \times 10^5, 2.34 \times 10^5]$
	$\chi = 9.80 \times 10^{-1}$	fitted	$\chi \in [-1.26 \times 10^{-1}, 2.09]$
	$\theta = 9.75 \times 10^{-2}$	fitted	$\theta \in [-1.83 \times 10^{-2}, 2.13 \times 10^{-1}]$
Period 2: Endemic phase May 10, 2020 - Jun 22, 2020	$a = 5.67 \times 10^2$	computed	
	$N_0 = 2.28 \times 10^5$	computed	
Period 3: Epidemic phase Jun 22, 2020 - Oct 02, 2020	$N_0 = 2.38 \times 10^3$	fitted	$N_0 \in [1.39 \times 10^3, 3.36 \times 10^3]$
	$N_{base} = 2.50 \times 10^5$	fitted	$N_{base} \in [2.48 \times 10^5, 2.53 \times 10^5]$
	$N_\infty = 9.89 \times 10^5$	fitted	$N_\infty \in [9.02 \times 10^5, 1.08 \times 10^6]$
	$\chi = 9.29 \times 10^{-2}$	fitted	$\chi \in [7.07 \times 10^{-2}, 1.15 \times 10^{-1}]$
	$\theta = 3.84 \times 10^{-1}$	fitted	$\theta \in [2.38 \times 10^{-1}, 5.29 \times 10^{-1}]$
Period 4: Endemic phase Oct 02, 2020 - Oct 18, 2020	$a = 1.09 \times 10^4$	computed	
	$N_0 = 8.14 \times 10^5$	computed	
Period 5: Epidemic phase Oct 18, 2020 - Dec 06, 2020	$N_0 = 1.68 \times 10^5$	fitted	$N_0 \in [-3.50 \times 10^4, 3.72 \times 10^5]$
	$N_{base} = 8.20 \times 10^5$	fitted	$N_{base} \in [6.12 \times 10^5, 1.03 \times 10^6]$
	$N_\infty = 9.85 \times 10^5$	fitted	$N_\infty \in [8.01 \times 10^5, 1.17 \times 10^6]$
	$\chi = 3.15 \times 10^{-1}$	fitted	$\chi \in [-1.05, 1.68]$
	$\theta = 2.02 \times 10^{-1}$	fitted	$\theta \in [-7.15 \times 10^{-1}, 1.12]$
Period 6: Endemic phase Dec 06, 2020 - Dec 26, 2020	$a = 9.15 \times 10^3$	computed	
	$N_0 = 1.72 \times 10^6$	computed	
Period 7: Epidemic phase Dec 26, 2020 - Feb 25, 2021	$N_0 = 5.94 \times 10^4$	fitted	$N_0 \in [3.86 \times 10^4, 8.02 \times 10^4]$
	$N_{base} = 1.84 \times 10^6$	fitted	$N_{base} \in [1.81 \times 10^6, 1.87 \times 10^6]$
	$N_\infty = 1.30 \times 10^6$	fitted	$N_\infty \in [1.28 \times 10^6, 1.32 \times 10^6]$
	$\chi = 1.30 \times 10^{-1}$	fitted	$\chi \in [9.90 \times 10^{-2}, 1.60 \times 10^{-1}]$
	$\theta = 7.84 \times 10^{-1}$	fitted	$\theta \in [5.50 \times 10^{-1}, 1.02]$

Table A7: *In this table we list the parameters of the phenomenological model which gives the best fit to the cumulative number of cases data in Spain from January 03 2020 to February 01 2021.*

United Kingdom

Period	Parameters value	Method	95% Confidence interval
Period 1: Epidemic phase Feb 15, 2020 - Jun 15, 2020	$N_0 = 2.65 \times 10^{-2}$	fitted	$N_0 \in [-8.82 \times 10^{-2}, 1.41 \times 10^{-1}]$
	$N_{base} = 1.12 \times 10^2$	fitted	$N_{base} \in [-4.82 \times 10^2, 7.06 \times 10^2]$
	$N_\infty = 2.86 \times 10^5$	fitted	$N_\infty \in [2.84 \times 10^5, 2.88 \times 10^5]$
	$\chi = 1.76$	fitted	$\chi \in [-1.46, 4.98]$
	$\theta = 2.76 \times 10^{-2}$	fitted	$\theta \in [-2.38 \times 10^{-2}, 7.90 \times 10^{-2}]$
Period 2: Endemic phase Jun 15, 2020 - Sep 01, 2020	$a = 9.43 \times 10^2$	computed	
	$N_0 = 2.70 \times 10^5$	computed	
Period 3: Epidemic phase Sep 01, 2020 - Nov 20, 2020	$N_0 = 7.85 \times 10^3$	fitted	$N_0 \in [3.63 \times 10^3, 1.21 \times 10^4]$
	$N_{base} = 3.36 \times 10^5$	fitted	$N_{base} \in [3.28 \times 10^5, 3.43 \times 10^5]$
	$N_\infty = 2.14 \times 10^6$	fitted	$N_\infty \in [1.93 \times 10^6, 2.36 \times 10^6]$
	$\chi = 2.41 \times 10^{-1}$	fitted	$\chi \in [2.16 \times 10^{-2}, 4.60 \times 10^{-1}]$
	$\theta = 1.32 \times 10^{-1}$	fitted	$\theta \in [-9.25 \times 10^{-3}, 2.74 \times 10^{-1}]$
Period 4: Endemic phase Nov 20, 2020 - Dec 10, 2020	$a = 1.61 \times 10^4$	computed	
	$N_0 = 1.48 \times 10^6$	computed	
Period 5: Epidemic phase Dec 10, 2020 - Feb 01, 2021	$N_0 = 2.26 \times 10^5$	fitted	$N_0 \in [1.16 \times 10^5, 3.35 \times 10^5]$
	$N_{base} = 1.58 \times 10^6$	fitted	$N_{base} \in [1.46 \times 10^6, 1.70 \times 10^6]$
	$N_\infty = 2.42 \times 10^6$	fitted	$N_\infty \in [2.34 \times 10^6, 2.51 \times 10^6]$
	$\chi = 8.57 \times 10^{-2}$	fitted	$\chi \in [5.14 \times 10^{-2}, 1.20 \times 10^{-1}]$
	$\theta = 1.08$	fitted	$\theta \in [4.85 \times 10^{-1}, 1.68]$

Table A8: *In this table we list the parameters of the phenomenological model which gives the best fit to the cumulative number of cases data in the United Kingdom from January 03 2020 to February 01 2021.*

A2 Plot of the multiple Bernoulli–Verhulst models fitted to each epidemic phase

In Figure A1, we present the details of the fit of the Bernoulli–Verhulst models to the successive epidemic waves in the 8 geographic areas considered. Each epidemic wave is associated with a different color.

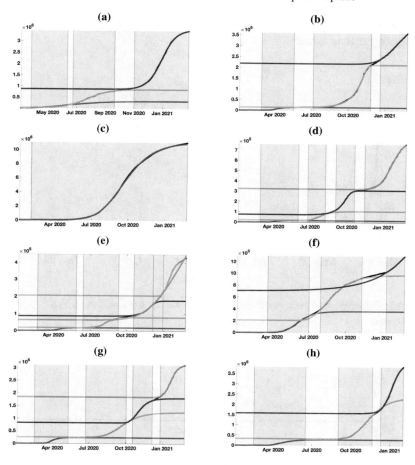

Fig. A1: *In this figure, we plot the cumulative number of cases (black dots) and the best fit of Bernoulli–Verhulst for each epidemic wave for (a) California; (b) France; (c) India; (d) Israel; (e) Japan; (f) Peru; (g) Spain; (h) United Kingdom.*

A3 Relative error of the fitted curve compared to the data in each geographic area

California

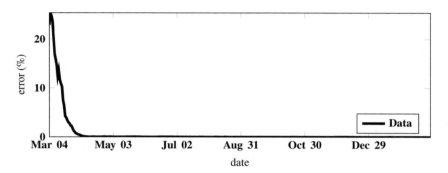

Fig. A2: *Relative error between the data and the model for California State, expressed in percent.*

France

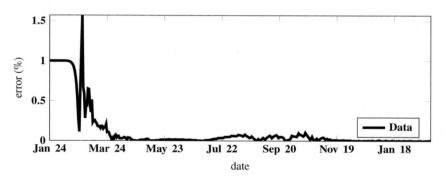

Fig. A3: *Relative error between the data and the model for France, expressed in percent.*

India

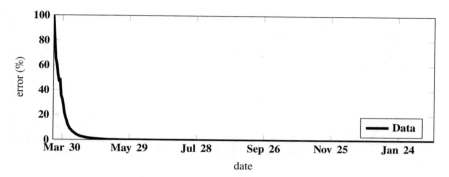

Fig. A4: *Relative error between the data and the model for India, expressed in percent.*

Israel

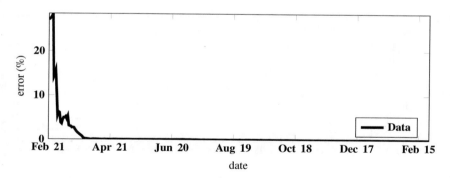

Fig. A5: *Relative error between the data and the model for Israel, expressed in percent.*

Japan

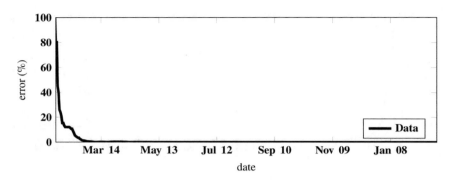

Fig. A6: *Relative error between the data and the model for Japan, expressed in percent.*

Peru

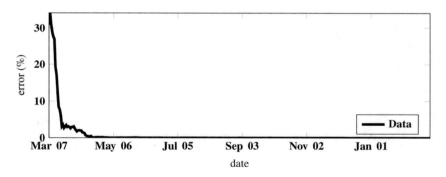

Fig. A7: *Relative error between the data and the model for Peru, expressed in percent.*

Spain

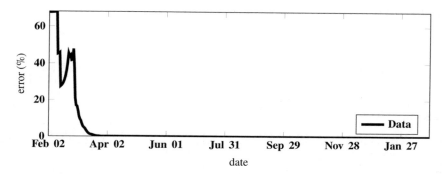

Fig. A8: *Relative error between the data and the model for Spain, expressed in percent.*

United Kingdom

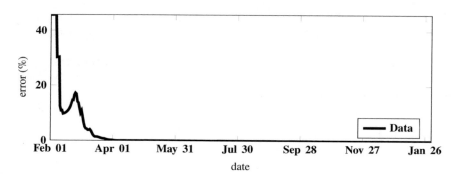

Fig. A9: *Relative error between the data and the model for the UK, expressed in percent.*

A4 Table of estimated parameters for the phenomenological model

California

Period	Parameters value	Method	95% Confidence interval
Period 1: Epidemic phase Mar 26, 2020 - Jun 11, 2020	$N_0 = 7.34 \times 10^3$	fitted	$N_0 \in [4.16 \times 10^3, 1.05 \times 10^4]$
	$N_{base} = 1.14 \times 10^{-5}$	fitted	$N_{base} \in [-4.33 \times 10^3, 4.33 \times 10^3]$
	$N_\infty = 3.24 \times 10^5$	fitted	$N_\infty \in [2.52 \times 10^5, 3.96 \times 10^5]$
	$\chi = 4.14 \times 10^4$	fitted	$\chi \in [7.74 \times 10^2, 8.20 \times 10^4]$
	$\theta = 4.62 \times 10^{-7}$	fitted	$\theta \in [2.39 \times 10^{-8}, 9.00 \times 10^{-7}]$
Period 2: Endemic phase Jun 11, 2020 - Jun 23, 2020	$a = 3.81 \times 10^3$	computed	
	$N_0 = 1.36 \times 10^5$	computed	
Period 3: Epidemic phase Jun 23, 2020 - Sep 20, 2020	$N_0 = 1.57 \times 10^5$	fitted	$N_0 \in [5.96 \times 10^4, 2.55 \times 10^5]$
	$N_{base} = 2.45 \times 10^4$	fitted	$N_{base} \in [-7.58 \times 10^4, 1.25 \times 10^5]$
	$N_\infty = 8.22 \times 10^5$	fitted	$N_\infty \in [7.36 \times 10^5, 9.08 \times 10^5]$
	$\chi = 5.54 \times 10^{-2}$	fitted	$\chi \in [5.32 \times 10^{-3}, 1.05 \times 10^{-1}]$
	$\theta = 7.18 \times 10^{-1}$	fitted	$\theta \in [-3.59 \times 10^{-2}, 1.47]$
Period 4: Endemic phase Sep 20, 2020 - Nov 01, 2020	$a = 3.66 \times 10^3$	computed	
	$N_0 = 7.76 \times 10^5$	computed	
Period 5: Epidemic phase Nov 01, 2020 - Feb 25, 2021	$N_0 = 6.27 \times 10^4$	fitted	$N_0 \in [4.95 \times 10^4, 7.59 \times 10^4]$
	$N_{base} = 8.67 \times 10^5$	fitted	$N_{base} \in [8.45 \times 10^5, 8.88 \times 10^5]$
	$N_\infty = 2.66 \times 10^6$	fitted	$N_\infty \in [2.64 \times 10^6, 2.67 \times 10^6]$
	$\chi = 6.36 \times 10^{-2}$	fitted	$\chi \in [5.73 \times 10^{-2}, 6.98 \times 10^{-2}]$
	$\theta = 1.02$	fitted	$\theta \in [8.79 \times 10^{-1}, 1.16]$

Table A9: *In this table we list the values of the parameters of the phenomenological model which give the best fit to the cumulative number of cases data in California from January 03 2020 to February 25 2021.*

France

Period	Parameters value	Method	95% Confidence interval
Period 1: Epidemic phase Feb 27, 2020 - May 17, 2020	$N_0 = 3.61 \times 10^{-4}$	fitted	$N_0 \in [-3.77, 3.77]$
	$N_{base} = 0.00$	fixed	
	$N_\infty = 1.43 \times 10^5$	fitted	$N_\infty \in [-1.58 \times 10^4, 3.01 \times 10^5]$
	$\chi = 1.17 \times 10^2$	fitted	$\chi \in [-1.09 \times 10^7, 1.09 \times 10^7]$
	$\theta = 7.29 \times 10^{-4}$	fitted	$\theta \in [-6.84 \times 10^1, 6.84 \times 10^1]$
Period 2: Endemic phase May 17, 2020 - Jul 05, 2020	$a = 3.14 \times 10^2$	computed	
	$N_0 = 1.39 \times 10^5$	computed	
Period 3: Epidemic phase Jul 05, 2020 - Nov 26, 2020	$N_0 = 1.50 \times 10^4$	fitted	$N_0 \in [1.36 \times 10^4, 1.65 \times 10^4]$
	$N_{base} = 1.40 \times 10^5$	fitted	$N_{base} \in [1.33 \times 10^5, 1.46 \times 10^5]$
	$N_\infty = 1.99 \times 10^6$	fitted	$N_\infty \in [1.97 \times 10^6, 2.01 \times 10^6]$
	$\chi = 3.68 \times 10^{-2}$	fitted	$\chi \in [3.60 \times 10^{-2}, 3.76 \times 10^{-2}]$
	$\theta = 6.55$	fitted	$\theta \in [5.52, 7.58]$
Period 4: Endemic phase Nov 26, 2020 - Dec 20, 2020	$a = 1.28 \times 10^4$	computed	
	$N_0 = 2.11 \times 10^6$	computed	
Period 5: Epidemic phase Dec 20, 2020 - Feb 25, 2021	$N_0 = 2.73 \times 10^5$	fitted	$N_0 \in [-2.43 \times 10^3, 5.48 \times 10^5]$
	$N_{base} = 2.15 \times 10^6$	fitted	$N_{base} \in [1.86 \times 10^6, 2.43 \times 10^6]$
	$N_\infty = 2.13 \times 10^6$	fitted	$N_\infty \in [1.88 \times 10^6, 2.39 \times 10^6]$
	$\chi = 5.88 \times 10^{-2}$	fitted	$\chi \in [-6.11 \times 10^{-2}, 1.79 \times 10^{-1}]$
	$\theta = 5.47 \times 10^{-1}$	fitted	$\theta \in [-9.19 \times 10^{-1}, 2.01]$

Table A10: *In this table we list the values of the parameters of the phenomenological model which give the best fit to the cumulative number of cases data in France from January 03 2020 to February 25 2021.*

India

Period	Parameters value	Method	95% Confidence interval
Period 1: Epidemic phase Feb 01, 2020 - Feb 25, 2021	$N_0 = 5.83 \times 10^2$	fitted	$N_0 \in [3.45 \times 10^2, 8.20 \times 10^2]$
	$N_{base} = 1.97 \times 10^4$	fitted	$N_{base} \in [5.36 \times 10^3, 3.39 \times 10^4]$
	$N_\infty = 1.10 \times 10^7$	fitted	$N_\infty \in [1.10 \times 10^7, 1.11 \times 10^7]$
	$\chi = 4.89 \times 10^{-2}$	fitted	$\chi \in [4.59 \times 10^{-2}, 5.20 \times 10^{-2}]$
	$\theta = 5.12 \times 10^{-1}$	fitted	$\theta \in [4.71 \times 10^{-1}, 5.54 \times 10^{-1}]$

Table A11: *In this table we list the values of the parameters of the phenomenological model which give the best fit to the cumulative number of cases data in India from January 03 2020 to February 25 2021.*

Israel

Period	Parameters value	Method	95% Confidence interval
Period 1: Epidemic phase Feb 27, 2020 - Jun 01, 2020	$N_0 = 1.08 \times 10^{-2}$	fitted	$N_0 \in [-3.85 \times 10^{-2}, 6.02 \times 10^{-2}]$
	$N_{base} = 4.27 \times 10^{1}$	fitted	$N_{base} \in [-3.36 \times 10^{1}, 1.19 \times 10^{2}]$
	$N_\infty = 1.71 \times 10^{4}$	fitted	$N_\infty \in [1.70 \times 10^{4}, 1.72 \times 10^{4}]$
	$\chi = 9.18 \times 10^{-1}$	fitted	$\chi \in [1.71 \times 10^{-1}, 1.67]$
	$\theta = 1.05 \times 10^{-1}$	fitted	$\theta \in [1.55 \times 10^{-2}, 1.94 \times 10^{-1}]$
Period 2: Endemic phase Jun 01, 2020 - Jun 25, 2020	$a = 2.04 \times 10^{2}$	computed	
	$N_0 = 1.70 \times 10^{4}$	computed	
Period 3: Epidemic phase Jun 25, 2020 - Aug 08, 2020	$N_0 = 2.48 \times 10^{3}$	fitted	$N_0 \in [3.43 \times 10^{2}, 4.61 \times 10^{3}]$
	$N_{base} = 1.95 \times 10^{4}$	fitted	$N_{base} \in [1.70 \times 10^{4}, 2.20 \times 10^{4}]$
	$N_\infty = 8.66 \times 10^{4}$	fitted	$N_\infty \in [7.78 \times 10^{4}, 9.55 \times 10^{4}]$
	$\chi = 2.93 \times 10^{-1}$	fitted	$\chi \in [-2.61 \times 10^{-1}, 8.48 \times 10^{-1}]$
	$\theta = 2.04 \times 10^{-1}$	fitted	$\theta \in [-2.43 \times 10^{-1}, 6.50 \times 10^{-1}]$
Period 4: Endemic phase Aug 08, 2020 - Sep 03, 2020	$a = 1.54 \times 10^{3}$	computed	
	$N_0 = 7.97 \times 10^{4}$	computed	
Period 5: Epidemic phase Sep 03, 2020 - Oct 20, 2020	$N_0 = 4.59 \times 10^{4}$	fitted	$N_0 \in [2.88 \times 10^{4}, 6.31 \times 10^{4}]$
	$N_{base} = 7.38 \times 10^{4}$	fitted	$N_{base} \in [5.53 \times 10^{4}, 9.23 \times 10^{4}]$
	$N_\infty = 2.35 \times 10^{5}$	fitted	$N_\infty \in [2.19 \times 10^{5}, 2.52 \times 10^{5}]$
	$\chi = 5.05 \times 10^{-2}$	fitted	$\chi \in [3.77 \times 10^{-2}, 6.34 \times 10^{-2}]$
	$\theta = 3.45$	fitted	$\theta \in [1.96, 4.93]$
Period 6: Endemic phase Oct 20, 2020 - Nov 14, 2020	$a = 8.90 \times 10^{2}$	computed	
	$N_0 = 3.04 \times 10^{5}$	computed	
Period 7: Epidemic phase Nov 14, 2020 - Feb 25, 2021	$N_0 = 3.16 \times 10^{3}$	fitted	$N_0 \in [2.16 \times 10^{3}, 4.17 \times 10^{3}]$
	$N_{base} = 3.23 \times 10^{5}$	fitted	$N_{base} \in [3.21 \times 10^{5}, 3.25 \times 10^{5}]$
	$N_\infty = 4.87 \times 10^{5}$	fitted	$N_\infty \in [4.79 \times 10^{5}, 4.95 \times 10^{5}]$
	$\chi = 8.28 \times 10^{-2}$	fitted	$\chi \in [7.22 \times 10^{-2}, 9.34 \times 10^{-2}]$
	$\theta = 7.06 \times 10^{-1}$	fitted	$\theta \in [5.69 \times 10^{-1}, 8.43 \times 10^{-1}]$

Table A12: *In this table we list the values of the parameters of the phenomenological model which give the best fit to the cumulative number of cases data in Israel from January 03 2020 to February 25 2021.*

Japan

Period	Parameters value	Method	95% Confidence interval
Period 1: Epidemic phase Feb 20, 2020 - May 27, 2020	$N_0 = 5.83$	fitted	$N_0 \in [1.91, 9.74]$
	$N_{base} = 3.25 \times 10^2$	fitted	$N_{base} \in [2.55 \times 10^2, 3.95 \times 10^2]$
	$N_\infty = 1.63 \times 10^4$	fitted	$N_\infty \in [1.62 \times 10^4, 1.64 \times 10^4]$
	$\chi = 1.48 \times 10^{-1}$	fitted	$\chi \in [1.30 \times 10^{-1}, 1.65 \times 10^{-1}]$
	$\theta = 8.29 \times 10^{-1}$	fitted	$\theta \in [6.88 \times 10^{-1}, 9.70 \times 10^{-1}]$
Period 2: Endemic phase May 27, 2020 - Jun 13, 2020	$a = 7.07 \times 10^1$	computed	
	$N_0 = 1.65 \times 10^4$	computed	
Period 3: Epidemic phase Jun 13, 2020 - Sep 10, 2020	$N_0 = 1.49 \times 10^2$	fitted	$N_0 \in [8.52 \times 10^1, 2.13 \times 10^2]$
	$N_{base} = 1.75 \times 10^4$	fitted	$N_{base} \in [1.73 \times 10^4, 1.78 \times 10^4]$
	$N_\infty = 6.02 \times 10^4$	fitted	$N_\infty \in [5.93 \times 10^4, 6.10 \times 10^4]$
	$\chi = 1.19 \times 10^{-1}$	fitted	$\chi \in [1.03 \times 10^{-1}, 1.35 \times 10^{-1}]$
	$\theta = 6.28 \times 10^{-1}$	fitted	$\theta \in [5.04 \times 10^{-1}, 7.52 \times 10^{-1}]$
Period 4: Endemic phase Sep 10, 2020 - Oct 18, 2020	$a = 5.36 \times 10^2$	computed	
	$N_0 = 7.27 \times 10^4$	computed	
Period 5: Epidemic phase Oct 18, 2020 - Dec 05, 2020	$N_0 = 6.33 \times 10^3$	fitted	$N_0 \in [4.64 \times 10^3, 8.01 \times 10^3]$
	$N_{base} = 8.68 \times 10^4$	fitted	$N_{base} \in [8.48 \times 10^4, 8.88 \times 10^4]$
	$N_\infty = 9.10 \times 10^4$	fitted	$N_\infty \in [7.75 \times 10^4, 1.05 \times 10^5]$
	$\chi = 5.60 \times 10^{-2}$	fitted	$\chi \in [4.74 \times 10^{-2}, 6.46 \times 10^{-2}]$
	$\theta = 2.58$	fitted	$\theta \in [1.00, 4.16]$
Period 6: Epidemic phase Dec 05, 2020 - Dec 30, 2020	$N_0 = 1.23 \times 10^5$	fitted	$N_0 \in [-2.43 \times 10^5, 4.90 \times 10^5]$
	$N_{base} = 3.43 \times 10^4$	fitted	$N_{base} \in [-3.33 \times 10^5, 4.01 \times 10^5]$
	$N_\infty = 3.49 \times 10^5$	fitted	$N_\infty \in [-2.92 \times 10^7, 2.99 \times 10^7]$
	$\chi = 1.78 \times 10^{-2}$	fitted	$\chi \in [-3.59 \times 10^{-2}, 7.15 \times 10^{-2}]$
	$\theta = 7.84$	fitted	$\theta \in [-1.28 \times 10^3, 1.30 \times 10^3]$
Period 7: Epidemic phase Dec 30, 2020 - Feb 25, 2021	$N_0 = 2.00 \times 10^4$	fitted	$N_0 \in [1.59 \times 10^3, 3.84 \times 10^4]$
	$N_{base} = 2.05 \times 10^5$	fitted	$N_{base} \in [1.85 \times 10^5, 2.25 \times 10^5]$
	$N_\infty = 2.29 \times 10^5$	fitted	$N_\infty \in [2.11 \times 10^5, 2.47 \times 10^5]$
	$\chi = 7.98 \times 10^{-1}$	fitted	$\chi \in [-2.54, 4.13]$
	$\theta = 9.61 \times 10^{-2}$	fitted	$\theta \in [-3.15 \times 10^{-1}, 5.07 \times 10^{-1}]$

Table A13: *In this table we list the values of the parameters of the phenomenological model which give the best fit to the cumulative number of cases data in Japan from January 03 2020 to February 25 2021.*

Peru

Period	Parameters value	Method	95% Confidence interval
Period 1: Epidemic phase Mar 20, 2020 - Jul 01, 2020	$N_0 = 8.36 \times 10^2$	fitted	$N_0 \in [2.63 \times 10^2, 1.41 \times 10^3]$
	$N_{base} = 3.00 \times 10^{-5}$	fitted	$N_{base} \in [-1.74 \times 10^3, 1.74 \times 10^3]$
	$N_\infty = 3.61 \times 10^5$	fitted	$N_\infty \in [3.44 \times 10^5, 3.79 \times 10^5]$
	$\chi = 1.08 \times 10^{-1}$	fitted	$\chi \in [7.59 \times 10^{-2}, 1.41 \times 10^{-1}]$
	$\theta = 4.20 \times 10^{-1}$	fitted	$\theta \in [2.41 \times 10^{-1}, 5.98 \times 10^{-1}]$
Period 2: Endemic phase Jul 01, 2020 - Jul 30, 2020	$a = 3.67 \times 10^3$	computed	
	$N_0 = 2.83 \times 10^5$	computed	
Period 3: Epidemic phase Jul 30, 2020 - Nov 10, 2020	$N_0 = 1.86 \times 10^5$	fitted	$N_0 \in [-2.61 \times 10^4, 3.98 \times 10^5]$
	$N_{base} = 2.03 \times 10^5$	fitted	$N_{base} \in [-1.11 \times 10^4, 4.18 \times 10^5]$
	$N_\infty = 7.69 \times 10^5$	fitted	$N_\infty \in [5.65 \times 10^5, 9.72 \times 10^5]$
	$\chi = 4.84 \times 10^{-1}$	fitted	$\chi \in [-6.23, 7.20]$
	$\theta = 5.95 \times 10^{-2}$	fitted	$\theta \in [-7.74 \times 10^{-1}, 8.93 \times 10^{-1}]$
Period 4: Endemic phase Nov 10, 2020 - Jan 11, 2021	$a = 1.80 \times 10^3$	computed	
	$N_0 = 9.16 \times 10^5$	computed	
Period 5: Epidemic phase Jan 11, 2021 - Feb 25, 2021	$N_0 = 3.23 \times 10^5$	fitted	
	$N_{base} = 7.04 \times 10^5$	fitted	
	$N_\infty = 7.00 \times 10^6$	fitted	
	$\chi = 1.36 \times 10^{-2}$	fitted	
	$\theta = 3.67 \times 10^1$	fitted	

Table A14: *In this table we list the values of the parameters of the phenomenological model which give the best fit to the cumulative number of cases data in Peru from January 03 2020 to February 25 2021.*

Spain

Period	Parameters value	Method	95% Confidence interval
Period 1: Epidemic phase Feb 15, 2020 - May 10, 2020	$N_0 = 5.19 \times 10^{-4}$	fitted	$N_0 \in [-5.00 \times 10^{-3}, 6.04 \times 10^{-3}]$
	$N_{base} = 5.77 \times 10^2$	fitted	$N_{base} \in [-4.50 \times 10^2, 1.60 \times 10^3]$
	$N_\infty = 2.32 \times 10^5$	fitted	$N_\infty \in [2.30 \times 10^5, 2.34 \times 10^5]$
	$\chi = 9.80 \times 10^{-1}$	fitted	$\chi \in [-1.26 \times 10^{-1}, 2.09]$
	$\theta = 9.75 \times 10^{-2}$	fitted	$\theta \in [-1.83 \times 10^{-2}, 2.13 \times 10^{-1}]$
Period 2: Endemic phase May 10, 2020 - Jun 22, 2020	$a = 5.67 \times 10^2$	computed	
	$N_0 = 2.28 \times 10^5$	computed	
Period 3: Epidemic phase Jun 22, 2020 - Oct 02, 2020	$N_0 = 2.38 \times 10^3$	fitted	$N_0 \in [1.39 \times 10^3, 3.36 \times 10^3]$
	$N_{base} = 2.50 \times 10^5$	fitted	$N_{base} \in [2.48 \times 10^5, 2.53 \times 10^5]$
	$N_\infty = 9.89 \times 10^5$	fitted	$N_\infty \in [9.02 \times 10^5, 1.08 \times 10^6]$
	$\chi = 9.29 \times 10^{-2}$	fitted	$\chi \in [7.07 \times 10^{-2}, 1.15 \times 10^{-1}]$
	$\theta = 3.84 \times 10^{-1}$	fitted	$\theta \in [2.38 \times 10^{-1}, 5.29 \times 10^{-1}]$
Period 4: Endemic phase Oct 02, 2020 - Oct 18, 2020	$a = 1.09 \times 10^4$	computed	
	$N_0 = 8.14 \times 10^5$	computed	
Period 5: Epidemic phase Oct 18, 2020 - Dec 06, 2020	$N_0 = 1.68 \times 10^5$	fitted	$N_0 \in [-3.50 \times 10^4, 3.72 \times 10^5]$
	$N_{base} = 8.20 \times 10^5$	fitted	$N_{base} \in [6.12 \times 10^5, 1.03 \times 10^6]$
	$N_\infty = 9.85 \times 10^5$	fitted	$N_\infty \in [8.01 \times 10^5, 1.17 \times 10^6]$
	$\chi = 3.15 \times 10^{-1}$	fitted	$\chi \in [-1.05, 1.68]$
	$\theta = 2.02 \times 10^{-1}$	fitted	$\theta \in [-7.15 \times 10^{-1}, 1.12]$
Period 6: Endemic phase Dec 06, 2020 - Dec 26, 2020	$a = 9.15 \times 10^3$	computed	
	$N_0 = 1.72 \times 10^6$	computed	
Period 7: Epidemic phase Dec 26, 2020 - Feb 25, 2021	$N_0 = 5.94 \times 10^4$	fitted	$N_0 \in [3.86 \times 10^4, 8.02 \times 10^4]$
	$N_{base} = 1.84 \times 10^6$	fitted	$N_{base} \in [1.81 \times 10^6, 1.87 \times 10^6]$
	$N_\infty = 1.30 \times 10^6$	fitted	$N_\infty \in [1.28 \times 10^6, 1.32 \times 10^6]$
	$\chi = 1.30 \times 10^{-1}$	fitted	$\chi \in [9.90 \times 10^{-2}, 1.60 \times 10^{-1}]$
	$\theta = 7.84 \times 10^{-1}$	fitted	$\theta \in [5.50 \times 10^{-1}, 1.02]$

Table A15: *In this table we list the values of the parameters of the phenomenological model which give the best fit to the cumulative number of cases data in Spain from January 03 2020 to February 01 2021.*

United Kingdom

Period	Parameters value	Method	95% Confidence interval
Period 1: Epidemic phase Feb 15, 2020 - Jun 15, 2020	$N_0 = 2.65 \times 10^{-2}$	fitted	$N_0 \in [-8.82 \times 10^{-2}, 1.41 \times 10^{-1}]$
	$N_{base} = 1.12 \times 10^2$	fitted	$N_{base} \in [-4.82 \times 10^2, 7.06 \times 10^2]$
	$N_\infty = 2.86 \times 10^5$	fitted	$N_\infty \in [2.84 \times 10^5, 2.88 \times 10^5]$
	$\chi = 1.76$	fitted	$\chi \in [-1.46, 4.98]$
	$\theta = 2.76 \times 10^{-2}$	fitted	$\theta \in [-2.38 \times 10^{-2}, 7.90 \times 10^{-2}]$
Period 2: Endemic phase Jun 15, 2020 - Sep 01, 2020	$a = 9.43 \times 10^2$	computed	
	$N_0 = 2.70 \times 10^5$	computed	
Period 3: Epidemic phase Sep 01, 2020 - Nov 20, 2020	$N_0 = 7.85 \times 10^3$	fitted	$N_0 \in [3.63 \times 10^3, 1.21 \times 10^4]$
	$N_{base} = 3.36 \times 10^5$	fitted	$N_{base} \in [3.28 \times 10^5, 3.43 \times 10^5]$
	$N_\infty = 2.14 \times 10^6$	fitted	$N_\infty \in [1.93 \times 10^6, 2.36 \times 10^6]$
	$\chi = 2.41 \times 10^{-1}$	fitted	$\chi \in [2.16 \times 10^{-2}, 4.60 \times 10^{-1}]$
	$\theta = 1.32 \times 10^{-1}$	fitted	$\theta \in [-9.25 \times 10^{-3}, 2.74 \times 10^{-1}]$
Period 4: Endemic phase Nov 20, 2020 - Dec 10, 2020	$a = 1.61 \times 10^4$	computed	
	$N_0 = 1.48 \times 10^6$	computed	
Period 5: Epidemic phase Dec 10, 2020 - Feb 01, 2021	$N_0 = 2.26 \times 10^5$	fitted	$N_0 \in [1.16 \times 10^5, 3.35 \times 10^5]$
	$N_{base} = 1.58 \times 10^6$	fitted	$N_{base} \in [1.46 \times 10^6, 1.70 \times 10^6]$
	$N_\infty = 2.42 \times 10^6$	fitted	$N_\infty \in [2.34 \times 10^6, 2.51 \times 10^6]$
	$\chi = 8.57 \times 10^{-2}$	fitted	$\chi \in [5.14 \times 10^{-2}, 1.20 \times 10^{-1}]$
	$\theta = 1.08$	fitted	$\theta \in [4.85 \times 10^{-1}, 1.68]$

Table A16: *In this table we list the values of the parameters of the phenomenological model which give the best fit to the cumulative number of cases data in the United Kingdom from January 03 2020 to February 01 2021.*

A5 Additional information for the results section

Period	Interpretation	Parameters value	Method
U_0	Number of unreported symptomatic infectious at time t_0	1	Fixed
R_0	Number of reported symptomatic infectious at time t_0	0	Fixed
$\tau(t)$	Transmission rate	Eqs (14.27)–(14.32)	Computed
f	Fraction of reported symptomatic infectious	0.8	Fixed
κ	Fraction of unreported symptomatic infectious capable to transmit the pathogen	1	Fixed
$1/\alpha$	Average duration of the exposed period	1 days	Fixed
$1/\nu$	Average duration of the asymptomatic infectious period	3 days	Fixed
$1/\eta$	Average duration of the symptomatic infectious period	7 days	Fixed

Table A17: *In this table we list the values of the parameters of the epidemic model used for the simulations.*

California

Period	Interpretation	Parameters value	Method
t_0	Time at which we started the epidemic model	Mar 26, 2020	Fixed
S_0	Number of susceptibles at time t_0	3.95×10^7	Fixed
E_0	Number of exposed at time t_0	7.91×10^2	Computed
I_0	Number of asymptotic infectious at time t_0	2.06×10^3	Computed

Table A18: *In this table we list the values of the parameters of the epidemic model used for the simulations.*

Compatibility condition between data and epidemic model

By using the Californian data for the first, the second and the third epidemic waves, we get from Eqs (14.59) and (14.60) the following estimates for the average duration of the exposed and asymptomatic infectious periods and the fraction of reported cases

First epidemic wave	$\frac{1}{\alpha}$ and $\frac{1}{\nu} \le \frac{1}{\chi\theta} = 5.23 \times 10^1$ days	$f \ge \frac{N_\infty}{S_0} = 8.21 \times 10^{-3}$
Second epidemic wave	$\frac{1}{\alpha}$ and $\frac{1}{\nu} \le \frac{1}{\chi\theta} = 2.52 \times 10^1$ days	$f \ge \frac{N_\infty}{S_0} = 2.08 \times 10^{-2}$
Third epidemic wave	$\frac{1}{\alpha}$ and $\frac{1}{\nu} \le \frac{1}{\chi\theta} = 1.54 \times 10^1$ days	$f \ge \frac{N_\infty}{S_0} = 6.72 \times 10^{-2}$

France

Period	Interpretation	Parameters value	Method
t_0	Time at which we started the epidemic model	Feb 27, 2020	Fixed
S_0	Number of susceptibles at time t_0	6.50×10^7	Fixed
E_0	Number of exposed at time t_0	4.27×10^1	Computed
I_0	Number of asymptomatic infectious at time t_0	6.30×10^1	Computed

Table A19: *In this table we list the values of the parameters of the epidemic model used for the simulations.*

> **Compatibility condition between data and epidemic model**
>
> By using the French data for the first, the second and the third epidemic waves, we get from Eqs (14.59) and (14.60) the following estimates for the average duration of the exposed and asymptomatic infectious periods and the fraction of reported cases
>
> | First epidemic wave | $\frac{1}{\alpha}$ and $\frac{1}{\nu} \leq \frac{1}{\chi\theta} = 1.17 \times 10^1$ days | $f \geq \frac{N_\infty}{S_0} = 2.19 \times 10^{-3}$ |
> |---|---|---|
> | Second epidemic wave | $\frac{1}{\alpha}$ and $\frac{1}{\nu} \leq \frac{1}{\chi\theta} = 4.15$ days | $f \geq \frac{N_\infty}{S_0} = 3.06 \times 10^{-2}$ |
> | Third epidemic wave | $\frac{1}{\alpha}$ and $\frac{1}{\nu} \leq \frac{1}{\chi\theta} = 3.11 \times 10^1$ days | $f \geq \frac{N_\infty}{S_0} = 3.28 \times 10^{-2}$ |

India

Figure 4 of the main text is devoted to the reproduction number of the model. The instantaneous reproduction number $t \rightarrow R_e(t)$ is decreasing from February 01, 2020 until February 25, 2021.

Period	Interpretation	Parameters value	Method
t_0	Time at which we started the epidemic model	Feb 01, 2020	Fixed
S_0	Number of susceptibles at time t_0	1.39×10^9	Fixed
E_0	Number of exposed at time t_0	4.29×10^1	Computed
I_0	Number of asymptomatic infectious at time t_0	1.12×10^2	Computed

Table A20: *In this table we list the values of the parameters of the epidemic model used for the simulations.*

> **Compatibility condition between data and epidemic model**
>
> By using the Indian data for the first single wave, we get from Eqs (14.59) and (14.60) the following estimates for the average duration of the exposed and asymptomatic infectious periods and the fraction of reported cases
>
> | First epidemic wave | $\frac{1}{\alpha}$ and $\frac{1}{\nu} \leq \frac{1}{\chi\theta} = 3.99 \times 10^1$ days | $f \geq \frac{N_\infty}{S_0} = 7.93 \times 10^{-3}$ |
> |---|---|---|

Israel

Period	Interpretation	Parameters value	Method
t_0	Time at which we started the epidemic model	Feb 27, 2020	Fixed
S_0	Number of susceptibles at time t_0	8.74×10^6	Fixed
E_0	Number of exposed at time t_0	4.16	Computed
I_0	Number of asymptomatic infectious at time t_0	6.25	Computed

Table A21: *In this table we list the values of the parameters of the epidemic model used for the simulations.*

Compatibility condition between data and epidemic model

By using the Israeli data for the first, the second, the third and the fourth epidemic waves, we get from Eqs (14.59) and (14.60) the following estimates for the average duration of the exposed and asymptomatic infectious periods and the fraction of reported cases

First epidemic wave	$\frac{1}{\alpha}$ and $\frac{1}{\nu} \leq \frac{1}{\chi\theta} = 1.04 \times 10^1$ days	$f \geq \frac{N_\infty}{S_0} = 1.95 \times 10^{-3}$
Second epidemic wave	$\frac{1}{\alpha}$ and $\frac{1}{\nu} \leq \frac{1}{\chi\theta} = 1.67 \times 10^1$ days	$f \geq \frac{N_\infty}{S_0} = 9.91 \times 10^{-3}$
Third epidemic wave	$\frac{1}{\alpha}$ and $\frac{1}{\nu} \leq \frac{1}{\chi\theta} = 5.74$ days	$f \geq \frac{N_\infty}{S_0} = 2.69 \times 10^{-2}$
Fourth epidemic wave	$\frac{1}{\alpha}$ and $\frac{1}{\nu} \leq \frac{1}{\chi\theta} = 1.71 \times 10^1$ days	$f \geq \frac{N_\infty}{S_0} = 5.57 \times 10^{-2}$

Japan

Period	Interpretation	Parameters value	Method
t_0	Time at which we started the epidemic model	Feb 20, 2020	Fixed
S_0	Number of susceptibles at time t_0	1.26×10^8	Fixed
E_0	Number of exposed at time t_0	2.61	Computed
I_0	Number of asymptomatic infectious at time t_0	5.45	Computed

Table A22: *In this table we list the values of the parameters of the epidemic model used for the simulations.*

Compatibility condition between data and epidemic model

By using the Japanese data for the first, the second, the third, the fourth and the fifth epidemic waves, we get from Eqs (14.59) and (14.60) the following estimates for the average duration of the exposed and asymptomatic infectious periods and the fraction of reported cases

First epidemic wave	$\frac{1}{\alpha}$ and $\frac{1}{\nu} \leq \frac{1}{\chi\theta} = 8.18$ days	$f \geq \frac{N_\infty}{S_0} = 1.29 \times 10^{-4}$
Second epidemic wave	$\frac{1}{\alpha}$ and $\frac{1}{\nu} \leq \frac{1}{\chi\theta} = 1.34 \times 10^1$ days	$f \geq \frac{N_\infty}{S_0} = 4.77 \times 10^{-4}$
Third epidemic wave	$\frac{1}{\alpha}$ and $\frac{1}{\nu} \leq \frac{1}{\chi\theta} = 6.92$ days	$f \geq \frac{N_\infty}{S_0} = 7.22 \times 10^{-4}$
Fourth epidemic wave	$\frac{1}{\alpha}$ and $\frac{1}{\nu} \leq \frac{1}{\chi\theta} = 7.17$ days	$f \geq \frac{N_\infty}{S_0} = 2.77 \times 10^{-3}$
Fifth epidemic wave	$\frac{1}{\alpha}$ and $\frac{1}{\nu} \leq \frac{1}{\chi\theta} = 1.30 \times 10^1$ days	$f \geq \frac{N_\infty}{S_0} = 1.82 \times 10^{-3}$

Peru

Period	Interpretation	Parameters value	Method
t_0	Time at which we started the epidemic model	Mar 20, 2020	Fixed
S_0	Number of susceptibles at time t_0	3.32×10^7	Fixed
E_0	Number of exposed at time t_0	1.64×10^2	Computed
I_0	Number of asymptomatic infectious at time t_0	3.85×10^2	Computed

Table A23: *In this table we list the values of the parameters of the epidemic model used for the simulations.*

Compatibility condition between data and epidemic model

By using the Peruvian data for the first, the second and the third epidemic waves, we get from Eqs (14.59) and (14.60) the following estimates for the average duration of the exposed and asymptomatic infectious periods and the fraction of reported cases

First epidemic wave	$\frac{1}{\alpha}$ and $\frac{1}{\nu} \leq \frac{1}{\chi\theta} = 2.20 \times 10^1$ days	$f \geq \frac{N_\infty}{S_0} = 1.09 \times 10^{-2}$
Second epidemic wave	$\frac{1}{\alpha}$ and $\frac{1}{\nu} \leq \frac{1}{\chi\theta} = 3.47 \times 10^1$ days	$f \geq \frac{N_\infty}{S_0} = 2.32 \times 10^{-2}$
Third epidemic wave	$\frac{1}{\alpha}$ and $\frac{1}{\nu} \leq \frac{1}{\chi\theta} = 2.01$ days	$f \geq \frac{N_\infty}{S_0} = 2.11 \times 10^{-1}$

Spain

Period	Interpretation	Parameters value	Method
t_0	Time at which we started the epidemic model	Feb 15, 2020	Fixed
S_0	Number of susceptibles at time t_0	3.95×10^7	Fixed
E_0	Number of exposed at time t_0	5.10	Computed
I_0	Number of asymptomatic infectious at time t_0	6.87	Computed

Table A24: *In this table we list the values of the parameters of the epidemic model used for the simulations.*

Compatibility condition between data and epidemic model

By using the Spanish data for the first, the second, the third and the fourth epidemic waves, we get from Eqs (14.59) and (14.60) the following estimates for the average duration of the exposed and asymptomatic infectious periods and the fraction of reported cases

First epidemic wave	$\frac{1}{\alpha}$ and $\frac{1}{\nu} \leq \frac{1}{\chi\theta} = 1.05 \times 10^1$ days	$f \geq \frac{N_\infty}{S_0} = 5.87 \times 10^{-3}$
Second epidemic wave	$\frac{1}{\alpha}$ and $\frac{1}{\nu} \leq \frac{1}{\chi\theta} = 2.81 \times 10^1$ days	$f \geq \frac{N_\infty}{S_0} = 2.50 \times 10^{-2}$
Third epidemic wave	$\frac{1}{\alpha}$ and $\frac{1}{\nu} \leq \frac{1}{\chi\theta} = 1.58 \times 10^1$ days	$f \geq \frac{N_\infty}{S_0} = 2.49 \times 10^{-2}$
Fourth epidemic wave	$\frac{1}{\alpha}$ and $\frac{1}{\nu} \leq \frac{1}{\chi\theta} = 9.84$ days	$f \geq \frac{N_\infty}{S_0} = 3.29 \times 10^{-2}$

United Kingdom

Period	Interpretation	Parameters value	Method
t_0	Time at which we started the epidemic model	Feb 15, 2020	Fixed
S_0	Number of susceptibles at time t_0	6.81×10^7	Fixed
E_0	Number of exposed at time t_0	3.41	Computed
I_0	Number of asymptomatic infectious at time t_0	5.15	Computed

Table A25: *In this table we list the values of the parameters of the epidemic model used for the simulations.*

Compatibility condition between data and epidemic model

By using the data from the United Kingdom for the first, the second and the third epidemic waves, we get from Eqs (14.59) and (14.60) the following estimates for the average duration of the exposed and asymptotic infectious periods and the fraction of reported cases

First epidemic wave	$\frac{1}{\alpha}$ and $\frac{1}{\nu} \leq \frac{1}{\chi\theta} = 2.06 \times 10^1$ days	$f \geq \frac{N_\infty}{S_0} = 4.20 \times 10^{-3}$
Second epidemic wave	$\frac{1}{\alpha}$ and $\frac{1}{\nu} \leq \frac{1}{\chi\theta} = 3.14 \times 10^1$ days	$f \geq \frac{N_\infty}{S_0} = 3.15 \times 10^{-2}$
Third epidemic wave	$\frac{1}{\alpha}$ and $\frac{1}{\nu} \leq \frac{1}{\chi\theta} = 1.08 \times 10^1$ days	$f \geq \frac{N_\infty}{S_0} = 3.56 \times 10^{-2}$

A6 Dependency with respect to the parameters for the French data

Influence of f on basic reproduction number:

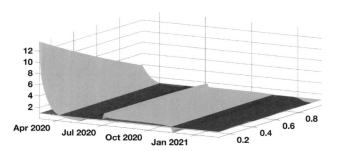

Fig. A10: *In this figure we plot $(t, f) \rightarrow R_e(t)$ when t varies from January 03 2020 to January 04 2021 and f varies from 0.1 to 1.*

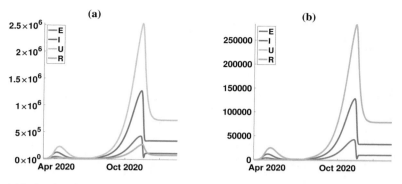

Fig. A11: *In this figure we explore the influence of the parameter f on the solution of model. The figure (a) corresponds to f = 0.1 and figure (b) corresponds to f = 1. The remaining parameters are unchanged.*

Influence of κ on basic reproduction number:

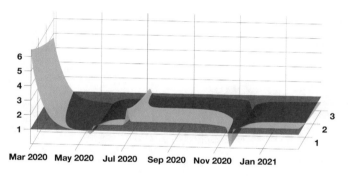

Fig. A12: *In this figure we plot $(t, \kappa) \rightarrow R_e(t)$ when t varies from January 03 2020 to January 04 2021 and κ varies from 0.1 to 3.*

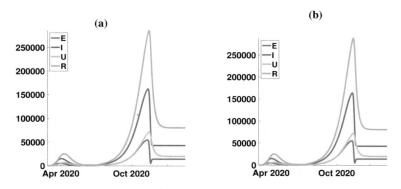

Fig. A13: *In this figure we explore the influence of the parameter f on the solution of model. The figure (a) corresponds to $\kappa = 0.1$ and figure (b) corresponds to $\kappa = 3$. The remaining parameters are unchanged.*

Influence of v on basic reproduction number:

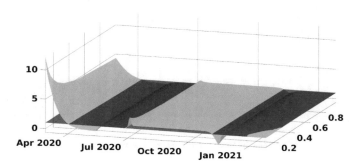

Fig. A14: *In this figure we plot $(t, v) \rightarrow R_e(t)$ when t varies from January 03 2020 to January 04 2021 and v varies from 0.1 to 1 (or equivalently $1/v$ varies from 10 days to 1 day).*

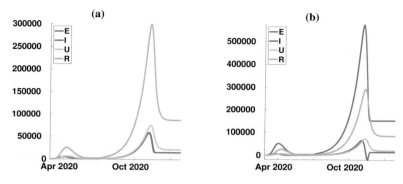

Fig. A15: *In this figure we explore the influence of the parameter $1/\nu$ on the solution of model. The figure (a) corresponds to $1/\nu = 1$ and figure (b) corresponds to $1/\nu = 10$. The remaining parameters are unchanged.*

Influence of η on basic reproduction number:

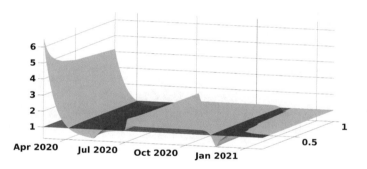

Fig. A16: *In this figure we plot $(t, \eta) \rightarrow R_e(t)$ when t varies from January 03 2020 to January 04 2021 and η varies from 0.1 to 1 (or equivalently $1/\eta$ varies from 10 days to 1 day).*

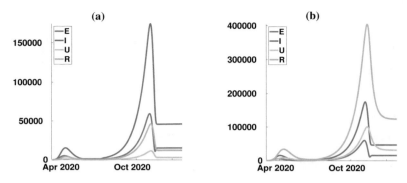

Fig. A17: *In this figure we explore the influence of the parameter f on the solution of model. The figure (a) corresponds to $1/\eta = 1$ days and figure (b) corresponds to $1/\eta = 10$ days. The remaining parameters are unchanged.*

Influence of α on basic reproduction number:

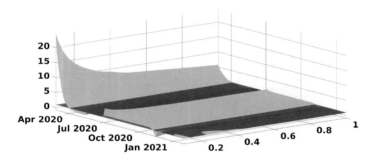

Fig. A18: *In this figure we plot $(t, \alpha) \rightarrow R_e(t)$ when t varies from January 03 2020 to January 04 2021 and α varies from 0.1 to 1 (or equivalently $1/\alpha$ varies from 10 days to 1 day).*

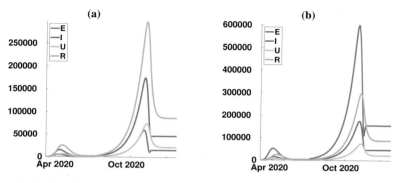

Fig. A19: *In this figure we explore the influence of the parameter f on the solution of model. The figure (a) corresponds to 1/α = 1 days and figure (b) corresponds to 1/α = 10 days. The remaining parameters are unchanged.*

A7 Upper bound of the duration for the exposed period and the asymptomatic infectious period

Let us finally mention that for each country and each epidemic wave we evaluated the parameter $1/(\chi\,\theta)$. In Figure A20 we plot the histogram of its estimated value and obtain a median value of 15.61 days. Therefore the length of exposure and the length of the asymptomatic infectious period should smaller than 15.61 days.

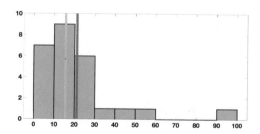

Fig. A20: *In this figure we plot the histogram for the estimated values $1/(\chi\,\theta)$. The red vertical line is mean value which is equal to 21 days. The yellow vertical line is median value which is equal to 15.61 days.*

(a)   **(b)**

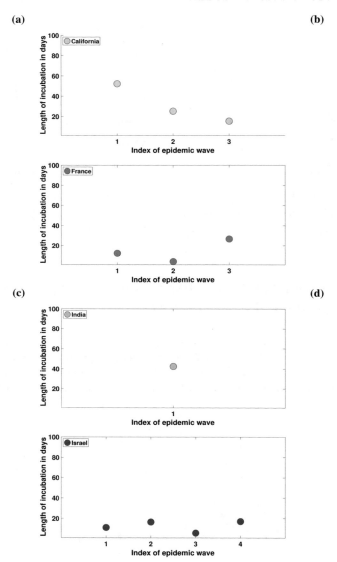

(c)   **(d)**

Fig. A21: *In this figure we plot the values of the parameter* $1/(\chi\,\theta)$ *estimated for each epidemic wave and for California (a), France (b), India (c), Israel (d). This parameter represents the maximal length of the incubation period. In each figure, we plot this parameter for each epidemic wave and for each country.*

(e)   **(f)**

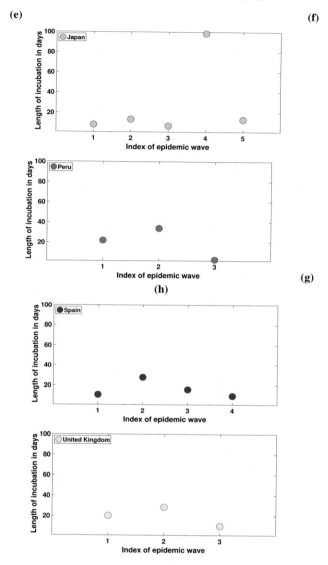

(g)

(h)

Fig. A22: *In this figure we plot the values of the parameter* $1/(\chi\,\theta)$ *estimated for each epidemic wave and for Japan (e), Peru (f), Spain (g) and United Kingdom (h). This parameter represents the maximal length of the incubation period. In each figure, we plot this parameter for each epidemic wave and for each country.*

In this section, we plot the estimated values of the parameter $1/(\chi\,\theta)$ for each epidemic period and each country considered in this study. The parameter corresponds to the upper bound of the length of the exposed period and asymptomatic infectious period. Indeed from the section devoted to the compatibility condition we know that the average duration of the exposed period should satisfy

$$1/\nu \le 1/(\chi\,\theta),$$

and the average duration of the asymptomatic infectious period should should satisfy

$$1/\alpha \le 1/(\chi\,\theta).$$

A8 Computing R_0

The basic reproduction number R_0 can be computed for the SEIUR model by the formula (see [88, 93])

$$R_0 = \rho(FV^{-1}),$$

where F is the matrix containing new infections and V contains the rates of transfer between classes:

$$F := \begin{pmatrix} 0 & \tau S & \tau\kappa S & 0 \\ 0 & 0 & 0 & 0 \\ 0 & 0 & 0 & 0 \\ 0 & 0 & 0 & 0 \end{pmatrix}, \qquad V := \begin{pmatrix} \alpha & 0 & 0 & 0 \\ -\alpha & \nu & 0 & 0 \\ 0 & -\nu(1-f) & \eta & 0 \\ 0 & \nu(1-f) & 0 & \eta \end{pmatrix},$$

see [88] and [93] for details. Therefore

$$V^{-1} = \begin{pmatrix} 1/\alpha & 0 & 0 & 0 \\ 1/\nu & 1/\nu & 0 & 0 \\ (1-f)/\eta & (1-f)/\eta & 1/\eta & 0 \\ f/\eta & f/\eta & 0 & 1/\eta \end{pmatrix},$$

$$FV^{-1} = \frac{\tau S}{\eta\nu} \begin{pmatrix} \eta+\kappa\nu(1-f) & \eta+\kappa\nu(1-f) & \kappa\nu & 0 \\ 0 & 0 & 0 & 0 \\ 0 & 0 & 0 & 0 \\ 0 & 0 & 0 & 0 \end{pmatrix}.$$

It follows that

$$R_0 = \frac{\tau S}{\eta\nu}\big(\eta+\kappa\nu(1-f)\big).$$

A9 Stochastic approach to effective reproductive ratio

We present the results obtained by applying the method described in the paper of Cori et al. [66]. Let us summarize the principle of the method. We consider the incidence data (i.e. the daily number of new reported cases) to correspond to infection events that have occurred in the past. For each new reported case, we reconstruct the time the infectious period started by sampling a Gamma distribution (i.e. the time from the infection to the moment at which the individual is reported follows a Gamma distribution). The parameters of this Gamma distribution are computed to match the differential equation framework. With $1/\mu = 10$ days, we took the average for the average of the Gamma distribution as well as its standard deviation. We denote by I_t the resulting number of individuals that begin their infectious period on the day t. As described in [66], we use a smoothing window of τ days ($\tau = 14$ days in this case). The resulting effective reproductive ratio R_t is then computed as

$$R_t = \frac{a + \sum_{s=t-\tau+1}^{t} I_s}{\frac{1}{b} + \sum_{s=t-\tau+1}^{t} \Lambda_s},$$

where a and b are a priori distributions on R_t (we took $a = 1$ and $b = 5$, as in [66]) and Λ_s is computed by the formula

$$\Lambda_s = \sum_{s=1}^{t} I_{t-s} w_s,$$

where w_s is the average infectiousness profile after time s. Following [66, Web Appendix 11], we used the formula for w_s

$$w_s = s F_{\Gamma,\alpha,\beta}(s) + (s-2) F_{\Gamma,\alpha,\beta}(s-2) - 2(s-1) F_{\Gamma,\alpha,\beta}(s-1)$$
$$+ \alpha\beta(2 F_{\Gamma,\alpha+1,\beta}(s-1) - F_{\Gamma,\alpha+1,\beta}(s-2) - F_{\Gamma,\alpha+1,\beta}(s)),$$

where $F_{\Gamma,\alpha,\beta}(s)$ is the cumulative density of a Gamma distribution of parameters (α, β):

$$F_{\Gamma,\alpha,\beta}(t) = \int_0^t \frac{1}{\Gamma(\alpha)\beta^\alpha} s^{\alpha-1} e^{-\frac{s}{\beta}} \, ds.$$

The parameters α and β are computed to match the Gamma distribution of the serial intervals which, in our case, have mean value and standard deviation $1/\mu = 10$ days, so that $\alpha = 1/\mu$ and $\beta = 1/\mu$.

Because of the sampling of random numbers involved in the computation of R_t, the procedure described above was repeated 100 times (each time drawing a new sequence of I_s from the daily number of new cases) and the final value of R_t presented in Figure 14.3 of the main text (green curves) is the average of the values obtained during these 100 simulations.

References

[1] Alfaro, M., Ducrot, A.: Population invasion with bistable dynamics and adaptive evolution: the evolutionary rescue. *Proc. Amer. Math. Soc.* **146**(11), 4787–4799 (2018). DOI 10.1090/proc/14150. URL https://doi.org/10.1090/proc/14150

[2] Alikakos, N.D., Fusco, G.: A dynamical systems proof of the Krein–Rutman theorem and an extension of the Perron theorem. *Proceedings of the Royal Society of Edinburgh Section A: Mathematics* **117**(3-4), 209–214 (1991)

[3] Allee, W.C.: *Animal Aggregations: A Study in General Sociology*. University of Chicago Press (1931)

[4] Allee, W.C., Bowen, E.S.: Studies in animal aggregations: Mass protection against colloidal silver among goldfishes. *Journal of Experimental Zoology* **61**(2), 185–207 (1932). DOI 10.1002/jez.1400610202. URL https://onlinelibrary.wiley.com/doi/abs/10.1002/jez.1400610202

[5] Amann, H.: Fixed point equations and nonlinear eigenvalue problems in ordered Banach spaces. *SIAM Rev.* **18**(4), 620–709 (1976). DOI 10.1137/1018114. URL https://doi.org/10.1137/1018114

[6] Ambrosio, L.: Geometric evolution problems, distance function and viscosity solutions. In: *Calculus of variations and partial differential equations (Pisa, 1996)*, pp. 5–93. Springer, Berlin (2000)

[7] Anderson, R.M., May, R.M.: *Infectious diseases of humans: dynamics and control*. Oxford University Press (1992)

[8] Aniţa, S.: *Analysis and control of age-dependent population dynamics, Mathematical Modelling: Theory and Applications*, vol. 11. Kluwer Academic Publishers, Dordrecht (2000). DOI 10.1007/978-94-015-9436-3. URL https://doi.org/10.1007/978-94-015-9436-3

[9] Anzolin, E., Amante, A.: First Italian dies of coronavirus as outbreak flares in north. *Reuters* (2020). February 21

[10] Arino, J., Brauer, F., van den Driessche, P., Watmough, J., Wu, J.: Simple models for containment of a pandemic. *Journal of the Royal Society Interface* **3**(8), 453–457 (2006). DOI 10.1098/rsif.2006.0112

[11] Arino, J., van den Driessche, P.: A multi-city epidemic model. *Mathematical Population Studies. An International Journal of Mathematical Demography*

10(3), 175–193 (2003). DOI 10.1080/08898480306720. URL `https://doi.org/10.1080/08898480306720`

[12] Arino, O., Hbid, M.L., Dads, E.A.: *Delay Differential Equations and Applications: Proceedings of the NATO Advanced Study Institute held in Marrakech, Morocco, 9-21 September 2002*, vol. 205. Springer Science & Business Media (2007)

[13] Aronson, D.G.: The asymptotic speed of propagation of a simple epidemic. In: *Nonlinear diffusion (NSF-CBMS Regional Conf. Nonlinear Diffusion Equations, Univ. Houston, Houston, Tex., 1976)*, pp. 1–23. Res. Notes Math., No. 14. Springer, Berlin (1977)

[14] Aronson, D.G., Weinberger, H.F.: Nonlinear diffusion in population genetics, combustion, and nerve pulse propagation. In: *Partial differential equations and related topics (Program, Tulane Univ., New Orleans, La., 1974)*, pp. 5–49. Lecture Notes in Math., Vol. 446. Springer, Berlin (1975)

[15] Attanayake, A.M.C.H., Perera, S.S.N., Jayasinghe, S.: Phenomenological Modelling of COVID-19 Epidemics in Sri Lanka, Italy, the United States, and Hebei Province of China. Computational and mathematical methods in medicine **2020** (2020). DOI 10.1155/2020/6397063

[16] Aubin, J.P.: *Viability theory*. Systems & Control: Foundations & Applications. Birkhäuser Boston, Inc., Boston, MA (1991)

[17] Ayoub, H.H., Chemaitelly, H., Mumtaz, G.R., Seedat, S., Awad, S.F., Makhoul, M., Abu-Raddad, L.J.: Characterizing key attributes of the epidemiology of COVID-19 in China: Model-based estimations. *medRxiv* (2020). DOI 10.1101/2020.04.08.20058214. URL `https://www.medrxiv.org/content/early/2020/04/11/2020.04.08.20058214`

[18] Ayoub, H.H., Chemaitelly, H., Seedat, S., Mumtaz, G.R., Makhoul, M., Abu-Raddad, L.J.: Age could be driving variable SARS-CoV-2 epidemic trajectories worldwide. *PLOS ONE* **15**(8), 1–11 (2020). DOI 10.1371/journal.pone.0237959. URL `https://doi.org/10.1371/journal.pone.0237959`

[19] Bacaër, N.: Approximation of the basic reproduction number R_0 for vector-borne diseases with a periodic vector population. *Bulletin of Mathematical Biology* **69**(3), 1067–1091 (2007)

[20] Bacaër, N.: Periodic matrix population models: growth rate, basic reproduction number, and entropy. *Bulletin of Mathematical Biology* **71**(7), 1781–1792 (2009)

[21] Bacaër, N., et al.: On the biological interpretation of a definition for the parameter r 0 in periodic population models. *Journal of Mathematical Biology* **65**(4), 601–621 (2012)

[22] Bailey, N.T.J.: *The mathematical theory of epidemics*. Hafner Publishing Co., New York (1957)

[23] Bakhta, A., Boiveau, T., Maday, Y., Mula, O.: Epidemiological Forecasting with Model Reduction of Compartmental Models. Application to the COVID-19 Pandemic. *Biology* **10**(1) (2021). DOI 10.3390/biology10010022. URL `https://www.mdpi.com/2079-7737/10/1/22`

[24] Bar-On, Y.M., Flamholz, A., Phillips, R., Milo, R.: Science Forum: SARS-CoV-2 (COVID-19) by the numbers. *eLife* **9**, e57309 (2020). DOI 10.7554/eLife.57309. URL https://doi.org/10.7554/eLife.57309

[25] Barreira, L., Valls, C.: *Stability of nonautonomous differential equations*, vol. 1926. Springer (2008)

[26] Bates, P.W., Lu, K.: A Hartman–Grobman theorem for the Cahn–Hilliard and phase-field equations. *J. Dynam. Differential Equations* **6**(1), 101–145 (1994). DOI 10.1007/BF02219190. URL https://doi.org/10.1007/BF02219190

[27] Bennett, J.J.R., Sherratt, J.A.: Long-distance seed dispersal affects the resilience of banded vegetation patterns in semi-deserts. *J. Theoret. Biol.* **481**, 151–161 (2019). DOI 10.1016/j.jtbi.2018.10.002. URL https://doi.org/10.1016/j.jtbi.2018.10.002

[28] Bernoulli, D.: Essai d'une nouvelle analyse de la petite Vérole, & des avantages de l'Inoculation pour la prévenir. *Mémoire Académie Royale des Sciences, Paris* (1760)

[29] Blower, S.: An attempt at a new analysis of the mortality caused by smallpox and of the advantages of inoculation to prevent it. Reviews in Medical Virology **14**(5), 275–288 (2004). DOI 10.1002/rmv.443. URL https://onlinelibrary.wiley.com/doi/abs/10.1002/rmv.443

[30] Bolker, B.M.: *Ecological models and data in R*. Princeton University Press, Princeton, NJ (2008)

[31] Bony, J.M.: Principe du maximum, inégalite de Harnack et unicité du problème de Cauchy pour les opérateurs elliptiques dégénérés. *Ann. Inst. Fourier (Grenoble)* **19**(fasc. 1), 277–304 xii (1969). URL http://www.numdam.org/item?id=AIF_1969__19_1_277_0

[32] Brauer, F., Castillo-Chávez, C.: *Mathematical models in population biology and epidemiology*, *Texts in Applied Mathematics*, vol. 40. Springer-Verlag, New York (2001). DOI 10.1007/978-1-4757-3516-1. URL https://doi.org/10.1007/978-1-4757-3516-1

[33] Brauer, F., Castillo-Chavez, C.: *Mathematical models in population biology and epidemiology*, *Texts in Applied Mathematics*, vol. 40, second edn. Springer, New York (2012). DOI 10.1007/978-1-4614-1686-9. URL https://doi.org/10.1007/978-1-4614-1686-9

[34] Brauer, F., Castillo-Chavez, C., Feng, Z.: *Mathematical models in epidemiology*, *Texts in Applied Mathematics*, vol. 69. Springer, New York (2019). DOI 10.1007/978-1-4939-9828-9. URL https://doi.org/10.1007/978-1-4939-9828-9. With a foreword by Simon Levin

[35] Brauer, F., Van den Driessche, P., Wu, J.: *Mathematical epidemiology*, vol. 1945. Springer (2008). DOI 10.1007/978-3-540-78911-6

[36] Brauer, F., Van den Driessche, P., Wu, J.: *Mathematical epidemiology*. Berlin, Germany: Springer (2008)

[37] Brezis, H.: On a characterization of flow-invariant sets. *Comm. Pure Appl. Math.* **23**, 261–263 (1970). DOI 10.1002/cpa.3160230211. URL https://doi.org/10.1002/cpa.3160230211

[38] Brezis, H.: *Functional analysis, Sobolev spaces and partial differential equations*. Springer Science & Business Media (2010)

[39] Brockmann, D., Hufnagel, L., Geisel, T.: The scaling laws of human travel. *Nature* **439**(7075), 462–465 (2006). DOI 10.1038/nature04292

[40] Brunner, H.: *Collocation methods for Volterra integral and related functional differential equations*, vol. 15. Cambridge University Press (2004)

[41] Burton, T.A.: *Volterra integral and differential equations*, vol. 202. Elsevier (2005)

[42] Busenberg, S., Cooke, K.: *Vertically transmitted diseases*, Biomathematics, vol. 23. Springer-Verlag, Berlin (1993). DOI 10.1007/978-3-642-75301-5. URL https://doi.org/10.1007/978-3-642-75301-5. Models and dynamics

[43] Busenberg, S., Cooke, K.: *Vertically transmitted diseases: models and dynamics*, vol. 23. Springer Science & Business Media (2012)

[44] Busenberg, S., Iannelli, M.: A degenerate nonlinear diffusion problem in age-structured population dynamics. *Nonlinear Anal.* **7**(12), 1411–1429 (1983). DOI 10.1016/0362-546X(83)90009-3. URL https://doi.org/10.1016/0362-546X(83)90009-3

[45] Bylicki, O., Paleiron, N., Janvier, F.: An Outbreak of Covid-19 on an Aircraft Carrier. *New Engl. J. Med.* **384**(10), 976–977 (2021). DOI 10.1056/NEJMc2034424

[46] Byrne, A.W., McEvoy, D., Collins, A.B., et al.: Inferred duration of infectious period of SARS-CoV-2: rapid scoping review and analysis of available evidence for asymptomatic and symptomatic COVID-19 cases. *BMJ Open* **10**(8) (2020). DOI 10.1136/bmjopen-2020-039856. URL https://bmjopen.bmj.com/content/10/8/e039856

[47] Cantrell, R.S., Cosner, C.: *Spatial ecology via reaction-diffusion equations*. Wiley Series in Mathematical and Computational Biology. John Wiley & Sons, Ltd., Chichester (2003). DOI 10.1002/0470871296. URL https://doi.org/10.1002/0470871296

[48] Cao, Q., Chen, Y.C., Chen, C.L., Chiu, C.H.: SARS-CoV-2 infection in children: Transmission dynamics and clinical characteristics. *Journal of the Formosan Medical Association* **119**(3), 670 (2020). DOI 10.1016/j.jfma.2020.02.009

[49] Castro, M., Ares, S., Cuesta, J.A., Manrubia, S.: The turning point and end of an expanding epidemic cannot be precisely forecast. *Proceedings of the National Academy of Sciences* **117**(42), 26190–26196 (2020). DOI 10.1073/pnas.2007868117. URL https://www.pnas.org/content/117/42/26190

[50] Caswell, H.: *Matrix population models*, vol. 1. Sinauer Sunderland, MA, USA (2000)

[51] Cazenave, T., Haraux, A.: *An introduction to semilinear evolution equations*, *Oxford Lecture Series in Mathematics and its Applications*, vol. 13. The Clarendon Press, Oxford University Press, New York (1998). Translated from the 1990 French original by Yvan Martel and revised by the authors

[52] Chen, D., Moulin, B., Wu, J.: *Analyzing and modeling spatial and temporal dynamics of infectious diseases.* Wiley Online Library (2015)

[53] Chicone, C.: *Ordinary differential equations with applications*, vol. 34. Springer Science & Business Media (2006)

[54] Chikina, M., Pegden, W.: Modeling strict age-targeted mitigation strategies for COVID-19. *PLOS ONE* **15**(7), 1–17 (2020). DOI 10.1371/journal.pone. 0236237. URL https://doi.org/10.1371/journal.pone.0236237

[55] Chowell, G., Diaz-Dueñas, P., Miller, J.C., Alcazar-Velazco, A., Hyman, J.M., Fenimore, P.W., Castillo-Chávez, C.: Estimation of the reproduction number of dengue fever from spatial epidemic data. *Math. Biosci.* **208**(2), 571–589 (2007). DOI 10.1016/j.mbs.2006.11.011. URL https://doi.org/10.1016/j.mbs.2006.11.011

[56] Chowell, G., Hengartner, N.W., Castillo-Chávez, C., Fenimore, P.W., Hyman, J.M.: The basic reproductive number of Ebola and the effects of public health measures: the cases of Congo and Uganda. *J. Theoret. Biol.* **229**(1), 119–126 (2004). DOI 10.1016/j.jtbi.2004.03.006. URL https://doi.org/10.1016/j.jtbi.2004.03.006

[57] Chu, J., Ducrot, A., Magal, P., Ruan, S.: Hopf bifurcation in a size-structured population dynamic model with random growth. *Journal of Differential Equations* **247**(3), 956–1000 (2009)

[58] Chueh, K.N., Conley, C.C., Smoller, J.A.: Positively invariant regions for systems of nonlinear diffusion equations. *Indiana University Mathematics Journal* **26**(2), 373–392 (1977)

[59] Chueshov, I.: Order-preserving random dynamical systems generated by a class of coupled stochastic semilinear parabolic equations. In: *International Conference on Differential Equations, Vol. 1, 2 (Berlin, 1999)*, pp. 711–716. World Sci. Publ., River Edge, NJ (2000)

[60] Chueshov, I.: Order-preserving skew-product flows and nonautonomous parabolic systems. *Acta Appl. Math.* **65**(1-3), 185–205 (2001). DOI 10.1023/A:1010604112317. URL https://doi.org/10.1023/A:1010604112317. Special issue dedicated to Antonio Avantaggiati on the occasion of his 70th birthday

[61] Chueshov, I.: *Monotone random systems theory and applications, Lecture Notes in Mathematics*, vol. 1779. Springer-Verlag, Berlin (2002). DOI 10.1007/b83277. URL https://doi.org/10.1007/b83277

[62] Chueshov, I.: *Monotone random systems theory and applications, Lecture Notes in Mathematics*, vol. 1779. Springer-Verlag, Berlin (2002). DOI 10.1007/b83277. URL https://doi.org/10.1007/b83277

[63] Ćmiel, A.M., Ćmiel, B.: A simple method to describe the COVID-19 trajectory and dynamics in any country based on Johnson cumulative density function fitting. Scientific reports **11**(1), 1–10 (2021). DOI 10.1038/s41598-021-97285-5

[64] Cohen, J.E., Newman, C.M.: The stability of large random matrices and their products. *The Annals of Probability* pp. 283–310 (1984)

[65] Coppel, W.A.: *Dichotomies in stability theory*, Lecture Notes in Mathematics, vol. 629. Springer (2006)

[66] Cori, A., Ferguson, N.M., Fraser, C., Cauchemez, S.: A new framework and software to estimate time-varying reproduction numbers during epidemics. *Am. J. Epidemiol.* **178**(9), 1505–1512 (2013). DOI 10.1093/aje/kwt133

[67] Cotta, R.M., Naveira-Cotta, C.P., Magal, P.: Mathematical Parameters of the COVID-19 Epidemic in Brazil and Evaluation of the Impact of Different Public Health Measures. *Biology* **9**(8) (2020). DOI 10.3390/biology9080220

[68] Cushing, J.M.: Periodic Lotka–Volterra competition equations. *Journal of Mathematical Biology* **24**(4), 381–403 (1986)

[69] Cushing, J.M.: *An introduction to structured population dynamics, CBMS-NSF Regional Conference Series in Applied Mathematics*, vol. 71. Society for Industrial and Applied Mathematics (SIAM), Philadelphia, PA (1998). DOI 10.1137/1.9781611970005. URL https://doi.org/10.1137/1.9781611970005

[70] Cushing, J.M.: *Integrodifferential equations and delay models in population dynamics*, vol. 20. Springer Science & Business Media (2013)

[71] Cushing, J.M.: *Integrodifferential equations and delay models in population dynamics*, vol. 20. Springer Science & Business Media (2013)

[72] Davies, N.G., Klepac, P., Liu, Y., Prem, K., Jit, M., Eggo, R.M.: Age-dependent effects in the transmission and control of COVID-19 epidemics. *Nature medicine* **26**(8), 1205–1211 (2020). DOI 10.1038/s41591-020-0962-9

[73] Debnath, L.: A short history of the Fibonacci and golden numbers with their applications. *Internat. J. Math. Ed. Sci. Tech.* **42**(3), 337–367 (2011). DOI 10.1080/0020739X.2010.543160. URL https://doi.org/10.1080/0020739X.2010.543160

[74] Deimling, K.: *Nonlinear functional analysis*. Springer-Verlag, Berlin (1985)

[75] Demetrius, L.: Primitivity conditions for growth matrices. *Mathematical Biosciences* **12**(1-2), 53–58 (1971)

[76] Demongeot, J., Flet-Berliac, Y., Seligmann, H.: Temperature decreases spread parameters of the new Covid-19 case dynamics. *Biology* **9**(5), 94 (2020). DOI 10.3390/biology9050094

[77] Demongeot, J., Griette, Q., Magal, P.: SI epidemic model applied to COVID-19 data in mainland China. *Royal Society Open Science* **7**(12), 201878 (2020). DOI 10.1098/rsos.201878

[78] Demongeot, J., Hansen, O., Taramasco, C.: Discrete dynamics of contagious social diseases: Example of obesity. *Virulence* **7**(2), 129–140 (2016). DOI 10.1080/21505594.2015.1082708. URL https://doi.org/10.1080/21505594.2015.1082708. PMID: 26375495

[79] Demongeot, J., Jelassi, M., Taramasco, C.: From susceptibility to frailty in social networks: The case of obesity. *Mathematical Population Studies* **24**(4), 219–245 (2017)

[80] Demongeot, J., Taramasco, C.: Evolution of social networks: the example of obesity. *Biogerontology* **15**(6), 611–626 (2014). DOI 10.1007/s10522-014-9542-z

[81] Desch, W., Schappacher, W.: Linearized stability for nonlinear semigroups. In: *Differential equations in Banach spaces (Bologna, 1985), Lecture Notes*

in Math., vol. 1223, pp. 61–73. Springer, Berlin (1986). DOI 10.1007/BFb0099183. URL https://doi.org/10.1007/BFb0099183

[82] Di Blasio, G.: Nonlinear age-dependent population diffusion. *J. Math. Biol.* **8**(3), 265–284 (1979). DOI 10.1007/BF00276312. URL https://doi.org/10.1007/BF00276312

[83] Di Blasio, G.: Mathematical analysis for an epidemic model with spatial and age structure. *Journal of Evolution Equations* **10**(4), 929–953 (2010)

[84] Diekmann, O.: Run for your life. a note on the asymptotic speed of propagation of an epidemic. *Journal of Differential Equations* **33**(1), 58–73 (1979)

[85] Diekmann, O., Gyllenberg, M.: Equations with infinite delay: blending the abstract and the concrete. *Journal of Differential Equations* **252**(2), 819–851 (2012)

[86] Diekmann, O., Heesterbeek, H., Britton, T.: *Mathematical tools for understanding infectious disease dynamics*. Princeton Series in Theoretical and Computational Biology. Princeton University Press, Princeton, NJ (2013)

[87] Diekmann, O., Heesterbeek, J.A.P.: *Mathematical epidemiology of infectious diseases: model building, analysis and interpretation*, vol. 5. John Wiley & Sons (2000)

[88] Diekmann, O., Heesterbeek, J.A.P., Metz, J.A.: On the definition and the computation of the basic reproduction ratio r_0 in models for infectious diseases in heterogeneous populations. *Journal of mathematical biology* **28**(4), 365–382 (1990)

[89] Diekmann, O., Van Gils, S.A., Lunel, S.M., Walther, H.O.: *Delay equations: functional-, complex-, and nonlinear analysis*, vol. 110. Springer Science & Business Media (2012)

[90] Dietz, K., Heesterbeek, J.A.P.: Daniel Bernoulli's epidemiological model revisited. *Math. Biosci.* **180**, 1–21 (2002). DOI 10.1016/S0025-5564(02)00122-0. John A. Jacquez memorial volume

[91] Dimarco, G., Perthame, B., Toscani, G., Zanella, M.: Kinetic models for epidemic dynamics with social heterogeneity. Journal of Mathematical Biology **83**(1), 1–32 (2021). DOI 10.1007/s00285-021-01630-1

[92] Dong, E., Du, H., Gardner, L.: An interactive web-based dashboard to track COVID-19 in real time. *Lancet Infect. Dis.* **20**(5), 533–534 (2020). DOI 10.1016/S1473-3099(20)30120-1. Data available at https://github.com/CSSEGISandData/COVID-19. Accessed June 9, 2021

[93] Van den Driessche, P., Watmough, J.: Reproduction numbers and sub-threshold endemic equilibria for compartmental models of disease transmission. *Mathematical Biosciences* **180**(1-2), 29–48 (2002)

[94] Driver, R.D.: *Ordinary and delay differential equations*, vol. 20. Springer Science & Business Media (2012)

[95] Ducrot, A., Le Foll, F., Magal, P., Murakawa, H., Pasquier, J., Webb, G.F.: An in vitro cell population dynamics model incorporating cell size, quiescence, and contact inhibition. *Mathematical Models and Methods in Applied Sciences* **21**(supp01), 871–892 (2011)

[96] Ducrot, A., Magal, P.: Travelling wave solutions for an infection-age structured model with diffusion. *Proc. Roy. Soc. Edinburgh Sect. A* **139**(3), 459–482 (2009)

[97] Ducrot, A., Magal, P.: A center manifold for second order semilinear differential equations on the real line and applications to the existence of wave trains for the gurtin–mccamy equation. *Transactions of the American Mathematical Society* **372**(5), 3487–3537 (2019)

[98] Ducrot, A., Magal, P.: Integrated semigroups and parabolic equations Part II: semilinear problems. *Ann. Sc. Norm. Super. Pisa Cl. Sci. (5)* **20**(3), 1071–1111 (2020)

[99] Ducrot, A., Magal, P., Nguyen, T., Webb, G.F.: Identifying the number of unreported cases in SIR epidemic models. *Math. Med. Biol.* **37**(2), 243–261 (2020). DOI 10.1093/imammb/dqz013. URL https://doi.org/10.1093/imammb/dqz013

[100] Ducrot, A., Magal, P., Prevost, K.: Integrated semigroups and parabolic equations. Part I: linear perturbation of almost sectorial operators. *J. Evol. Equ.* **10**(2), 263–291 (2010). DOI 10.1007/s00028-009-0049-z. URL https://doi.org/10.1007/s00028-009-0049-z

[101] Ducrot, A., Magal, P., Ruan, S.: Travelling wave solutions in multigroup age-structured epidemic models. *Archive for rational mechanics and analysis* **195**(1), 311–331 (2010)

[102] Ducrot, A., Magal, P., Ruan, S.: Projectors on the generalized eigenspaces for partial differential equations with time delay. In: *Infinite Dimensional Dynamical Systems*, pp. 353–390. Springer (2013)

[103] Dulac, H.: Recherches sur les points singuliers des équations différentielles. Gauthier-Villars (1903)

[104] Engel, K.J., Nagel, R.: *One-parameter semigroups for linear evolution equations, Graduate Texts in Mathematics*, vol. 194. Springer-Verlag, New York (2000)

[105] Engel, K.J., Nagel, R.: *A short course on operator semigroups*. Springer Science & Business Media (2006)

[106] Faranda, D., Castillo, I.P., Hulme, O., Jezequel, A., Lamb, J.S.W., Sato, Y., Thompson, E.L.: Asymptotic estimates of SARS-CoV-2 infection counts and their sensitivity to stochastic perturbation. Chaos: An Interdisciplinary Journal of Nonlinear Science **30**(5), 051107 (2020). DOI 10.1063/5.0008834. URL https://doi.org/10.1063/5.0008834

[107] Fife, P.C., Mcleod, J.B.: The approach of solutions of nonlinear diffusion equations to travelling wave solutions. *Bull. Amer. Math. Soc.* **81**(6), 1076–1078 (1975). DOI 10.1090/S0002-9904-1975-13922-X. URL https://doi.org/10.1090/S0002-9904-1975-13922-X

[108] Fisher, R.A.: The wave of advance of advantageous genes. *Annals of Eugenics* **7**(4), 355–369 (1937). DOI 10.1111/j.1469-1809.1937.tb02153.x. URL http://dx.doi.org/10.1111/j.1469-1809.1937.tb02153.x

[109] Floquet, G.: Sur les équations différentielles linéaires à coefficients périodiques. *Annales scientifiques de l'École normale supérieure* **12**, 47–88 (1883)

[110] Foote, R.L.: Regularity of the distance function. *Proc. Amer. Math. Soc.* **92**(1), 153–155 (1984). DOI 10.2307/2045171. URL https://doi.org/ 10.2307/2045171

[111] Frobenius, G.F.: Ueber matrizen aus positiven elementen, sitzungsber. *Preus. Akad. Wiss Berlin* pp. 471–476 (1908)

[112] Frobenius, G.F.: Über matrizen aus positiven elementen, 2?, sitzungsber. *Königl. Preuss. Akad. Wiss* pp. 514–518 (1909)

[113] Fu, X., Griette, Q., Magal, P.: A cell–cell repulsion model on a hyperbolic Keller–Segel equation. *Journal of mathematical biology* **80**(7), 2257–2300 (2020)

[114] Gantmacher, F.R.: *The theory of matrices*, vol. 2. Chelsea Pub Co., New York (1959)

[115] Garnier, J., Roques, L., Hamel, F.: Success rate of a biological invasion in terms of the spatial distribution of the founding population. *Bull. Math. Biol.* **74**(2), 453–473 (2012). DOI 10.1007/s11538-011-9694-9. URL https: //doi.org/10.1007/s11538-011-9694-9

[116] Garroni, M.G., Langlais, M.: Age-dependent population diffusion with external constraint. *Journal of Mathematical Biology* **14**(1), 77–94 (1982)

[117] Gaudart, J., Ghassani, M., Mintsa, J., Rachdi, M., Waku, J., Demongeot, J.: Demography and diffusion in epidemics: malaria and black death spread. *Acta Biotheoretica* **58**(2), 277–305 (2010). DOI 10.1007/s10441-010-9103-z

[118] Gavin, H.P.: The levenberg-marquardt algorithm for nonlinear least squares curve-fitting problems. Department of Civil and Environmental Engineering, Duke University pp. 1–19 (2019)

[119] Gopalsamy, K.: *Stability and oscillations in delay differential equations of population dynamics*, vol. 74. Springer Science & Business Media (2013)

[120] Greenhalgh, S.: Missile science, population science: the origins of China's one-child policy. *The China Quarterly* **182**, 253–276 (2005)

[121] Greenhalgh, S.: *Just one child: Science and policy in Deng's China.* Univ of California Press (2008)

[122] Griette, Q., Demongeot, J., Magal, P.: A robust phenomenological approach to investigate COVID-19 data for France. Mathematics in Applied Sciences and Engineering (2021). DOI 10.5206/mase/14031

[123] Griette, Q., Demongeot, J., Magal, P.: What can we learn from COVID-19 data by using epidemic models with unidentified infectious cases? *MBE* **19**(1), 537–594 (2021). DOI 10.3934/mbe.2022025

[124] Griette, Q., Liu, Z., Magal, P.: Estimating the end of the first wave of epidemic for COVID-19 outbreak in mainland China. *medRxiv* (2020). DOI 10.1101/2020.04.14.20064824. URL https://www.medrxiv.org/ content/early/2020/07/06/2020.04.14.20064824

[125] Griette, Q., Magal, P.: Clarifying predictions for COVID-19 from testing data: The example of New York State. *Infectious Disease Modelling* **6**, 273–283 (2021). DOI 10.1016/j.idm.2020.12.011. URL https://www. sciencedirect.com/science/article/pii/S2468042721000026

[126] Griette, Q., Magal, P., Seydi, O.: Unreported cases for age dependent COVID-19 outbreak in Japan. *Biology* **9**(6), 132 (2020)

[127] Griette, Q., Magal, P., Seydi, O.: Unreported cases for age dependent COVID-19 outbreak in Japan. *Biology* **9**(6), 132 (2020). DOI 10.3390/biology9060132

[128] Gripenberg, G., Londen, S.O., Staffans, O.: *Volterra integral and functional equations*. 34. Cambridge University Press (1990)

[129] Grobman, D.M.: Homeomorphism of systems of differential equations. *Dokl. Akad. Nauk SSSR* **128**, 880–881 (1959)

[130] Gronwall, T.H.: Note on the derivatives with respect to a parameter of the solutions of a system of differential equations. *Ann. of Math. (2)* **20**(4), 292–296 (1919). DOI 10.2307/1967124. URL https://doi.org/10.2307/1967124

[131] Guan, W.j., Ni, Z.y., Hu, Y., Liang, W.h., Ou, C.q., He, J.x., Liu, L., Shan, H., Lei, C.l., Hui, D.S., Du, B., Li, L.j., Zeng, G., Yuen, K.Y., Chen, R.c., Tang, C.l., Wang, T., Chen, P.y., Xiang, J., Li, S.y., Wang, J.l., Liang, Z.j., Peng, Y.x., Wei, L., Liu, Y., Hu, Y.h., Peng, P., Wang, J.m., Liu, J.y., Chen, Z., Li, G., Zheng, Z.j., Qiu, S.q., Luo, J., Ye, C.j., Zhu, S.y., Zhong, N.s.: Clinical Characteristics of Coronavirus Disease 2019 in China. *New England Journal of Medicine* **382**(18), 1708–1720 (2020). DOI 10.1056/NEJMoa2002032. URL https://doi.org/10.1056/NEJMoa2002032

[132] Guillon, P., Clément, M., et al.: Inhibition of the interaction between the SARS-CoV Spike protein and its cellular receptor by anti-histo-blood group antibodies. *Glycobiology* **18**(12), 1085–1093 (2008). DOI 10.1093/glycob/cwn093. URL https://doi.org/10.1093/glycob/cwn093

[133] Gurtin, M.E.: A system of equations for age-dependent population diffusion. *Journal of Theoretical Biology* **40**(2), 389–392 (1973). DOI 10.1016/0022-5193(73)90139-2. URL https://www.sciencedirect.com/science/article/pii/0022519373901392

[134] Gurtin, M.E., MacCamy, R.C.: Product solutions and asymptotic behavior for age-dependent, dispersing populations. *Math. Biosci.* **62**(2), 157–167 (1982). DOI 10.1016/0025-5564(82)90080-3. URL https://doi.org/10.1016/0025-5564(82)90080-3

[135] Győri, I., Györi, I., Gyori, I., Ladas, G., Ladas, G.: *Oscillation theory of delay differential equations: With applications*. Clarendon Press (1991)

[136] Hadeler, K.P.: Parameter identification in epidemic models. *Mathematical Biosciences* **229**(2), 185 – 189 (2011). DOI 10.1016/j.mbs.2010.12.004. URL http://www.sciencedirect.com/science/article/pii/S0025556410001859

[137] Hale, J.K.: Functional differential equations. In: *Analytic theory of differential equations*, pp. 9–22. Springer (1971)

[138] Hale, J.K.: Retarded functional differential equations: basic theory. In: *Theory of Functional Differential Equations*, pp. 36–56. Springer (1977)

[139] Hale, J.K.: Retarded equations with infinite delays. In: *Functional Differential Equations and Approximation of Fixed Points*, pp. 157–193. Springer (1979)

[140] Hale, J.K.: *Ordinary differential equations*, second edn. Robert E. Krieger Publishing Co., Inc., Huntington, N.Y. (1980)

[141] Hale, J.K., Lunel, S.M.V.: *Introduction to functional differential equations*, vol. 99. Springer Science & Business Media (2013)

[142] Hale, J.K., Somolinos, A.S.: Competition for fluctuating nutrient. *J. Math. Biol.* **18**(3), 255–280 (1983). DOI 10.1007/BF00276091. URL https://doi.org/10.1007/BF00276091

[143] Harris, G., Martin, C.: The roots of a polynomial vary continuously as a function of the coefficients. Proc. Amer. Math. Soc. **100**(2), 390–392 (1987). DOI 10.2307/2045978. URL https://doi.org/10.2307/2045978

[144] Harris, G., Martin, C.: Large roots yield large coefficients. An addendum to: "The roots of a polynomial vary continuously as a function of the coefficients" [Proc. Amer. Math. Soc. **100** (1987), no. 2, 390–392; MR0884486 (88h:30006)]. Proc. Amer. Math. Soc. **102**(4), 993–994 (1988). DOI 10.2307/2047347. URL https://doi.org/10.2307/2047347

[145] Hartman, P.: A lemma in the theory of structural stability of differential equations. *Proc. Amer. Math. Soc.* **11**, 610–620 (1960). DOI 10.2307/2034720. URL https://doi.org/10.2307/2034720

[146] Hartman, P.: On invariant sets and on a theorem of Ważewski. *Proc. Amer. Math. Soc.* **32**, 511–520 (1972). DOI 10.2307/2037848. URL https://doi.org/10.2307/2037848

[147] Hartung, F., Krisztin, T., Walther, H.O., Wu, J.: Functional differential equations with state-dependent delays: theory and applications. In: *Handbook of differential equations: ordinary differential equations*, vol. 3, pp. 435–545. Elsevier (2006)

[148] Hassard, B.D., Kazarinoff, N.D., Wan, Y.H.: *Theory and Applications of Hopf Bifurcaton*. Cambridge Univ. Press, Cambridge (1981)

[149] Henry, D.: *Geometric theory of semilinear parabolic equations, Lecture Notes in Mathematics*, vol. 840. Springer-Verlag, Berlin-New York (1981)

[150] Hethcote, H.W.: The mathematics of infectious diseases. *SIAM review* **42**(4), 599–653 (2000)

[151] Hilker, F.M., Langlais, M., Malchow, H.: The Allee effect and infectious diseases: extinction, multistability, and the (dis-) appearance of oscillations. *The American Naturalist* **173**(1), 72–88 (2009)

[152] Hille, E.: *Functional Analysis and Semi-Groups*. American Mathematical Society Colloquium Publications, Vol. 31. American Mathematical Society, New York (1948)

[153] Hino, Y., Murakami, S., Naito, T.: *Functional differential equations with infinite delay*. Springer (2006)

[154] Hino, Y., Murakami, S., Naito, T., Van Minh, N.: A variation-of-constants formula for abstract functional differential equations in the phase space. *Journal of Differential Equations* **179**(1), 336–355 (2002)

[155] Hirsch, M.W., Smale, S., Devaney, R.L.: *Differential equations, dynamical systems, and an introduction to chaos*, third edn. Elsevier/Academic Press, Amsterdam (2013). DOI 10.1016/B978-0-12-382010-5.00001-4. URL https://doi.org/10.1016/B978-0-12-382010-5.00001-4

[156] Hirsch, M.W., Smith, H.L.: Monotone dynamical systems. In: *Handbook of differential equations: ordinary differential equations*, vol. 2, pp. 239–357. Elsevier (2006)

[157] Hofbauer, J., Sigmund, K.: *Evolutionary games and population dynamics*. Cambridge University Press, Cambridge (1998). DOI 10.1017/CBO9781139173179. URL https://doi.org/10.1017/CBO9781139173179

[158] Hofbauer, J., So, J.W.: Multiple limit cycles for three dimensional Lotka–Volterra equations. *Applied Mathematics Letters* **7**(6), 65–70 (1994)

[159] Holshue, M.L., DeBolt, C., Lindquist, S., Lofy, K.H., Wiesman, J., Bruce, H., Spitters, C., Ericson, K., Wilkerson, S., Tural, A., Diaz, G., Cohn, A., Fox, L., Patel, A., Gerber, S.I., Kim, L., Tong, S., Lu, X., Lindstrom, S., Pallansch, M.A., Weldon, W.C., Biggs, H.M., Uyeki, T.M., Pillai, S.K.: First Case of 2019 Novel Coronavirus in the United States. *New Engl. J. Med.* **382**(10), 929–936 (2020). DOI 10.1056/NEJMoa2001191

[160] Hopf, E.: Abzweigung einer periodischen Lösung von einer stationären eines Differential systems. *Ber. Verh. Sächs. Akad. Wiss. Leipzig Math.-Nat. Kl.* **95**(1), 3–22 (1943)

[161] Horn, R.A., Johnson, C.R.: *Matrix analysis*. Cambridge University Press (2012)

[162] Hsieh, Y., Chang H. Lee, J.: SARS Epidemiology Modeling. Emerging Infectious Diseases **10**(6), 1165–1167 (2004). DOI 10.3201/eid1006.031023

[163] Hsieh, Y.H.: Richards model: a simple procedure for real-time prediction of outbreak severity. In: *Modeling and dynamics of infectious diseases*, Ser. *Contemp. Appl. Math. CAM*, vol. 11, pp. 216–236. Higher Ed. Press, Beijing (2009)

[164] Hsu, S.B., Waltman, P.: Analysis of a model of two competitors in a chemostat with an external inhibitor. *SIAM Journal on Applied Mathematics* **52**(2), 528–540 (1992)

[165] Huo, X., Chen, J., Ruan, S.: Estimating asymptomatic, undetected and total cases for the COVID-19 outbreak in Wuhan: a mathematical modeling study. *BMC Infect. Dis.* **21**(1), 1–18 (2021). DOI 10.1007/s11538-017-0284-3

[166] Iannelli, M.: Mathematical theory of age-structured population dynamics. *Giardini Editori e Stampatori in Pisa* (1995). URL https://ci.nii.ac.jp/naid/10010355596/en/

[167] Iannelli, M., Pugliese, A.: *An Introduction to Mathematical Population Dynamics: Along the Trail of Volterra and Lotka*, Unitext, vol. 79. Springer (2015)

[168] Inaba, H.: On a new perspective of the basic reproduction number in heterogeneous environments. *Journal of mathematical biology* **65**(2), 309–348 (2012)

[169] Inaba, H.: *Age-structured population dynamics in demography and epidemiology*. Springer (2017)

[170] Jones, T.C., Biele, G., Mühlemann, B., Veith, T., Schneider, J., Beheim-Schwarzbach, J., Bleicker, T., Tesch, J., Schmidt, M.L., Sander, L.E., Kurth, F., Menzel, P., Schwarzer, R., Zuchowski, M., Hofmann, J., Krumbholz, A., Stein, A., Edelmann, A., Corman, V.M., Drosten, C.: Estimating infectiousness throughout SARS-CoV-2 infection course. *Science* (2021).

DOI 10.1126/science.abi5273. URL https://science.sciencemag.org/content/early/2021/05/24/science.abi5273

[171] Kang, H., Ruan, S.: Nonlinear age-structured population models with nonlocal diffusion and nonlocal boundary conditions. *Journal of Differential Equations* **278**, 430–462 (2021)

[172] Kato, T.: *Perturbation theory for linear operators*. Classics in Mathematics. Springer-Verlag, Berlin (1995). Reprint of the 1980 edition

[173] Kawasuji, H., Takegoshi, Y., Kaneda, M., Ueno, A., Miyajima, Y., Kawago, K., Fukui, Y., Yoshida, Y., Kimura, M., Yamada, H., Sakamaki, I., Tani, H., Morinaga, Y., Yamamoto, Y.: Transmissibility of COVID-19 depends on the viral load around onset in adult and symptomatic patients. PLOS ONE **15**(12), 1–8 (2020). DOI 10.1371/journal.pone.0243597. URL https://doi.org/10.1371/journal.pone.0243597

[174] Keeling, M.J., Rohani, P.: *Modeling infectious diseases in humans and animals*. Princeton University Press, Princeton, NJ (2008)

[175] Kendall, D.G.: Discussion of 'Measles periodicity and community size' by M.S. Bartlett. *J. Roy. Stat. Soc. A* **120**, 64–76 (1957)

[176] Kermack, W.O., McKendrick, A.G.: A contribution to the mathematical theory of epidemics. *Proceedings of the Royal Society of London A: Mathematical, Physical and Engineering Sciences* **115**(772), 700–721 (1927). DOI 10.1098/rspa.1927.0118. URL http://rspa.royalsocietypublishing.org/content/115/772/700

[177] Kermack, W.O., McKendrick, A.G.: Contributions to the mathematical theory of epidemics. II. The problem of endemicity. *Proceedings of the Royal Society of London A: Mathematical, Physical and Engineering Sciences* **138**(834), 55–83 (1932). DOI 10.1098/rspa.1932.0171. URL http://rspa.royalsocietypublishing.org/content/138/834/55

[178] Kermack, W.O., McKendrick, A.G.: Contributions to the mathematical theory of epidemics. III. Further studies of the problem of endemicity. *Proceedings of the Royal Society of London A: Mathematical, Physical and Engineering Sciences* **141**(843), 94–122 (1933). DOI 10.1098/rspa.1933.0106. URL http://rspa.royalsocietypublishing.org/content/141/843/94

[179] Keyfitz, N.: *Applied mathematical demography*. Springer (2005)

[180] Keyfitz, N., Caswell, H.: *Applied Mathematical Demography*. Statistics for Biology and Health. Springer, New York, NY (2005). DOI 10.1007/b139042

[181] Khan, K., McNabb, S.J., Memish, Z.A., Eckhardt, R., Hu, W., Kossowsky, D., Sears, J., Arino, J., Johansson, A., Barbeschi, M., McCloskey, B., Henry, B., Cetron, M., Brownstein, J.S.: Infectious disease surveillance and modelling across geographic frontiers and scientific specialties. *The Lancet Infectious Diseases* **12**(3), 222–230 (2012). DOI 10.1016/S1473-3099(11)70313-9. URL https://www.sciencedirect.com/science/article/pii/S1473309911703139

[182] Kim, S.E., Jeong, H.S., Yu, Y., Shin, S.U., Kim, S., Oh, T.H., Kim, U.J., Kang, S.J., Jang, H.C., Jung, S.I., et al.: Viral kinetics of SARS-CoV-2 in asymptomatic carriers and presymptomatic patients. International Journal of Infectious Diseases **95**, 441–443 (2020). DOI 10.1016/j.ijid.2020.04.

083. URL https://www.sciencedirect.com/science/article/pii/
S120197122030299X

[183] Kimura, M.: "stepping stone" model of population. *Annual Report of the National Institute of Genetics Japan* **3**, 62–63 (1953)

[184] Kimura, M., Weiss, G.H.: The stepping stone model of population structure and the decrease of genetic correlation with distance. *Genetics* **49**(4), 561 (1964)

[185] Kingsland, S.: Alfred J. Lotka and the origins of theoretical population ecology. *Proceedings of the National Academy of Sciences* **112**(31), 9493–9495 (2015). DOI 10.1073/pnas.1512317112

[186] Kolmanovskii, V.B., Nosov, V.R.: *Stability of functional differential equations*, vol. 180. Elsevier (1986)

[187] Kolmogorov, A.N., Petrovski, I.G., Piskunov, N.S.: Étude de l'équation de la diffusion avec croissance de la quantité de matière et son application à un problème biologique. *Bull. Univ. Moskow, Ser. Internat., Sec. A* **1**, 1–25 (1937)

[188] Kot, M.: *Elements of mathematical ecology*. Cambridge University Press, Cambridge (2001). DOI 10.1017/CBO9780511608520. URL https://doi.org/10.1017/CBO9780511608520

[189] Krasnoselskii, M.A.: *Positive solutions of operator equations*. Translated from the Russian by Richard E. Flaherty; edited by Leo F. Boron. P. Noordhoff Ltd. Groningen (1964)

[190] Krasnoselskii, M.A.: *The operator of translation along the trajectories of differential equations*. Translations of Mathematical Monographs, Vol. 19. American Mathematical Society, Providence, R.I. (1968). Translated from the Russian by Scripta Technica

[191] Krein, M.G., Rutman, M.A.: Linear operators leaving invariant a cone in a Banach space. *Uspekhi Matematicheskikh Nauk* **3**(1), 3–95 (1948)

[192] Krisztin, T., Wu, J.: Monotone semiflows generated by neutral equations with different delays in neutral and retarded parts. *Acta Math. Univ. Comenian. (N.S.)* **63**(2), 207–220 (1994)

[193] Kuang, Y.: *Delay differential equations*. University of California Press (2012)

[194] Kucharski, A.J., Russell, T.W., Diamond, C., Liu, Y., Edmunds, J., Funk, S., Eggo, R.M., Sun, F., Jit, M., Munday, J.D., et al.: Early dynamics of transmission and control of COVID-19: a mathematical modelling study. *The Lancet infectious diseases* **20**(5), 553–558 (2020). DOI 10.1016/S1473-3099(20)30144-4

[195] Ladde, G.S., Lakshmikantham, V.: *Random differential inequalities*, *Mathematics in Science and Engineering*, vol. 150. Academic Press, Inc. [Harcourt Brace Jovanovich, Publishers], New York-London (1980)

[196] Lakshmikantham, V.: *Theory of integro-differential equations*, vol. 1. CRC press (1995)

[197] Langlais, M.: A nonlinear problem in age-dependent population diffusion. *SIAM J. Math. Anal.* **16**(3), 510–529 (1985). DOI 10.1137/0516037. URL https://doi.org/10.1137/0516037

[198] Langlais, M.: Large time behavior in a nonlinear age-dependent population dynamics problem with spatial diffusion. *J. Math. Biol.* **26**(3), 319–346 (1988). DOI 10.1007/BF00277394. URL https://doi.org/10.1007/BF00277394

[199] Leslie, P.H.: On the use of matrices in certain population mathematics. *Biometrika* **33**, 183–212 (1945). DOI 10.1093/biomet/33.3.183. URL https://doi.org/10.1093/biomet/33.3.183

[200] Leslie, P.H.: Some further notes on the use of matrices in population mathematics. *Biometrika* **35**, 213–245 (1948). DOI 10.1093/biomet/35.3-4.213. URL https://doi.org/10.1093/biomet/35.3-4.213

[201] Li, R., Pei, S., Chen, B., Song, Y., Zhang, T., Yang, W., Shaman, J.: Substantial undocumented infection facilitates the rapid dissemination of novel coronavirus (SARS-CoV-2). *Science* **368**(6490), 489–493 (2020). DOI 10.1126/science.abb3221. URL https://science.sciencemag.org/content/368/6490/489

[202] Li, T.Y., Yorke, J.A.: Period three implies chaos. *Amer. Math. Monthly* **82**(10), 985–992 (1975). DOI 10.2307/2318254. URL https://doi.org/10.2307/2318254

[203] Li, X.Z., Yang, J., Martcheva, M.: *Age Structured Epidemic Modeling*, vol. 52. Springer Nature (2020)

[204] Lian, Z., Lu, K.: *Lyapunov exponents and invariant manifolds for random dynamical systems in a Banach space*. American Mathematical Soc. (2010)

[205] Liu, Z., Magal, P.: Functional differential equation with infinite delay in a space of exponentially bounded and uniformly continuous functions. *arXiv preprint* arXiv:1811.12014 (2018)

[206] Liu, Z., Magal, P., Ruan, S.: Projectors on the generalized eigenspaces for functional differential equations using integrated semigroups. *Journal of Differential Equations* **244**(7), 1784–1809 (2008)

[207] Liu, Z., Magal, P., Seydi, O., Webb, G.: Understanding unreported cases in the COVID-19 epidemic outbreak in Wuhan, China, and the importance of major public health interventions. *Biology* **9**(3), 50 (2020). DOI 10.3390/biology9030050

[208] Liu, Z., Magal, P., Seydi, O., Webb, G.F.: A COVID-19 epidemic model with latency period. *Infectious Disease Modelling* **5**, 323–337 (2020). DOI 10.1016/j.idm.2020.03.003. URL https://www.sciencedirect.com/science/article/pii/S2468042720300099

[209] Liu, Z., Magal, P., Seydi, O., Webb, G.F.: A model to predict COVID-19 epidemics with applications to South Korea, Italy, and Spain. *SIAM News* **53**(4) (2020)

[210] Liu, Z., Magal, P., Seydi, O., Webb, G.F.: Predicting the cumulative number of cases for the COVID-19 epidemic in China from early data. *Mathematical Biosciences and Engineering* **17**(4), 3040–3051 (2020). DOI 10.3934/mbe.2020172

[211] Liu, Z., Magal, P., Webb, G.F.: Predicting the number of reported and unreported cases for the COVID-19 epidemics in China, South Korea, Italy, France, Germany and United Kingdom. *Journal of Theoretical Biology*

509, 110501 (2021). DOI 10.1016/j.jtbi.2020.110501. URL https://www.sciencedirect.com/science/article/pii/S0022519320303568

[212] London, W.P., Yorke, J.A.: Recurrent outbreaks of measles, chickenpox and mumps: I. Seasonal variation in contact rates. *American Journal of Epidemiology* **98**(6), 453–468 (1973). DOI 10.1093/oxfordjournals.aje.a121575

[213] Lotka, A.J.: Relation between birth rates and death rates. *Science* **26**(653), 21–22 (1907)

[214] Lotka, A.J.: Contribution to the theory of periodic reactions. *The Journal of Physical Chemistry* **14**(3), 271–274 (1910). DOI 10.1021/j150111a004

[215] Lotka, A.J.: Analytical note on certain rhythmic relations in organic systems. *Proceedings of the National Academy of Sciences* **6**(7), 410–415 (1920). DOI 10.1073/pnas.6.7.410

[216] Lotka, A.J.: Undamped oscillations derived from the law of mass action. *Journal of the American Chemical Society* **42**(8), 1595–1599 (1920)

[217] Lotka, A.J.: *Elements of physical biology*. Williams & Wilkins Co, Baltimore (1925)

[218] Lou, Y., Xiao, D., Zhou, P.: Qualitative analysis for a Lotka–Volterra competition system in advective homogeneous environment. *Discrete & Continuous Dynamical Systems* **36**(2), 953 (2016)

[219] Lu, X., Zhang, L., Du, H., Zhang, J., Li, Y.Y., Qu, J., Zhang, W., Wang, Y., Bao, S., Li, Y., Wu, C., Liu, H., Liu, D., Shao, J., Peng, X., Yang, Y., Liu, Z., Xiang, Y., Zhang, F., Silva, R.M., Pinkerton, K.E., Shen, K., Xiao, H., Xu, S., Wong, G.W.: SARS-CoV-2 Infection in Children. *New England Journal of Medicine* **382**(17), 1663–1665 (2020). DOI 10.1056/NEJMc2005073. URL https://doi.org/10.1056/NEJMc2005073. PMID: 32187458

[220] Ma, S., Zhang, J., et al.: Epidemiological parameters of coronavirus disease 2019: a pooled analysis of publicly reported individual data of 1155 cases from seven countries. *medRxiv* (2020). DOI 10.1101/2020.03.21.20040329. URL https://www.medrxiv.org/content/early/2020/03/24/2020.03.21.20040329

[221] Ma, Z., Magal, P.: Global asymptotic stability for gurtin-maccamy's population dynamics model. *Proc of AMS (to appear)* (2021)

[222] Ma, Z., Zhou, Y., Wu, J.: *Modeling and dynamics of infectious diseases*, vol. 11. World Scientific (2009)

[223] Macdonald, G.: Epidemiological basis of malaria control. *Bulletin of the World Health Organization* **15**(3-5), 613 (1956)

[224] Macdonald, G., et al.: The analysis of the sporozoite rate. *Tropical Diseases Bulletin* **49**(6) (1952)

[225] Macdonald, G., et al.: The epidemiology and control of malaria. *The Epidemiology and Control of Malaria* (1957)

[226] MacDonald, N., MacDonald, N.: *Biological delay systems: linear stability theory*. Cambridge University Press (2008)

[227] Magal, P.: Compact attractors for time-periodic age-structured population models. *Electron. J. Differential Equations* pp. No. 65, 35 (2001)

[228] Magal, P.: Global stability for differential equations with homogeneous non-linearity and application to population dynamics. *Discrete & Continuous Dynamical Systems-B* **2**(4), 541 (2002)

[229] Magal, P., McCluskey, C.: Two-group infection age model including an application to nosocomial infection. *SIAM J. Appl. Math.* **73**(2), 1058–1095 (2013). DOI 10.1137/120882056

[230] Magal, P., McCluskey, C.C., Webb, G.F.: Lyapunov functional and global asymptotic stability for an infection-age model. *Appl. Anal.* **89**(7), 1109–1140 (2010). DOI 10.1080/00036810903208122

[231] Magal, P., Noussair, A., Webb, G., Wu, Y.: Modeling epidemic outbreaks in geographical regions: Seasonal influenza in puerto rico. *Discrete & Continuous Dynamical Systems-S* **13**(12), 3535 (2020)

[232] Magal, P., Ruan, S.: *Center manifolds for semilinear equations with non-dense domain and applications to Hopf bifurcation in age structured models*. American Mathematical Soc. (2009)

[233] Magal, P., Ruan, S.: On semilinear Cauchy problems with non-dense domain. *Adv. Differential Equations* **14**(11-12), 1041–1084 (2009)

[234] Magal, P., Ruan, S.: Sustained oscillations in an evolutionary epidemiological model of influenza A drift. *Proceedings of the Royal Society A: Mathematical, Physical and Engineering Sciences* **466**(2116), 965–992 (2010)

[235] Magal, P., Ruan, S.: Susceptible-infectious-recovered models revisited: from the individual level to the population level. *Math. Biosci.* **250**, 26–40 (2014). DOI 10.1016/j.mbs.2014.02.001. URL https://doi.org/10.1016/j.mbs.2014.02.001

[236] Magal, P., Ruan, S.: *Theory and applications of abstract semilinear Cauchy problems*. Springer (2018)

[237] Magal, P., Ruan, S., et al.: On integrated semigroups and age structured models in L^p spaces. *Differential and Integral Equations* **20**(2), 197–239 (2007)

[238] Magal, P., Ruan, S., et al.: On semilinear cauchy problems with non-dense domain. *Advances in Differential Equations* **14**(11/12), 1041–1084 (2009)

[239] Magal, P., Seydi, O., Wang, F.B.: Monotone abstract non-densely defined cauchy problems applied to age structured population dynamic models. *Journal of Mathematical Analysis and Applications* **479**(1), 450–481 (2019)

[240] Magal, P., Seydi, O., Wang, F.B.: Positively invariant subset for non-densely defined cauchy problems. *Journal of Mathematical Analysis and Applications* **494**(2), 124600 (2021)

[241] Magal, P., Webb, G.: The parameter identification problem for SIR epidemic models: identifying unreported cases. *J. Math. Biol.* **77**(6-7), 1629–1648 (2018). DOI 10.1007/s00285-017-1203-9. URL https://doi.org/10.1007/s00285-017-1203-9

[242] Magal, P., Zhang, Z.: Competition for light in forest population dynamics: From computer simulator to mathematical model. *Journal of Theoretical Biology* **419**, 290–304 (2017)

[243] Magal, P., Zhang, Z.: A system of state-dependent delay differential equation modeling forest growth I: semiflow properties. *Journal of Evolution Equations* **18**(4), 1853–1888 (2018)

[244] Magal, P., Zhang, Z.: A system of state-dependent delay differential equation modelling forest growth II: boundedness of solutions. *Nonlinear Analysis: Real World Applications* **42**, 334–352 (2018)

[245] Mallet-Paret, J., Nussbaum, R.D.: Generalizing the Krein–Rutman theorem, measures of noncompactness and the fixed point index. *Journal of Fixed Point Theory and Applications* **7**(1), 103–143 (2010)

[246] Malthus, T.R.: *An essay on the principle of population*. The Works of Thomas Robert Malthus, London, Pickering & Chatto Publishers (1798)

[247] Martcheva, M.: *An introduction to mathematical epidemiology*, *Texts in Applied Mathematics*, vol. 61. Springer (2015)

[248] Martin, R.H.: Differential equations on closed subsets of a banach space. *Transactions of the American Mathematical Society* **179**, 399–414 (1973)

[249] Martin, R.H.: A maximum principle for semilinear parabolic systems. *Proc. Amer. Math. Soc.* **74**(1), 66–70 (1979). DOI 10.2307/2042107. URL https://doi.org/10.2307/2042107

[250] Martin, R.H., Smith, H.L.: Abstract functional-differential equations and reaction-diffusion systems. *Transactions of the American Mathematical Society* **321**(1), 1–44 (1990)

[251] Matsunaga, H., Murakami, S., Nagabuchi, Y., Van Minh, N.: Center manifold theorem and stability for integral equations with infinite delay. *Funkcialaj Ekvacioj* **58**(1), 87–134 (2015)

[252] Mazurek, J.: The evaluation of COVID-19 prediction precision with a Lyapunov-like exponent. PLOS ONE **16**(5), 1–9 (2021). DOI 10.1371/journal.pone.0252394. URL https://doi.org/10.1371/journal.pone.0252394

[253] McKendrick, A.G., Pai, M.K.: Xlv.—the rate of multiplication of microorganisms: a mathematical study. *Proceedings of the Royal Society of Edinburgh* **31**, 649–655 (1912)

[254] Meinsma, G.: Elementary proof of the Routh–Hurwitz test. *Systems Control Lett.* **25**(4), 237–242 (1995). DOI 10.1016/0167-6911(94)00089-E. URL https://doi.org/10.1016/0167-6911(94)00089-E

[255] Meyer-Nieberg, P.: *Banach lattices*. Universitext. Springer-Verlag, Berlin (1991). DOI 10.1007/978-3-642-76724-1. URL https://doi.org/10.1007/978-3-642-76724-1

[256] Minc, H.: *Nonnegative matrices*. Wiley-Interscience Series in Discrete Mathematics and Optimization. John Wiley & Sons, Inc., New York (1988)

[257] Mizumoto, K., Kagaya, K., Zarebski, A., Chowell, G.: Estimating the asymptomatic proportion of coronavirus disease 2019 (COVID-19) cases on board the Diamond Princess cruise ship, Yokohama, Japan, 2020. *Eurosurveillance* **25**(10), 2000180 (2020). DOI 10.2807/1560-7917.ES.2020.25.10.2000180

[258] Mohammed, S.E.A., Salah-El Din, A.M.: *Stochastic functional differential equations*, *Research Notes in Mathematics*, vol. 99. Pitman Advanced Publishing Program (1984)

[259] Mossong, J., Hens, N., Jit, M., Beutels, P., Auranen, K., Mikolajczyk, R., Massari, M., Salmaso, S., Tomba, G.S., Wallinga, J., Heijne, J., Sadkowska-Todys, M., Rosinska, M., Edmunds, W.J.: Social Contacts and Mixing Patterns

Relevant to the Spread of Infectious Diseases. *PLOS Medicine* **5**(3), 1–1 (2008). DOI 10.1371/journal.pmed.0050074. URL https://doi.org/10.1371/journal.pmed.0050074

[260] de Mottoni, P., Schiaffino, A.: Competition systems with periodic coefficients: a geometric approach. *J. Math. Biol.* **11**(3), 319–335 (1981). DOI 10.1007/BF00276900. URL https://doi.org/10.1007/BF00276900

[261] Munasinghe, L., Asai, Y., Nishiura, H.: Quantifying heterogeneous contact patterns in Japan: a social contact survey. *Theoretical Biology and Medical Modelling* **16**(1), 1–10 (2019). DOI 10.1186/s12976-019-0102-8

[262] Murray, J.D.: *Mathematical biology, Biomathematics*, vol. 19. Springer-Verlag, Berlin (1989). DOI 10.1007/978-3-662-08539-4. URL https://doi.org/10.1007/978-3-662-08539-4

[263] Murray, J.D.: *Mathematical biology. I An introduction, Interdisciplinary Applied Mathematics*, vol. 17, third edn. Springer-Verlag, New York (2002)

[264] Murray, J.D.: *Mathematical biology. II Spatial models and biomedical applications, Interdisciplinary Applied Mathematics*, vol. 18, third edn. Springer-Verlag, New York (2003)

[265] Nagumo, M.: Über die Lage der Integralkurven gewöhnlicher Differentialgleichungen. *Proc. Phys.-Math. Soc. Japan (3)* **24**, 551–559 (1942)

[266] Newman, M.E.J.: The structure and function of complex networks. *SIAM Rev.* **45**(2), 167–256 (2003). DOI 10.1137/S003614450342480. URL https://doi.org/10.1137/S003614450342480

[267] Nishiura, H., Kobayashi, T., Yang, Y., Hayashi, K., Miyama, T., Kinoshita, R., Linton, N.M., Jung, S.m., Yuan, B., Suzuki, A., et al.: The rate of under-ascertainment of novel coronavirus (2019-nCoV) infection: estimation using Japanese passengers data on evacuation flights. *J. Clin. Med.* (2020). DOI 10.3390/jcm9020419

[268] Nussbaum, R.D.: Eigenvectors of nonlinear positive operators and the linear krein–rutman theorem. In: *Fixed point theory*, pp. 309–330. Springer (1981)

[269] Okubo, A., et al.: *Diffusion and ecological problems: mathematical models*. Springer-Verlag, Berlin-Heidelberg-New York (1980)

[270] Omori, R., Mizumoto, K., Nishiura, H.: Ascertainment rate of novel coronavirus disease (COVID-19) in Japan. *Int. J. Infect. Dis.* **96**, 673–675 (2020). DOI 10.1016/j.ijid.2020.04.080. URL https://www.sciencedirect.com/science/article/pii/S1201971220302927

[271] Palatella, L., Vanni, F., Lambert, D.: A phenomenological estimate of the true scale of CoViD-19 from primary data. Chaos, Solitons & Fractals **146**, 110854 (2021). DOI 10.1016/j.chaos.2021.110854. URL https://www.sciencedirect.com/science/article/pii/S0960077921002071

[272] Pan, A., Liu, L., Wang, C., Guo, H., Hao, X., Wang, Q., Huang, J., He, N., Yu, H., Lin, X., Wei, S., Wu, T.: Association of Public Health Interventions With the Epidemiology of the COVID-19 Outbreak in Wuhan, China. *JAMA* **323**(19), 1915–1923 (2020). DOI 10.1001/jama.2020.6130. URL https://doi.org/10.1001/jama.2020.6130

[273] Pavel, N.H., Motreanu, D.: *Tangency, flow invariance for differential equations, and optimization problems*, Pure and Applied Mathematics, vol. 219. CRC Press (1999)

[274] Pazy, A.: *Semigroups of linear operators and applications to partial differential equations*, Applied Mathematical Sciences, vol. 44. Springer Science & Business Media (2012)

[275] Perron, O.: Zur Theorie der Matrices. *Math. Ann.* **64**(2), 248–263 (1907). DOI 10.1007/BF01449896. URL https://doi.org/10.1007/BF01449896

[276] Perthame, B.: *Transport equations in biology*. Frontiers in Mathematics. Birkhäuser Verlag, Basel (2007)

[277] Perthame, B.: *Parabolic equations in biology*. Lecture Notes on Mathematical Modelling in the Life Sciences. Springer, Cham (2015). DOI 10.1007/978-3-319-19500-1. URL https://doi.org/10.1007/978-3-319-19500-1. Growth, reaction, movement and diffusion

[278] Pianka, E.R.: *Evolutionary ecology*. Eric R. Pianka (2011)

[279] Poincaré, H.: Sur le problème des trois corps et les équations de la dynamique. *Acta mathematica* **13**(1), A3–A270 (1890)

[280] Polyanin, A.D., Manzhirov, A.V.: *Handbook of integral equations*. CRC press (2008)

[281] Prem, K., Cook, A.R., Jit, M.: Projecting social contact matrices in 152 countries using contact surveys and demographic data. *PLOS Computational Biology* **13**(9), 1–21 (2017). DOI 10.1371/journal.pcbi.1005697. URL https://doi.org/10.1371/journal.pcbi.1005697

[282] Prem, K., Liu, Y., Russell, T.W., Kucharski, A.J., Eggo, R.M., Davies, N., Flasche, S., Clifford, S., Pearson, C.A., Munday, J.D., et al.: The effect of control strategies to reduce social mixing on outcomes of the COVID-19 epidemic in Wuhan, China: a modelling study. *The Lancet Public Health* **5**(5), e261–e270 (2020). DOI 10.1016/S2468-2667(20)30073-6

[283] Protter, M.H., Weinberger, H.F.: *Maximum principles in differential equations*. Springer Science & Business Media (2012)

[284] Qiu, J.: Covert coronavirus infections could be seeding new outbreaks. *Nature (Lond.)* (2020). DOI 10.1038/d41586-020-00822-x

[285] Qiu, Y., Chen, X., Shi, W.: Impacts of social and economic factors on the transmission of coronavirus disease 2019 (COVID-19) in China. *Journal of Population Economics* **33**, 1127–1172 (2020). DOI 10.1007/s00148-020-00778-2

[286] Quandt, J.: On the Hartman–Grobman theorem for maps. *J. Differential Equations* **64**(2), 154–164 (1986). DOI 10.1016/0022-0396(86)90085-9. URL https://doi.org/10.1016/0022-0396(86)90085-9

[287] Redheffer, R.M., Walter, W.L.: Flow-invariant sets and differential inequalities in normed spaces. *Applicable Analysis* **5**(2), 149–161 (1975). DOI 10.1080/00036817508839117. URL https://doi.org/10.1080/00036817508839117

[288] Redheffer, R.M., Walter, W.L.: Invariant sets for systems of partial differential equations. I. Parabolic equations. *Archive for Rational Mechan-*

ics and Analysis **67**(1), 41–52 (1978). DOI 10.1007/BF00280826. URL https://doi.org/10.1007/BF00280826

[289] Richards, F.J.: A flexible growth function for empirical use. *Journal of Experimental Botany* **10**(2), 290–301 (1959)

[290] Ricker, W.E.: Stock and recruitment. *Journal of the Fisheries Board of Canada* **11**(5), 559–623 (1954). DOI 10.1139/f54-039

[291] Roda, W.C., Varughese, M.B., Han, D., Li, M.Y.: Why is it difficult to accurately predict the COVID-19 epidemic? *Infectious Disease Modelling* **5**, 271 – 281 (2020). DOI 10.1016/j.idm.2020.03.001. URL http://www.sciencedirect.com/science/article/pii/S2468042720300075

[292] Rodrigues, H.M., Solà-Morales, J.: On the Hartman-Grobman theorem with parameters. *J. Dynam. Differential Equations* **22**(3), 473–489 (2010). DOI 10.1007/s10884-010-9160-7. URL https://doi.org/10.1007/s10884-010-9160-7

[293] Roff, D.: *Evolution of life histories: theory and analysis*. Springer Science & Business Media (1993)

[294] Roosa, K., Lee, Y., Luo, R., Kirpich, A., Rothenberg, R., Hyman, J., Yan, P., Chowell, G.: Real-time forecasts of the COVID-19 epidemic in China from February 5th to February 24th, 2020. Infectious Disease Modelling **5**, 256–263 (2020). DOI 10.1016/j.idm.2020.02.002. URL https://www.sciencedirect.com/science/article/pii/S2468042720300051

[295] Roques, L., Klein, E.K., Papaix, J., Sar, A., Soubeyrand, S.: Impact of lockdown on the epidemic dynamics of COVID-19 in France. *Frontiers in Medicine* **7**, 274 (2020). DOI 10.3389/fmed.2020.00274

[296] Roques, L., Klein, E.K., Papaix, J., Sar, A., Soubeyrand, S.: Using early data to estimate the actual infection fatality ratio from COVID-19 in France. *Biology* **9**(5), 97 (2020). DOI 10.3390/biology9050097

[297] Ross, R.: Some quantitative studies in epidemiology. *Nature* **87**, 466–467 (1911). DOI 10.1038/087466a0

[298] Ross, R.: An Application of the Theory of Probabilities to the Study of a priori Pathometry. Part I. *Proceedings of the Royal Society of London A: Mathematical, Physical and Engineering Sciences* **92**(638), 204–230 (1916). DOI 10.1098/rspa.1916.0007. URL http://rspa.royalsocietypublishing.org/content/92/638/204

[299] Ross, R., Hudson, H.P.: An Application of the Theory of Probabilities to the Study of a priori Pathometry. Part II. *Proceedings of the Royal Society of London A: Mathematical, Physical and Engineering Sciences* **93**(650), 212–225 (1917). DOI 10.1098/rspa.1917.0014. URL http://rspa.royalsocietypublishing.org/content/93/650/212

[300] Ross, R., Hudson, H.P.: An Application of the Theory of Probabilities to the Study of a priori Pathometry. Part III. *Proceedings of the Royal Society of London A: Mathematical, Physical and Engineering Sciences* **93**(650), 225–240 (1917). DOI 10.1098/rspa.1917.0015. URL http://rspa.royalsocietypublishing.org/content/93/650/225

[301] Rothe, C., Schunk, M., Sothmann, P., Bretzel, G., Froeschl, G., Wallrauch, C., Zimmer, T., Thiel, V., Janke, C., Guggemos, W., et al.: Transmission of

2019-nCoV infection from an asymptomatic contact in Germany. *New Engl. J. Med.* **382**(10), 970–971 (2020). DOI 10.1056/NEJMc2001468

[302] Rothe, F.: Convergence to travelling fronts in semilinear parabolic equations. *Proceedings of the Royal Society of Edinburgh Section A: Mathematics* **80**(3-4), 213–234 (1978)

[303] Ruan, S.: Spatial-temporal dynamics in nonlocal epidemiological models. In: *Mathematics for life science and medicine*, pp. 97–122. Springer (2007)

[304] Rudin, W.: *Real and complex analysis*, third edn. McGraw-Hill Book Co., New York (1987)

[305] Sattenspiel, L., Dietz, K.: A structured epidemic model incorporating geographic mobility among regions. *Mathematical Biosciences* **128**(1-2), 71–91 (1995). DOI 10.1016/0025-5564(94)00068-B

[306] Schaaf, R.: *Global solution branches of two-point boundary value problems*, *Lecture Notes in Mathematics*, vol. 1458. Springer-Verlag, Berlin (1990). DOI 10.1007/BFb0098346. URL https://doi.org/10.1007/BFb0098346

[307] Schaefer, H.H.: Banach lattices. In: *Banach Lattices and Positive Operators*, pp. 46–153. Springer (1974)

[308] Schneider, H., Vidyasagar, M.: Cross-positive matrices. *SIAM J. Numer. Anal.* **7**, 508–519 (1970). DOI 10.1137/0707041. URL https://doi.org/10.1137/0707041

[309] Scire, J., Nadeau, S.A., Vaughan, T.G., Gavin, B., Fuchs, S., Sommer, J., Koch, K.N., Misteli, R., Mundorff, L., Götz, T., et al.: Reproductive number of the COVID-19 epidemic in Switzerland with a focus on the Cantons of Basel-Stadt and Basel-Landschaft. *Swiss Med. Wkly.* **150**(19-20), w20271 (2020). DOI 10.4414/smw.2020.20271

[310] Sell, G.R.: The floquet problem for almost periodic linear differential equations. In: *Ordinary and Partial Differential Equations*, pp. 239–251. Springer (1974)

[311] Seneta, E.: *Non-negative matrices and Markov chains*. Springer Science & Business Media (2006)

[312] Sharkovsky, O.M.: Coexistence of cycles of a continuous map of the line into itself. *Urain. Mat. Zh.* **16**(1), 61–71 (1964)

[313] Sharkovsky, O.M., Kolyada, S.F., Sivak, A.G., Fedorenko, V.V.: *Dynamics of one-dimensional maps*, *Mathematics and its Applications*, vol. 407. Kluwer Academic Publishers Group, Dordrecht (1997). DOI 10.1007/978-94-015-8897-3. URL https://doi.org/10.1007/978-94-015-8897-3. Translated from the 1989 Russian original by Sivak, P. Malyshev and D. Malyshev and revised by the authors

[314] Sharpe, F.R., Lotka, A.J.: L. a problem in age-distribution. *The London, Edinburgh, and Dublin Philosophical Magazine and Journal of Science* **21**(124), 435–438 (1911)

[315] Shen, W., Yi, Y.: Almost automorphic and almost periodic dynamics in skew-product semiflows. *Mem. Amer. Math. Soc.* **136**(647), x+93 (1998). DOI 10.1090/memo/0647. URL https://doi.org/10.1090/memo/0647

[316] Shigesada, N., Kawasaki, K.: *Biological invasions: theory and practice*. Oxford University Press, UK (1997)

[317] Singh, R., Adhikari, R.: Age-structured impact of social distancing on the covid-19 epidemic in india. *arXiv preprint* arXiv:2003.12055 (2020)

[318] Singh, R.K., Rani, M., Bhagavathula, A.S., Sah, R., Rodriguez-Morales, A.J., Kalita, H., Nanda, C., Sharma, S., Sharma, Y.D., Rabaan, A.A., Rahmani, J., Kumar, P.: Prediction of the COVID-19 Pandemic for the Top 15 Affected Countries: Advanced Autoregressive Integrated Moving Average (ARIMA) Model. JMIR Public Health Surveill **6**(2), e19115 (2020). DOI 10.2196/19115

[319] Skellam, J.G.: Random dispersal in theoretical populations. *Biometrika* **38**(1-2), 196 (1951). DOI 10.1093/biomet/38.1-2.196. URL +http://dx.doi.org/10.1093/biomet/38.1-2.196

[320] Smirnova, A., deCamp, L., Chowell, G.: Forecasting epidemics through non-parametric estimation of time-dependent transmission rates using the SEIR model. *Bulletin of Mathematical Biology* **81**(11), 4343–4365 (2019). DOI 10.1007/s11538-017-0284-3. URL https://doi.org/10.1007/s11538-017-0284-3

[321] Smith, H.L.: Periodic competitive differential equations and the discrete dynamics of competitive maps. *J. Differential Equations* **64**(2), 165–194 (1986). DOI 10.1016/0022-0396(86)90086-0. URL https://doi.org/10.1016/0022-0396(86)90086-0

[322] Smith, H.L.: Periodic solutions of periodic competitive and cooperative systems. *SIAM J. Math. Anal.* **17**(6), 1289–1318 (1986). DOI 10.1137/0517091. URL https://doi.org/10.1137/0517091

[323] Smith, H.L.: Reduction of structured population models to threshold-type delay equations and functional differential equations: a case study. *Mathematical Biosciences* **113**(1), 1–23 (1993)

[324] Smith, H.L.: A structured population model and a related functional differential equation: Global attractors and uniform persistence. *Journal of Dynamics and Differential Equations* **6**(1), 71–99 (1994)

[325] Smith, H.L.: Planar competitive and cooperative difference equations. *J. Differ. Equations Appl.* **3**(5-6), 335–357 (1998). DOI 10.1080/10236199708808108. URL https://doi.org/10.1080/10236199708808108

[326] Smith, H.L.: *Monotone Dynamical Systems: An Introduction to the Theory of Competitive and Cooperative Systems: An Introduction to the Theory of Competitive and Cooperative Systems.* No. 41 in Mathematical Surveys and Monographs. American Mathematical Soc. (2008)

[327] Smith, H.L.: *An introduction to delay differential equations with applications to the life sciences*, vol. 57. Springer New York (2011)

[328] Smith, H.L., Thieme, H.R.: *Dynamical systems and population persistence, Graduate Studies in Mathematics*, vol. 118. American Mathematical Society, Providence, RI (2011). DOI 10.1090/gsm/118. URL https://doi.org/10.1090/gsm/118

[329] Smith, H.L., Waltman, P.: *The theory of the chemostat: dynamics of microbial competition, Cambridge Studies in Mathematical Biology*, vol. 13. Cambridge University Press (1995)

[330] Smoller, J.: Shock waves and reaction-diffusion equations, volume 258 of. *Grundlehren der Mathematischen Wissenschaften* [Fundamental Principles of Mathematical Sciences] (1983)

[331] Song, J.: Some developments in mathematical demography and their application to the People's Republic of China. *Theoretical Population Biology* **22**(3), 382–391 (1982)

[332] Song, J., Kong, D., Yu, J.: Population system control. *Mathematical and Computer Modelling* **11**, 11–16 (1988)

[333] Takác, P.: A short elementary proof of the Krein–Rutman theorem. *Houston Journal of Mathematics* **20**(1), 93–98 (1994)

[334] Tang, B., Wang, X., Li, Q., Bragazzi, N.L., Tang, S., Xiao, Y., Wu, J.: Estimation of the transmission risk of the 2019-nCoV and its implication for public health interventions. *Journal of Clinical Medicine* **9**(2), 462 (2020)

[335] Thieme, H.R.: Density-dependent regulation of spatially distributed populations and their asymptotic speed of spread. *J. Math. Biol.* **8**(2), 173–187 (1979). DOI 10.1007/BF00279720. URL https://doi.org/10.1007/BF00279720

[336] Thieme, H.R.: *Asymptotic estimates of the solutions of nonlinear integral equations and asymptotic speeds for the spread of populations.* Walter de Gruyter, Berlin/New York Berlin, New York (1979)

[337] Thieme, H.R.: Semiflows generated by Lipschitz perturbations of non-densely defined operators. *Differential Integral Equations* **3**(6), 1035–1066 (1990)

[338] Thieme, H.R.: *Mathematics in Population Biology.* Princeton Series in Theoretical and Computational Biology. Princeton University Press, Princeton, NJ (2003)

[339] Thieme, H.R.: Spectral bound and reproduction number for infinite-dimensional population structure and time heterogeneity. *SIAM Journal on Applied Mathematics* **70**(1), 188–211 (2009)

[340] Thieme, H.R.: Spectral bound and reproduction number for infinite-dimensional population structure and time heterogeneity. *SIAM Journal on Applied Mathematics* **70**(1), 188–211 (2009)

[341] To, K.K.W., Tsang, O.T.Y., Leung, W.S., Tam, A.R., Wu, T.C., Lung, D.C., Yip, C.C.Y., Cai, J.P., Chan, J.M.C., Chik, T.S.H., et al.: Temporal profiles of viral load in posterior oropharyngeal saliva samples and serum antibody responses during infection by SARS-CoV-2: an observational cohort study. *The Lancet Infectious Diseases* **20**(5), 565–574 (2020). DOI 10.1016/S1473-3099(20)30196-1

[342] Tsoularis, A., Wallace, J.: Analysis of logistic growth models. *Mathematical Biosciences* **179**(1), 21–55 (2002)

[343] Tuljapurkar, S.: *Population Dynamics in Variable Environments. Lecture Notes in Biomathematics.* Springer, Berlin, Heidelberg (1990). DOI 10.1007/978-3-642-51652-8

[344] Turchin, P.: *Complex population dynamics: a theoretical/empirical synthesis, Monographs in Population Biology*, vol. 35. Princeton University Press, Princeton, NJ (2003)

[345] Uhl, R.: Ordinary differential inequalities and quasimonotonicity in ordered topological vector spaces. *Proc. Amer. Math. Soc.* **126**(7), 1999–2003 (1998). DOI 10.1090/S0002-9939-98-04311-1. URL https://doi.org/ 10.1090/S0002-9939-98-04311-1

[346] Usher, M.: A matrix model for forest management. *Biometrics* pp. 309–315 (1969). DOI 10.2307/2528791

[347] Verhulst, P.F.: Notice sur la loi que la population poursuit dans son accroissement. *Correspondance Mathématique et Physique* **vol.X**, 113–121 (1838)

[348] Verity, R., Okell, L.C., Dorigatti, I., Winskill, P., Whittaker, C., Imai, N., Cuomo-Dannenburg, G., Thompson, H., Walker, P.G., Fu, H., et al.: Estimates of the severity of coronavirus disease 2019: a model-based analysis. *The Lancet infectious diseases* **20**(6), 669–677 (2020). DOI 10.1016/S1473-3099(20)30243-7

[349] Volkmann, P.: Gewöhnliche Differentialungleichungen mit quasimonoton wachsenden Funktionen in topologischen Vektorräumen. *Math. Z.* **127**, 157–164 (1972). DOI 10.1007/BF01112607. URL https://doi.org/ 10.1007/BF01112607

[350] Volterra, V.: Fluctuations in the abundance of a species considered mathematically 1. *Nature* (1926). DOI 10.1038/118558a0

[351] Volterra, V.: *Variazioni e fluttuazioni del numero d'individui in specie animali conviventi.* C. Ferrari (1927)

[352] Volterra, V.: *Leçons sur la théorie mathématique de la lutte pour la vie.* Gauthier-Villars et cie. (1931)

[353] Volterra, V.: *Theory of functionals and of integral and integro-differential equations.* Dover (1959)

[354] Walker, P., Whittaker, C., Watson, O., Baguelin, M., Ainslie, K., Bhatia, S., Bhatt, S., Boonyasiri, A., et al.: The global impact of COVID-19 and strategies for mitigation and suppression. *Imperial Report* **12** (2020). DOI 10.25561/77735

[355] Walter, W.: *Differential and integral inequalities.* Ergebnisse der Mathematik und ihrer Grenzgebiete, Band 55. Springer-Verlag, New York-Berlin (1970). Translated from the German by Lisa Rosenblatt and Lawrence Shampine

[356] Walter, W.: Ordinary differential inequalities in ordered Banach spaces. *J. Differential Equations* **9**, 253–261 (1971). DOI 10.1016/0022-0396(71)90079-9. URL https://doi.org/10.1016/0022-0396(71)90079-9

[357] Waltman, P.: *Competition models in population biology.* SIAM (1983)

[358] Wang, P., Zheng, X., Li, J., Zhu, B.: Prediction of epidemic trends in COVID-19 with logistic model and machine learning technics. Chaos, Solitons & Fractals **139**, 110058 (2020). DOI 10.1016/j.chaos.2020. 110058. URL https://www.sciencedirect.com/science/article/ pii/S0960077920304550

[359] Wang, W., Ruan, S.: Simulating the SARS outbreak in Beijing with limited data. *J. Theoret. Biol.* **227**(3), 369–379 (2004). DOI 10.1016/j.jtbi.2003.11. 014. URL https://doi.org/10.1016/j.jtbi.2003.11.014

[360] Wang, W., Zhao, X.Q.: Threshold dynamics for compartmental epidemic models in periodic environments. *Journal of Dynamics and Differential Equations* **20**(3), 699–717 (2008)

[361] Wang, X., Wu, J., Yang, Y.: Richards model revisited: validation by and application to infection dynamics. *J. Theoret. Biol.* **313**, 12–19 (2012). DOI 10.1016/j.jtbi.2012.07.024

[362] Wang, Y., Jiang, J.: The general properties of discrete-time competitive dynamical systems. *J. Differential Equations* **176**(2), 470–493 (2001). DOI 10.1006/jdeq.2001.3989. URL https://doi.org/10.1006/jdeq.2001.3989

[363] Webb, G.F.: *Theory of nonlinear age-dependent population dynamics, Monographs and Textbooks in Pure and Applied Mathematics*, vol. 89. Marcel Dekker, Inc., New York (1985)

[364] Webb, G.F.: Population models structured by age, size, and spatial position. In: *Structured population models in biology and epidemiology*, pp. 1–49. Springer (2008)

[365] Wei, W.E., Li, Z., Chiew, C.J., Yong, S.E., Toh, M.P., Lee, V.J.: Presymptomatic transmission of SARS-CoV-2—Singapore, january 23–march 16, 2020. *Morbidity and Mortality Weekly Report* **69**(14), 411 (2020). DOI 10.15585/mmwr.mm6914e1

[366] Weinberger, H.F.: Long-time behavior of a class of biological models. *SIAM J. Math. Anal.* **13**(3), 353–396 (1982). DOI 10.1137/0513028. URL https://doi.org/10.1137/0513028

[367] WHO: Report of the WHO-China Joint Mission on Coronavirus Disease 2019 (COVID-19). Tech. rep., WHO (2020). URL https://www.who.int/docs/default-source/coronaviruse/who-china-joint-mission-on-covid-19-final-report.pdf

[368] WHO, Disease Outbreak News. Novel coronavirus – China. January 12, 2020. Tech. rep., WHO (2020). URL https://www.who.int/emergencies/disease-outbreak-news/item/2020-DON233

[369] WHO, Disease Outbreak News. Pneumonia of unknown cause–China. January 5, 2020. Tech. rep., WHO (2020). URL https://www.who.int/emergencies/disease-outbreak-news/item/2020-DON229

[370] Data from WHO. Accessed: June 30, 2021. Tech. rep., WHO (2021). URL https://covid19.who.int/WHO-COVID-19-global-data.csv

[371] Wright, S.: Isolation by distance. *Genetics* **28**(2), 114 (1943)

[372] Wu, J.: *Theory and applications of partial functional differential equations*, vol. 119. Springer Science & Business Media (2012)

[373] Wu, J.H.: Global dynamics of strongly monotone retarded equations with infinite delay. *J. Integral Equations Appl.* **4**(2), 273–307 (1992). DOI 10.1216/jiea/1181075685. URL https://doi.org/10.1216/jiea/1181075685

[374] Wu, J.T., Leung, K., Bushman, M., Kishore, N., Niehus, R., de Salazar, P.M., Cowling, B.J., Lipsitch, M., Leung, G.M.: Estimating clinical severity of COVID-19 from the transmission dynamics in Wuhan, China. *Nature medicine* **26**(4), 506–510 (2020). DOI 10.1038/s41591-020-0822-7

[375] Wu, J.T., Leung, K., Leung, G.M.: Nowcasting and forecasting the potential domestic and international spread of the 2019-nCoV outbreak originating in Wuhan, China: a modelling study. *The Lancet* **395**(10225), 689–697 (2020). DOI 10.1016/S0140-6736(20)30260-9

[376] Yang, Z., Zeng, Z., Wang, K., et al.: Modified SEIR and AI prediction of the epidemics trend of COVID-19 in China under public health interventions. *Journal of Thoracic Disease* **12**(3) (2020). DOI 10.21037/jtd.2020.02.64. URL http://jtd.amegroups.com/article/view/36385

[377] Yorke, J.A.: Invariance for ordinary differential equations. *Mathematical systems theory* **1**(4), 353–372 (1967)

[378] Yorke, J.A., London, W.P.: Recurrent outbreaks of measles, chickenpox and mumps: II. Systematic differences in contact rates and stochastic effects. *American Journal of Epidemiology* **98**(6), 469–482 (1973). DOI 10.1093/oxfordjournals.aje.a121576

[379] Yosida, K.: On the differentiability and the representation of one-parameter semi-group of linear operators. *Journal of the Mathematical Society of Japan* **1**(1), 15–21 (1948)

[380] Yosida, K.: *Functional analysis*. Classics in Mathematics. Springer-Verlag, Berlin (1995). DOI 10.1007/978-3-642-61859-8. URL https://doi.org/10.1007/978-3-642-61859-8. Reprint of the sixth (1980) edition

[381] Z, H., C, S., C, X., et al.: Clinical characteristics of 24 asymptomatic infections with COVID-19 screened among close contacts in Nanjing, China. *Sci. China Life Sci* **63**, 706–711 (2020). DOI 10.1007/s11427-020-1661-4

[382] Zeberg, H., Pääbo, S.: The major genetic risk factor for severe COVID-19 is inherited from Neanderthals. *Nature* (2020). DOI https://doi.org/10.1038/s41586-020-2818-3

[383] Zeeman, E.C.: Classification of quadratic carrying simplices in two-dimensional competitive Lotka–Volterra systems. *Nonlinearity* **15**(6), 1993 (2002)

[384] Zeeman, E.C., Zeeman, M.L.: An n-dimensional competitive Lotka–Volterra system is generically determined by the edges of its carrying simplex. *Nonlinearity* **15**(6), 2019 (2002)

[385] Zeeman, E.C., Zeeman, M.L.: From local to global behavior in competitive Lotka–Volterra systems. *Transactions of the American Mathematical Society* pp. 713–734 (2003)

[386] Zeeman, M.L., van den Driessche, P.: Three-dimensional competitive Lotka–Volterra systems with no periodic orbits. *SIAM Journal on Applied Mathematics* **58**(1), 227–234 (1998)

[387] Zhang, W., Lu, K., Zhang, W.: Differentiability of the conjugacy in the Hartman–Grobman theorem. *Trans. Amer. Math. Soc.* **369**(7), 4995–5030 (2017). DOI 10.1090/tran/6810. URL https://doi.org/10.1090/tran/6810

[388] Zhao, X.Q.: *Dynamical systems in population biology, CMS Books in Mathematics/Ouvrages de Mathématiques de la SMC*, vol. 16. Springer-Verlag, New York (2003). DOI 10.1007/978-0-387-21761-1. URL https://doi.org/10.1007/978-0-387-21761-1

[389] Zhao, X.Q.: *Dynamical systems in population biology*, second edn. CMS Books in Mathematics/Ouvrages de Mathématiques de la SMC. Springer, Cham (2017). DOI 10.1007/978-3-319-56433-3. URL https://doi.org/10.1007/978-3-319-56433-3

[390] Zhou, F., Yu, T., Du, R., Fan, G., Liu, Y., Liu, Z., Xiang, J., Wang, Y., Song, B., Gu, X., et al.: Clinical course and risk factors for mortality of adult inpatients with COVID-19 in Wuhan, China: a retrospective cohort study. *The Lancet* **395**(10229), 1054–1062 (2020). DOI 10.1016/S0140-6736(20)30566-3

[391] Zhou, G., Yan, G.: Severe acute respiratory syndrome epidemic in Asia. *Emerg. Infect. Dis.* **9**(12), 1608–1610 (2003)

[392] Zhou, P., Xiao, D.: Global dynamics of a classical Lotka–Volterra competition–diffusion–advection system. *Journal of Functional Analysis* **275**(2), 356–380 (2018)

[393] Zou, L., Ruan, F., Huang, M., Liang, L., Huang, H., Hong, Z., Yu, J., Kang, M., Song, Y., Xia, J., Guo, Q., Song, T., He, J., Yen, H.L., Peiris, M., Wu, J.: SARS-CoV-2 Viral Load in Upper Respiratory Specimens of Infected Patients. *New England Journal of Medicine* **382**(12), 1177–1179 (2020). DOI 10.1056/NEJMc2001737. URL https://doi.org/10.1056/NEJMc2001737. PMID: 32074444

[394] Zou, Y., Pan, S., Zhao, P., Han, L., Wang, X., Hemerik, L., Knops, J., van der Werf, W.: Outbreak analysis with a logistic growth model shows COVID-19 suppression dynamics in China. PLOS ONE **15**(6), 1–10 (2020). DOI 10.1371/journal.pone.0235247. URL https://doi.org/10.1371/journal.pone.0235247

Index

© The Author(s), under exclusive license to Springer Nature Switzerland AG 2022

A. Ducrot et al., *Differential Equations and Population Dynamics I*, Lecture Notes on
Mathematical Modelling in the Life Sciences, https://doi.org/10.1007/978-3-030-98136-5

Printed in the United States
by Baker & Taylor Publisher Services